MENOPAUSE:
Your Management *Your* Way ...
Now and for the *Rest of Your Life*

Barbara Taylor, M.D.

Copyright © 2008 Barbara Taylor, M.D.
All rights reserved.

ISBN: 1-4392-0795-X
ISBN-13: 9781439207956

Visit www.booksurge.com to order additional copies.

Acknowledgements

My greatest thanks goes to the many wonderful patients with whom I have worked over the years. They have taught me how to help them. I have listened to their requests, and it is they who have suggested repeatedly that I should write a book. They have given me positive feedback about my way of explaining things, and I have used the same conversational style in this book as I have with them. They have helped me to help you.

An extra special thanks goes to all the women who have attended my seminars based on this book. They have enabled me to test the value of the material and my presentation style prior to publishing the book. The seminars have been, and continue to be, tremendously rewarding and fun for me and for those who attend.

I wish to thank Christina Tottle, who drew multiple illustrations for this book. Christina is a dear friend, a phenomenal yoga instructor, and a loving spirit. She has improved the quality of my life and my book more deeply than she can imagine.

I extend special love and appreciation to my adoring husband, George Walther, whose support is endless. An author himself, George gives me his assistance when I need it, gives me space and independence when I don't, and never lets me forget that he loves me thoroughly.

Many thanks go to my publishers, who enabled me to produce *my* book *my* way so that you could manage *your* menopause *your* way.

Dedication

This book is dedicated to each unique, spectacular,
powerful woman who reads it.
It is dedicated to **you.**
You deserve the opportunity to manage
your menopause **your** way.
And you shall have it.

Menopause:
Your Management *Your* Way ... Now and for the *Rest of Your Life*

CONDENSED TABLE OF CONTENTS

Easing In. 1
Tools and Tables 3
    Worksheet. 5
    Tables 19
Section I: Introduction 29
    Chapter 1: An Introduction
       to the Mystery of "Menopause". 37
    Chapter 2: An Orientation to
       the Parts and Processes of Menopause. 47
    Chapter 3: Terminology:
       The Language of Menopause. 67
    Chapter 4: "How Will I Know
       When Menopause Comes a Knockin'?". 75
Section II: The Decision-Making
  Process and the Options. 81
    Chapter 5: The Balancing Act. 83
    Chapter 6: Options: Medical,
       Non-medical, and Everything in Between 91
    Chapter 7: Categories of
       Hormones and Their Sources. 107
    Chapter 8: Dosage Dictionary 153

Section III: Signs, Symptoms, and Diseases of Menopause and Aging Along With All the Management Options 159

   Introduction 161

   Chapter 9: Periods With a Personality Change 163

   Chapter 10: Hot Flashes 167

   Chapter 11: Night Sweats 177

   Chapter 12: Insomnia 183

   Chapter 13: Fatigue 195

   Chapter 14: Forgetfulness 203

   Chapter 15: Mood Swings, Irritability, and Depression 209

   Chapter 16: Cravings for Sweets, Carbohydrates, Alcohol 219

   Chapter 17: Breast Pain 221

   Chapter 18: Joint Stiffness and Joint Pain 223

   Chapter 19: Dry Skin 233

   Chapter 20: Hair Loss on the Scalp 239

   Chapter 21: Hair Growth in Undesirable Locations 245

   Chapter 22: Vaginal Dryness 249

   Chapter 23: Urinary Problems 255

   Chapter 24: Weight Gain 271

   Chapter 25: Decreased or Increased Sex Drive 277

   Chapter 26: Acne 285

   Chapter 27: Headaches 289

   Chapter 28: Heart Attack 295

   Chapter 29: Osteoporosis 313

   Chapter 30: Breast Cancer 345

   Chapter 31: Uterine Cancer 377

   Chapter 32: Ovarian Cancer 393

   Chapter 33: Alzheimer's Disease 401

Section IV: Research Studies
and For the Guys...........................409
   Chapter 34: "What About the
      Research Studies?"......................411
   Chapter 35: For the Guys...................437
   References 449
   Cited References by Chapter: 449
   General References 463
   Index....................................471
   About the Author.........................544

Menopause:
Your Management *Your* Way ...
Now and for the *Rest of Your Life*

EXTENDED TABLE OF CONTENTS

Easing In 1
Tools and Tables 3
    Worksheet 5
    Tables 19
Section I: Introduction 29
    It Doesn't Have To Be This Way 31
Chapter 1: An Introduction to
the Mystery of "Menopause" 37
    The Longest Female Phase 37
    Information Sources 38
    More Than Just The Golden Rule 40
    You Decide 41
    Empowerment 45
Chapter 2: An Orientation to the Parts
and Processes of Menopause 47
    Puberty in Reverse 48
    Anatomy 51
    "I'm Not Sure Which Surgical
        Procedure I've Had." 57
    Surgical and Premature Menopause 64
Chapter 3: Terminology:
The Language of Menopause 67
    Hormones 67

    It's Just a Phase. 70
Chapter 4: "How Will I Know When
    Menopause Comes a Knockin'?" 75
    Signs and Symptoms of Menopause 75
    "Do I Need a Lab Test to Confirm Menopause?" 78
        Blood FSH Level. 79
        Salivary Hormone Levels 80
        Timing. 80
Section II: The Decision-Making Process and the Options . . 81
    Chapter 5: The Balancing Act 83
    Principles 83
    The Balancing Scale 84
    Possible Options 85
    Questions to Ask Yourself 86
    Categories of Management Options. 86
    "Do I Want to Assume a Management Position?" 87
Chapter 6: Options: Medical, Non-medical, and
    Everything in Between. 91
    Diet and Lifestyle. 91
    Foundation. 91
        Basic Principles for Utilizing Alternative and
            Complementary Medicine Options 94
        Basic Principles for Utilizing
            Hormonal Options 94
        Botanical and Herbal Therapy 95
            Definitions 95
        Manufacture and Regulation
            of Botanicals and Herbs 97
        "Natural" Versus "Synthetic" Hormones. 99
            "Natural". 99
            "Synthetic" 101
            Summary. 102

  Bioidentical Hormones 102
  Acupuncture. 105
  Hypnosis 105
Chapter 7: Categories of Hormones
and Their Sources 107
  Estrogen 108
    Symptoms of Abnormal Estrogen Levels 108
      Symptoms of Estrogen Deficiency 108
      Symptoms of Estrogen Excess. 108
    Categories of Estrogen. 109
      Introduction to Botanical and
      Herbal Sources of Estrogen 109
        Phytoestrogens 109
        Foods as Hormonal Sources
        of Estrogen 116
          Soy. 116
          Flaxseed 117
          Bioflavonoids 118
      Botanical and Herbal Estrogen. 118
        Dong Quai (*Angelica sinensis*) 118
        Chasteberry (*Vitex agnus-castus*) 119
        Black Cohosh (*Cimicifuga racemosa*) . . . 119
        Licorice Root (*Glycyrrhiza glabra*) 121
        St. John's Wort
         (*Hypericum perforatum*) 121
        Valerian (*Valeriana officinalis*) 121
        Hops (*Humulus lupulus*) 122
        False Unicorn Root
         (*Veratum luteum*) 122
        Motherwort (*Leonurus cardiaca*) 123
        Joyful Change 123
        Chai Hu Long Gu Muli Wang 123

  Bioidentical Estrogen 123
  Synthetic Estrogen 126
   Estrogen Pills 126
   Estrogen Shots 127
   Estrogen Vaginal Rings 127
   Estrogen Skin Patches 127
   Estrogen Vaginal Creams 128
   Estrogen Gels 129
   Estrogen Vaginal Tablets 130
   Estrogen Pellets 130
  Selective Estrogen Receptor Modulators
   (SERMs) 130
   Tamoxifen (Nolvadex) 131
   Raloxifene (Evista) 132
   Bisphosphonates (Fosamax,
    Actonel, and Boniva) 133
   Tibolone 134
Progesterone 135
 Symptoms of Abnormal Progesterone Levels . . . 135
  Symptoms of Progesterone Deficiency 135
  Symptoms of Progesterone Excess 135
 Categories of Progesterone 136
  Botanical and Herbal Progesterone 137
   Chasteberry (*Vitex agnus-castus*) 137
   Wild Yam (*Dioscorea villosa*) 137
  Bioidentical Progesterone 138
   U.S.P. (United States Pharmacopeia)
    Progesterone (ProGest, Prometrium,
    Crinone) 139
   Progesterone Cream 139
  Synthetic Progesterone 139
   Progesterone Gel 139

Progesterone Pills 140
Progesterone Shots 140
Progesterone-Only Birth
    Control Pills 140
Progesterone-Containing
    Intrauterine Device (IUD) 141

Synthetic Estrogen Plus Progesterone 141
Variables 141
Low Dose Birth Control Pills 142
Low Dose Birth Control
    Skin Patches 145
Cyclic Estrogen Plus Progesterone 146
Continuous Estrogen
    Plus Progesterone 147
HRT Skin Patches Containing
    Estrogen and Progesterone 148

Testosterone 149
Symptoms of Abnormal Testosterone Levels . . . 149
Symptoms of Testosterone Deficiency 149
Symptoms of Testosterone Excess 149
Categories of Testosterone 149
Botanical and Herbal Testosterone 149
Cayenne (*Capsicum species*) 149
Cubeb (*Piper cubeba*) 150
Damiana (*Turnera diffusa*) 150
Bioidentical Testosterone 151
Dehydroepiandrosterone (DHEA) . . . 151
Testosterone Cream 151
Synthetic Testosterone 152

Chapter 8:   Dosage Dictionary 153
The Metric System
    (Systeme International or SI) 154

        The U.S. System (Imperial System) 155
Section III: Signs, Symptoms, and Diseases
of Menopause and Aging Along With All
the Management Options. 159
    Introduction 161
    Chapter 9: Periods With a Personality Change 163
        Management Options 165
            Hormonal Medication Options. 165
    Chapter 10: Hot Flashes 167
        Incidence 167
        Descriptive Aspects 167
        Triggers. 168
        Variables Affecting Hot Flashes 168
        Causes of Hot Flashes 169
        Management Options 170
            Diet and Lifestyle Options. 170
                Reduce Hot Flash Triggers 170
                Keep Cool. 170
                Regular Exercise 170
                Stress Reduction. 171
                Paced Respiration 171
            Vitamin and Mineral Options 171
                Vitamin E 171
            Botanical and Herbal Options. 171
                Phytoestrogens. 172
                Black Cohosh (*Cimicifuga racemosa*) 173
                Evening Primrose (*Oenothera biennis*) 173
                Dong Quai (*Angelica sinensis*) 173
            Hormonal Medication Options. 174
                Estrogen 174
                Progesterone 174
                Tibolone. 174

- Non-hormonal Medication Options 175
  - SSRI Antidepressants. 175
  - Neurontin (Gabapentin). 175
  - Bellergal 175
  - Antihypertensive Agents 176
  - Veralipride 176

Chapter 11: Night Sweats 177
- Description 177
- Management Options 177
  - Diet and Lifestyle Options. 177
    - Control Your Sleep Environment 177
  - Vitamin and Mineral Options 178
    - Vitamin E 178
  - Botanical and Herbal Options. 178
    - Phytoestrogens. 179
    - Black Cohosh (*Cimicifuga racemosa*) 179
    - Evening Primrose (*Oenothera biennis*) 180
    - Dong Quai (*Angelica sinensis*) 180
  - Hormonal Medication Options. 180
    - Estrogen 180
    - Progesterone 181
    - Tibolone. 181
  - Non-hormonal Medication Options 181
    - SSRI Antidepressants. 181
    - Neurontin (Gabapentin). 182
    - Bellergal 182
    - Antihypertensive Agents 182
    - Veralipride 182

Chapter 12: Insomnia 183
Description 183
Hormones, Aging, and Sleep 183
Consequences 185
Management Options 186
Diet and Lifestyle Options 186
Dietary Measures 186
Sleep Hygiene 186
Stimulus Control Measures 186
Sleep Routines 187
Sleep Restriction 187
Regular Exercise 187
Relaxation 187
Vitamin and Mineral Options 188
Melatonin and 5-HTP 188
Botanical and Herbal Options 188
Kava Kava (*Piper methysticum*) 188
Valerian (*Valeriana officinalis*) 188
Hops (*Humulus lupulus*) 189
Passion Flower (*Passiflora incarnata*) 189
Others 189
Hormonal Medication Options 189
Progesterone 189
Non-hormonal Medication Options 190
Sedative Hypnotic Medications 190
Benzodiazepines 190
Imidazopyridines 191
Antidepressant Medications 192
Tricyclic Antidepressants 192
SSRI Antidepressants 192

   Over the Counter Medications 193
    Antihistamines. 193
Chapter 13: Fatigue. 195
 Description. 195
 Management Options 196
  Diet and Lifestyle Options. 196
   Exercise 196
  Vitamin and Mineral Options 197
   Melatonin and 5-HTP 197
  Botanical and Herbal Options. 197
   Kava Kava *(Piper methysticum)*. 197
   Valerian (*Valeriana officinalis*) 198
   Hops (*Humulus lupulus*) 198
   Passion Flower (*Passiflora incarnata*). 198
   Others. 198
  Hormonal Medication Options. 199
   Progesterone 199
  Non-hormonal Medication Options 199
   Sedative Hypnotic Medications. 200
    Benzodiazepines 200
    Imidazopyridines. 201
   Antidepressant Medications 202
    Tricyclic Antidepressants 202
    SSRI Antidepressants 202
  Over the Counter Medications 202
   Antihistamines. 202
Chapter 14: Forgetfulness. 203
 Description. 203
 Management Options 204
  Diet and Lifestyle Options. 204

  Diet 204
   Alcohol Restriction 205
   Smoking Cessation. 205
  Vitamin and Mineral Options 205
  Botanical and Herbal Options. 206
   Ginkgo (*Ginkgo biloba*) 206
   Gotu Kola (*Centella asiatica*) 206
  Hormonal Medication Options. 206
   Estrogen 206
   Progesterone 207
   Testosterone 207
Chapter 15: Mood Swings, Irritability,
 and Depression 209
  Description. 209
   Mood Swings. 209
   Irritability 209
   Depression 210
    Incidence 210
    Mechanisms 210
  Management Options 212
   Diet and Lifestyle Options. 213
    Diet. 213
    Regular Exercise 213
   Vitamin and Mineral Options 213
    Vitamin Deficiencies 213
    5-Hydroxytryptophan (5-HTP) 214
    Inositol 214
    S-adenosyl-L-methionine (SAMe) 214
   Botanical and Herbal Options. 215
    St. John's Wort (*Hypericum perforatum*) 215
    California Poppy (*Eschscholtzia californica*) . . 216

  Valerian Root (*Valeriana officinalis*) 216
  Others 216
 Hormonal Medication Options 217
  Estrogen 217
  Testosterone 217
 Non-hormonal Medication Options 217
  SSRI Antidepressants 218
  Tricyclic Antidepressants 218

Chapter 16: Cravings for Sweets,
 Carbohydrates, Alcohol 219
 Cravings and Hormones 219
 Management Options 220

Chapter 17: Breast Pain 221
 Description 221
 Management Options 221

Chapter 18: Joint Stiffness and Joint Pain 223
 Description 223
 Management Options 225
  Diet and Lifestyle Options 225
   Exercise 225
   Heat 226
   Diet 226
    Oligomeric Proanthocyanidins (OPCs) . . . 227
   Weight 227
  Vitamin and Mineral Options 228
   Glucosamine 228
   Chondroitin Sulfate 228
   Glucosamine Chondroitin Sulfate 228
   Methylsulfonylmethane (MSM) 229
   S-Adenosyl-L-Methionine (SAMe) 229
  Botanical and Herbal Options 229

        Feverfew (*Tanacetum parthenium*) 229
        Aloe (*Aloe vera*) 230
    Hormonal Medication Options 230
    Non-hormonal Medication Options 231
        Acetominophen 231
        Nonsteroidal Anti-Inflammatory
        Drugs (NSAIDs) 231
        Steroids 232

Chapter 19: Dry Skin 233
    Description 233
    Skin Anatomy 233
    Management Options 235
        Diet and Lifestyle Options 235
            Sun Protection 235
            Water 235
            Diet 236
            Lotion 236
        Vitamin and Mineral Options 237
            Antioxidant Vitamins 237
        Botanical and Herbal Options 237
            Green Tea (*Camellia sinensis*) 237
        Hormonal Medication Options 238
            Estrogen 238
            Progesterone 238

Chapter 20: Hair Loss on the Scalp 239
    Hair Phases 239
    Management Options 240
        Diet and Lifestyle Options 240
            Weight Control 240
            Reduce Hair Manipulation 241
        Vitamin and Mineral Options 241

- Multivitamin 241
  - Hair Growth Vitamins and Minerals. 241
- Botanical and Herbal Options. 242
- Hormonal Medication Options. 242
  - Estrogen 242
  - Birth Control Pills 242
- Non-hormonal Medication Options 242
  - Dexamethasone 242
  - Spironolactone. 243
  - Minoxidil (Rogaine) 243

Chapter 21: Hair Growth in Undesirable Locations 245
- Description. 245
- Management Options 246
  - Mechanical Options. 246
    - Waxing 246
    - Electrolysis 246
    - Laser 247
  - Hormonal Medication Options. 247
    - Estrogen 247
    - Birth Control Pills 247
  - Non-hormonal Medication Options 247
    - Spironolactone. 247
    - Dexamethasone 247
    - Eflornithine Hydrochloride (Vaniqa Cream). 248

Chapter 22: Vaginal Dryness. 249
- Vaginal Anatomy 249
- Management Options 250
  - Diet and Lifestyle Options. 250
    - Sexual Activity 250

- Diet 251
  - Soy 251
- Mechanical Options 251
  - Lubricants 251
  - Moisturizers 252
- Vitamin and Mineral Options 252
  - Vitamin E 252
- Botanical and Herbal Options 252
- Hormonal Medication Options 252
  - Estrogen 252
  - Testosterone 254
  - Tibolone 254

Chapter 23: Urinary Problems 255
- Anatomy 255
- Urinary Tract Infections (UTIs) 256
  - Cause 256
  - Symptoms 257
  - Management Options 257
    - Diet and Lifestyle Options 257
- Urinary Incontinence 260
  - Incidence 260
  - Causes 260
  - Types of Incontinence 261
    - Stress Urinary Incontinence (SUI) 261
    - Urge Incontinence 261
  - Management Options 262
    - Diet and Lifestyle Options 262
      - Kegel Exercises 262
      - Dietary Habits 263
      - Stop Smoking 263
      - Weight Reduction 264

   Behavior Modification 264
  Vitamin and Mineral Options. 265
  Hormonal Medication Options 266
   Estrogen. 266
  Non-hormonal Medication Options. 266
   Tolterodine (Detrol). 266
   Anticholinergics 266
   Antispasmodics 267
   Tricyclic Antidepressants 267
   SSRI Antidepressants 267
  Incontinence Devices 267
  Injectable Substances. 268
  Surgical Procedures. 268
  Electrical Stimulation Techniques 269
  Acupuncture 269
  Hypnosis. 269
Chapter 24: Weight Gain 271
 Cause 271
 Body Mass Index (BMI) 272
 Management Options 273
  Diet and Lifestyle Options. 273
   Diet. 273
   Exercise 274
  Non-hormonal Medication Options 276
Chapter 25: Decreased or Increased Sex Drive. 277
 Description. 277
 Categories. 279
 Management Options 280
  Diet and Lifestyle Options. 280
   Make Sex Exciting 280
  Botanical and Herbal Options. 280

Cayenne (*Capsicum species*)................280
Damiana (*Turnera diffusa*)................281
Cubeb (*Piper cubeba*)................281
Chasteberry (*Vitex agnus-castus*)................281
Hormonal Medication Options................281
Estrogen................281
Testosterone................282
Progesterone................284
Non-hormonal Medication Options................284

Chapter 26: Acne................285
Sequence of Events................285
Management Options................286
Diet and Lifestyle Options................286
Diet................286
Ideal Body Weight................286
Hygiene................287
Vitamin and Mineral Options................287
Botanical and Herbal Options................287
Tea Tree Oil (*Medaleuca alternifolia*)................287
Hormonal Medication Options................287
Birth Control Pills................287
Estrogen................288
Non-hormonal Medication Options................288
Vitamin A Formulations................288
Benzoyl Peroxide................288
Antibiotics................288

Chapter 27: Headaches................289
Description................289
Management Options................290
Diet and Lifestyle Options................290
Stress Reduction................290

- Diet 290
  - Soy 290
- Botanical and Herbal Options. 290
  - Feverfew (*Tanacetum parthenium*) 290
- Hormonal Medication Options. 291
  - Birth Control Pills or Patchs 291
  - Cyclic or Continuous Hormone Replacement Therapy. 291
  - Progesterone 291
- Non-hormonal Medication Options 292
  - Nonsteroidal Anti-inflammatory Drugs (NSAIDs) 292
  - Antihypertensive Agents 292
  - Vasoconstrictors 292

Chapter 28: Heart Attack 295
- Statistics 295
- Causes. 295
- Symptoms. 297
- Risk Factors 298
- Management Options 300
  - Diet and Lifestyle Options. 300
    - Diet. 300
    - Exercise 301
    - Weight Control. 302
    - No Smoking 303
    - Limited Alcohol. 304
    - Dental Hygiene 304
  - Vitamin and Mineral Options 305
    - Calcium and Magnesium. 305
    - Potassium and Sodium 305
    - Vitamins B6, B12, and B9 306

- Vitamin C ... 306
- Vitamin E ... 306
- Vitamin B3 ... 307
- Coenzyme Q10 ... 307
- L-Carnitine ... 308
- Alpha Lipoic Acid (ALA) ... 308
- Homocysteine ... 308
- Botanical and Herbal Options ... 309
  - Hawthorne ... 309
  - Phytoestrogens ... 309
- Hormonal Medication Options ... 309
  - Estrogen ... 310
  - Progesterone ... 311
- Non-hormonal Medication Options ... 311
  - Statins ... 311
  - Aspirin ... 312
- Final Note ... 312
- Stroke ... 312
- Blood Clots (Thrombosis) ... 312

Chapter 29: Osteoporosis ... 313
- Definition ... 313
- Rates of Loss ... 314
- Symptoms ... 314
- Epidemiology and Prognosis ... 315
- Bone Architecture ... 316
- Risk Factors ... 317
- Calcium ... 320
- Bone Density ... 321
  - Bone Density Tests ... 321
    - Guidelines for Bone Density Testing ... 323

- T Score ... 324
- Z Score ... 326
- Urine Testing ... 326
- Management Options ... 327
  - Diet and Lifestyle Options ... 327
    - Prevent Falls ... 327
    - Exercise ... 329
    - Balance is Key ... 329
    - Smoking Cessation ... 330
    - Sun Exposure ... 331
  - Diet ... 331
    - Limit Caffeine ... 331
    - Limit Alcohol ... 332
    - Soy ... 332
    - Flaxseed ... 333
    - Protein ... 333
    - No Soft Drinks ... 333
    - Vitamin D Foods ... 333
    - Calcium-Rich Foods ... 334
  - Vitamin and Mineral Options ... 334
    - Calcium ... 334
    - Magnesium ... 335
    - Vitamin D ... 335
    - Vitamin B9 ... 336
    - Other Vitamins ... 336
    - Trace Minerals ... 336
  - Botanical and Herbal Options ... 336
    - Phytoestrogens ... 336
    - Green Tea (*Camellia sinensis*) ... 337
  - Hormonal Medication Options ... 337
    - Estrogen ... 337

> Testosterone 338
> Progesterone 338
> Calcitonin (Miacalcin) 338
> Teriparatide 339
> Non-hormonal Medication Options 339
>> Selective Estrogen Receptor Modulators
>> (SERMs) 340
>>> Tamoxifen (Nolvadex) 340
>>> Raloxifene (Evista) 340
>>> Bisphosphonates 341
>>>> Alendronate (Fosamax) 342
>>>> Risedronate (Actonel) 342
>>>> Ibandronate Sodium (Boniva) 342
>> Which SERM to Choose? 342

Chapter 30: Breast Cancer 345
> Statistics 345
> Risk Factors 345
> Management Options 349
>> Focus on Risks 349
>> Diet and Lifestyle Options 351
>>> No Smoking 351
>>> Exercise 352
>>> Weight Control 352
>>> Diet 353
>>> Limit Alcohol Intake 354
>> Hormonal Medication Options 354
>>> Estrogen 354
>>>> Does Estrogen Cause Breast Cancer? . 354
>>>>> Research and Facts 354
>>>>>> Consistency 355

- Dose Relationships............356
- Estrogen Alone Versus Estrogen Plus Progesterone............356
- Persistence............356
- Type of Breast Cancer............357
- Growth Rate............358
- Caution............358
- Progesterone............360
- Postmenopausal Hormone Replacment Therapy (HRT)............360
- Non-hormonal Medication Options............360
- Tamoxifen (Nolvadex)............360
- Aromatase Inhibitors............361
- Self Breast Examination............362
  - How to Check Your Breasts............363
    - Positions............363
      - Lying Down............363
      - Sitting or Standing in Front of a Mirror............365
    - Exclusions............366
  - When to Check Your Breasts............366
    - Cyclers............366
    - Non-Cyclers............368
    - Exclusions............369
  - What to Feel for When You Check Your Breasts............369
    - Ban on the Word "Lump"............369
    - Rocks or Pebbles............370
    - Time Investment............372
- Mammograms............372
  - Guidelines............372

  Limitations 373
Chapter 31: Uterine Cancer. 377
 Incidence 377
 Anatomy. 377
 The Effect of Estrogen on the Uterus 378
 Irregular Vaginal Bleeding 380
 Risk Factors 381
 Management Options 382
  Diet and Lifestyle Options. 382
   Weight Control. 382
   Diet. 383
  Botanical and Herbal Options. 383
   Chasteberry (*Vitex agnus-castus*) 383
   Wild Yam (*Dioscorea villosa*) 384
  Hormonal Medication Options. 385
   Beware of Estrogen Alone 385
  Cyclic Versus Continuous Estrogen Plus
   Progesterone 386
  Cyclic Regimen of Estrogen Plus
   Progesterone 387
  Low Dose Birth Control Pills
   or Skin Patches 387
  Cyclic Hormone Replacement
   Therapy (Cyclic HRT) 389
  Continuous Regimen of Estrogen Plus
   Progesterone (Continuous HRT) . . 391
  Progressive Estrogen Plus Progesterone
   Regimens. 392
Chapter 32: Ovarian Cancer. 393
 Incidence and Risk Factors 393
 Symptoms. 395
 Diagnosis 396
 Management Options 398

  Diet and Lifestyle Options 398
    Diet 398
    Weight Control 398
    Avoidance of Talc 398
  Hormonal Medication Options 399
    Birth Control Pills 399
  Preventive Surgery 399
Chapter 33: Alzheimer's Disease 401
  Description 401
  Alzheimer's and Estrogen 402
  Risk Factors 402
  Management Options 403
    Diet and Lifestyle Options 403
      Diet 403
      Exercise 403
      Play Mind Games 404
    Vitamin and Mineral Options 404
      Vitamin B1 404
      Vitamin B3 405
      Vitamin C 405
      Vitamin B6, Magnesium, and Zinc 405
      Vitamin E 405
      Lecithin 405
    Botanical and Herbal Options 406
      Ginkgo (*Ginkgo biloba*) 406
    Hormonal Medication Options 406
      Estrogen 406
      Dehydroepiandrosterone (DHEA) 407
  Summary 407
Section IV: Research Studies
and For the Guys 409

Chapter 34: "What About the Research Studies?" 411
    Introduction 411
    Types of Research Studies 411
    Significance of Research Results 412
    Factors Which Affect Research Studies. 414
    Postmenopausal Hormone History 414
    Women's Health Initiative (WHI) 422
        Purpose. 422
        Two Arms of the Study. 423
            Estrogen Plus Progesterone Arm 423
            Estrogen Alone Arm 423
        Analysis of the Estrogen Plus
            Progesterone Arm 423
            Risks. 425
            Benefits 425
        Analysis of the Estrogen Alone Arm 427
        The Bottom Line of the
            Estrogen Alone Arm. 427
        Limitations of the WHI Study 428
        Interpretation of Results 431
        Lesson. 431
        New Recommendations. 432

Chapter 35: For the Guys. 437
    Menopause in a Flash 437
        Anatomy 437
        Estrogen 438
        Phases of Menopause. 438
        Signs and Symptoms of Menopause 439
    Male Menopause 441
        Male Reproduction 441
        The Male Aging Process. 441

    Testosterone 442
    Emotional and Psychological Issues 442
    Male Mid-life Crisis. 442
  Men In Support of Menopause. 443
    Flashback. 443
    Whose Role is More Difficult? 443
    Knowledge and Preparation 444
    Sex and Romance. 445
    No Two Women Are Alike 446
    Options Galore. 446
References 449
  Cited References by Chapter: 449
  General References 463
Index 471
About the Author 544

Easing In

You're about to embark on a very long and very important journey. You're going on a trip that will take a very long time, and requires thorough preparation. You want to know as much as possible beforehand about what to expect. And even if you've already begun the journey, you welcome any information you can acquire along the way to make the journey smoother and more pleasant.

Where are you going? Well, you're going through menopause. Not only that, you're embarking on the rest of your life. You may have consulted pregnancy books to guide you when you were expecting. Well, now that you're *beyond* expecting, you have this book to guide you through menopause and beyond.

You see, menopause is *more* than just a transition. It's a right of passage. Once there, though, you'll live the rest of your life as a menopausal woman. Maybe you never thought of it that way before.

Transitioning into the last (and longest) phase of your life is a big deal. It isn't a quick, easy, process that is the same from one woman to another. It involves many complicated processes. I've written this book to guide you through *your* menopause so that you can manage it *your* way. In order to give you everything you need along the way, I've made sure to explain the basics, and I've even give you technical information where necessary.

Rushing through the information or glossing over it wouldn't be fair to you. So, as you read through this book, recognize it for what it is. It's thorough, detailed, and yet, down-to-earth. Don't let it overwhelm you. At times, the information will seem pretty deep. When it is, just keep reading. It won't stay that way.

As you read through the book, you'll fill in your own worksheet. That will narrow your focus and simplify the information. Don't expect to know how to fill in the worksheet before reading the material. The worksheet is located at the front of the book so that you can tear it out and fill in the designated part when I give you the signal to do so.

Think of this as your guidebook for your journey through the rest of your life. You'll refer to it often as you encounter new things along the way. Happy travels and happy reading.

Tools and Tables

The first two items in this book consist of tools to help you in navigating your way through this book in particular, and through menopause in general.

The **worksheet** will allow you to summarize all the information in the book as it pertains to you. You will see notations in the book entitled "Worksheet Timeout" indicating which worksheet questions to answer. If you answer the questions at the indicated times, you'll have adequate knowledge to answer them correctly. When you complete the worksheet, you'll have a personal, tailored document to help you focus on your unique needs and preferences. Detach the worksheet from the book, and refer to it as you read the book. You may even wish to make a few copies of the worksheet because, unless you're a robot, your personal situation will change over the course of your remaining life. You'll want to revisit the worksheet as you manage your menopause for the rest of your life.

The **tables** are a summary of all the symptoms and diseases pertinent to menopause, and all the management options available for each. The table encompasses five pages, one for each category of management options. These include:

    Diet and Lifestyle
    Vitamins and Minerals
    Botanicals and Herbs
    Hormonal Medications
    Non-hormonal Medications

MENOPAUSE

You'll find these tables useful *after* you've read the book. That's when you'll have the knowledge base to use them. As indicated in the legend on each page of the tables, the symbols are as follows:

A "+" means that the option will improve, prevent, or have a desirable effect on the symptom or disease.

A "-" means that the option will worsen, cause, or have an undesirable effect on the symptom or disease.

A "0" means that the option will have no effect on the symptom or disease.

A "@" means that the option can have a positive effect, a negative effect, or no effect at all on the symptom or disease. In other words, it's unpredictable.

A "n/a" means that the option is not applicable to the symptom or disease.

A "?" means that the option has an unknown effect on the symptom or disease.

Detach the tables from the book. You'll find them handy when you're at your physician's office, in the health food store, in the vitamin shop, or in a restaurant. It's easy to compare and contrast options for various symptoms and diseases. The best thing to do is to laminate them. That way, you'll preserve them for long term use.

Menopause:
Your Management *Your* Way ...
Now and for the *Rest of Your Life*

WORKSHEET

1. Your age:

2. Do you have a uterus?
       Uterus present   Uterus absent

   Do you have at least one ovary?
       Ovary present   Ovaries absent

   Was your menopause premature?
       After age 45   Before age 45

   Was your menopause natural or surgical?
       Natural   Surgical

3. Which are you?
       Peri-menopausal   Post-menopausal

   At what age did you begin peri-menopause? _____

   At what age did you become post-menopausal? _____

Worksheet

4. What symptoms do you have?
    - Periods with a personality change
    - Hot flashes
    - Night sweats
    - Insomnia
    - Fatigue
    - Forgetfulness
    - Mood swings
    - Irritability
    - Depression
    - Cravings for sweets, carbohydrates, alcohol
    - Breast pain
    - Joint stiffness or joint pain
    - Dry skin
    - Hair loss on your scalp
    - Hair growth in undesirable locations
    - Vaginal dryness
    - Urinary tract infections
    - Urinary incontinence
    - Weight gain
    - Decreased sex drive
    - Acne
    - Headaches

5. What are your risks for a heart attack?
    - Previous heart attack
    - Smoking
    - High lousy LDL
    - Low healthy HDL
    - High triglycerides
    - Obesity
    - Truncal obesity
    - High blood pressure
    - Diabetes
    - Sedentary life style
    - Gum disease
    - High homocysteine
    - Depression
    - Family history

WORKSHEET

6. What are your risks for osteoporosis?
   - Race (White > Asian > Black)
   - Naturally blonde hair
   - Thin body habitus
   - Family members with osteoporosis or fractures
   - Premature menopause (before age 45)
   - Tendency to fall
   - Sedentary lifestyle
   - Smoking
   - Diet high in caffeine
   - Excessive alcohol
   - Chronic excessive exercise
   - Anorexia or bulimia
   - Diabetes
   - Thyroid disease
   - Vitamin D deficiency
   - Lack of sun exposure
   - Meds for thyroid disease
   - Use of steroids
   - Meds: Immunosuppressants
     - Blood thinners
     - Anticonvulsants
     - Valium
     - Librium
     - Ativan
     - Lithium
     - Tamoxifen **before menopause**

Worksheet

7. What are your risks for breast cancer?
   - Previous breast cancer yourself
   - Family history (maternal first degree relatives)
   - Your age _____
   - First full term pregnancy after age 30
   - Few pregnancies
   - First period before age 12
   - Menopause after age 55
   - Smoking
   - Sedentary lifestyle
   - Obesity
   - High fat diet
   - Benign breast disease
   - Regular alcohol consumption
   - Exposure to intense radiation
   - Dense breasts

8. What are your risks for uterine cancer?
   (Ignore if you have no uterus)
   - Age over 45
   - Obesity
   - Excess estrogen from other sources not balanced with progesterone

9. What are your risks for ovarian cancer?
   - Genetics
   - Personal history of breast cancer
   - Age (middle-age, post-menopausal, or elderly) _____
   - Obesity
   - First period before age 12
   - No pregnancies
   - First pregnancy after age 30
   - Menopause after age 51
   - Infertility
   - Infertility drugs
   - Talcum powder use in your genital area
   - High fat diet
   - Low fiber diet

Worksheet

10. What are your risks for Alzheimer's?
    Age over 65
    Genetics (positive family history)
    Previous traumatic head injury
    Lower educational level
    High blood pressure
    High cholesterol
    Low levels of folate

11. What is your body type?
    Thin from head to toe
    Pudgy from head to toe
    Very solid and muscular
    Fat accumulation in the torso/belly
    Fat accumulation in the hips/thighs
    Underweight
    Ideal weight
    Overweight
    Obese
    Morbidly obese
    Height _____
    Weight _____
    BMI _____

12. Describe your diet:

Fat	High	Med	Low
Meat	High	Med	Low
Sugar	High	Med	Low
Caffeine	High	Med	Low
Processed food	High	Med	Low
Fiber	High	Med	Low
Fruit	High	Med	Low
Veggies	High	Med	Low
Soy	High	Med	Low

Worksheet

13. Describe your lifestyle:

Exercise	Hours/week	Intensity
Aerobic		High/Low
Resistance		High/Low
Balance/Core		High/Low
Flexibility/Yoga		High/Low

Alcohol:
   Number of drinks:
      ____ per day
      ____ per week

Smoking:
   Number of cigarettes:
      ____ per day
      ____ per week

14. What are your personal preferences?
    - Do nothing
    - Short-term management
    - Long-term management
    - Short- and long-term management

15. What category(ies) do you prefer?
    - Diet and lifestyle
    - Vitamins and minerals
    - Botanicals and herbs
    - Hormonal medications
        - Natural
        - Bioidentical
        - Synthetic
    - Non-hormonal medications
    - Acupuncture
    - Hypnosis

WORKSHEET

Your Balancing Act

Your History   <u>Positives</u>   <u>Negatives</u>
Questions # 1 - 3

Your Symptoms   <u>Positives</u>   <u>Negatives</u>
Question # 4

Your Risk Factors   <u>Positives</u>   <u>Negatives</u>
Questions # 5 - 10

Your Body and Lifestyle <u>Positives</u>   <u>Negatives</u>
Questions # 11 – 13

Your Preferences   <u>Positives</u>   <u>Negatives</u>
Questions # 14 – 15

Diet and Lifestyle Options

Alzheimer's Disease	Ovarian Cancer	Uterine Cancer	Breast Cancer	Osteoporosis	Stroke	Blood Clots	Heart Attack	Headaches	Acne	Decreased Sex Drive	Weight Gain	Incontinence	Urinary Tract Infection	Vaginal Dryness	Hair Growth	Hair Loss	Dry Skin	Joint Pain	Breast Pain	Cravings	Depression	Irritability	Mood Swings	Forgetfulness	Fatigue	Insomnia	Night Sweats	Hot Flashes	Irregular Periods	
n/a	n/a	n/a	n/a	n/a	n/a	n/a	n/a	n/a	+/o	?	?	?	+/o	?	?	?	?	?	?	?	?	?	?	?	?	?	?	?	?	Acupuncture
o	+	o	o	o	o	o	o	o	o	o	o	o	o	o	o	o	o	o	o	o	o	o	o	o	o	o	o	o	o	Avoid Talc & Talcum Powder
o	o	o	o	+	o	o	o	o	o	o	o	o	o	o	o	o	o	+/o	o	o	o	o	o	o	o	o	o	o	o	Balance
o	o	o	o	o	o	o	o	o	o	o	+	+/o	o	o	o	o	o	o	o	o	o	o	o	o	o	o	o	o	o	Bladder Training
o	o	o	o	o	o	o	o	o	o	o	o	+	o	o	o	o	o	o	o	o	o	o	o	o	o	o	o	o	o	Cranberry Juice
o	o	o	o	o	o	o	+	o	o	o	o	o	o	o	o	o	o	o	o	o	o	o	o	o	o	o	o	o	o	Dental Hygiene
o	o	o	o	+	o	o	o	o	o	o	+/o	o	o	o	o	o	o	+/o	o	o	o	o	o	o	o	o	o	o	o	Don't Fall
o	o	o	o	o	+/o	o	o	o	+	o	+	+	+	o	o	o	+	+/o	o	+/o	o	o	o	o	o	o	+/o	+/o	o	Drinking Water
+	+/o	+/o	+	+	+	+	+	+	o	+/o	+	+/o	o	o	o	o	o	+	o	o	+	+	+	+/o	+	+	+	+	+/o	Exercise
+/o	+/o	+	+	+/o	+	+	o	+/o	+/o	+/o	+/o	+/o	+/o	+	o	+/o	+/o	+/o	+/o	+/o	+/o	+/o	+/o	+/o	+/o	+/o	+/o	+/o	+/o	Flaxseed
o	o	o	o	o	o	o	o	o	o	+	o	o	o	o	o	o	o	o	+	o	+/o	+/o	+	+	o	o	o	o	o	Frequent Meals
o	o	o	o	+	o	o	o	o	o	o	o	o	o	o	o	o	o	o	o	o	o	o	o	o	o	o	o	o	o	Garlic
o	o	o	o	o	o	o	o	o	o	o	o	+	+	o	o	o	o	+/o	o	o	o	o	o	o	o	o	o	o	o	Good Hygiene
o	o	o	o	o	o	+	+	o	+	o	o	o	o	o	o	o	o	+	o	o	o	o	o	o	o	o	o	o	o	Green Tea
+/o	+	+/o	+	+/o	o	+	+	+	o	o	+	o	o	o	o	o	o	+/o	+	+/o	+	+	o	o	o	o	o	o	o	High Fiber Diet
+/o	+/o	+/o	+/o	+	o	+/o	+/o	o	o	o	o	o	o	o	o	o	o	+/o	o	+/o	o	+	+	o	o	o	o	o	o	High Protein Diet
o	o	o	o	o	o	o	o	o	o	o	+/o	o	o	o	o	o	o	o	o	+/o	o	o	o	o	o	o	o	o	o	Hypnosis
o	o	o	o	o	o	o	o	o	o	o	o	+	o	o	o	o	o	o	o	o	o	o	o	o	o	o	o	o	o	Incontinence Devices
o	o	o	o	o	o	o	o	o	o	+	o	+	o	o	o	o	o	o	o	o	o	o	o	o	o	o	o	o	o	Kegel Exercises
+/o	o	o	+	+	?	+	+	o	o	+/o	+	+	+	o	o	o	o	+/o	+	o	+	+	+	+/o	+	+	+	o	Limited/No Alcohol
o	o	o	o	o	o	o	o	o	o	o	o	o	o	o	o	o	+	o	o	o	o	o	o	o	o	o	o	o	o	Lotion
+/o	+/o	+/o	+	+/o	o	+/o	+	o	+/o	o	+	o	o	o	o	o	o	o	o	+	+	+	o	o	o	o	o	o	Low Carbohydrate Diet
o	+	+/o	+	+/o	o	+	+	o	+/o	o	+	o	o	o	o	o	o	+/o	o	+/o	+	+	o	o	o	o	o	o	Low Fat Diet
o	+	+/o	o	+/o	+	o	+	o	o	+	+	o	o	o	o	o	o	+	o	+	+	+	o	o	+/o	o	o	o	o	Low Sugar Diet
o	o	o	o	+	?	o	o	o	o	o	+	+	o	o	o	o	+	+/o	o	+	+	+	o	+	+	+	+	o	No Caffeine
+/o	+/o	+/o	+	+	+/o	+	+	o	o	+	o	o	o	o	o	o	+	o	o	o	o	o	o	+	o	o	+/o	+/o	o	No Smoking
+/o	+/o	+/o	o	+	o	+/o	+/o	o	+/o	o	+	o	+/o	o	o	o	o	+/o	o	+/o	o	+	+	o	o	o	o	o	o	No Soft Drinks
+	+/o	+/o	+/o	+/o	o	+	+/o	o	+/o	o	+	o	o	o	o	o	+/o	o	+/o	o	o	+	+	+/o	o	o	o	o	o	No Processed Foods
o	o	o	o	o	o	o	o	o	o	o	o	o	o	o	+	+	o	o	o	o	o	o	o	o	o	o	o	o	o	OPCs/Flavonoids
o	o	o	o	o	+	o	o	+	o	+	o	o	o	o	o	o	o	o	o	o	+/o	o	o	o	o	o	+	+	o	Paced Respiration
o	o	o	o	o	o	o	o	+/o	o	+/o	+/o	o	+/o	o	o	o	o	+/o	o	o	+/o	+/o	+/o	o	+	+	+/o	+/o	o	Relaxation
o	o	o	o	o	o	o	o	o	o	+/o	o	o	o	+	o	o	o	o	o	o	o	o	o	o	o	o	o	o	o	Sexual Intercourse
+/o	+/o	+	+	+	+	+	+	o	+/o	+/o	o	+/o	+/o	o	+	o	+	+	+/o	+/o	+/o	+/o	+	+	+	+/o	+/o	+	+/o	Soy
o	o	o	o	o	+	o	+/o	+	o	+/o	+/o	+/o	o	o	+/o	o	+/o	+/o	o	+/o	+	+	+	+	+	+	+	+	+/o	Stress Reduction
o	o	o	o	+	o	o	o	o	o	o	o	o	o	o	o	o	-	o	o	o	o	o	o	o	o	o	o	o	o	Sun Exposure
o	+	+	+	o	+/o	+	+	o	+	+/o	+	+/o	o	o	+/o	o	+	o	o	o	o	o	o	o	+/o	+/o	+/o	+/o	o	Weight Loss/Ideal Weight
o	o	o	o	o	o	o	o	o	+/o	o	o	o	+	+	o	o	o	o	o	o	o	o	o	o	o	o	o	o	o	Vaginal Moisture/Lubrication

Legend

- **+** Means: Improves the Situation, Prevents the Situation, or Produces a Desirable Effect.
- **-** Means: Worsens the Situation, Causes the Situation, or Produces an Undesirable Effect.
- **o** Means: Has No Effect on the Situation.
- **n/a** Means: Not Applicable.
- **?** Means: Unknown Effect.
- **@** Means that any result (+,-,0) is possible

VITAMIN AND MINERAL OPTIONS

Alzheimer's Disease	Ovarian Cancer	Uterine Cancer	Breast Cancer	Osteoporosis	Stroke	Blood Clots	Heart Attack	Headaches	Acne	Decreased Sex Drive	Weight Gain	Incontinence	Urinary Tract Infection	Vaginal Dryness	Hair Growth	Hair Loss	Dry Skin	Joint Pain	Breast Pain	Cravings	Depression	Irritability	Mood Swings	Forgetfulness	Fatigue	Insomnia	Night Sweats	Hot Flashes	Irregular Periods	
o	o	o	o	o	+	+	+	o	o	o	o	o	o	o	o	o	+	+	o	o	o	o	o	o	o	o	o	o	o	Alpha Lipoic Acid
o	o	o	o	o	o	o	o	o	o	o	o	o	o	o	o	+	o	o	o	o	+	+	+	o	o	o	o	o	o	Biotin
o	o	o	o	+	o	o	o	o	o	o	o	o	o	o	o	o	o	o	o	o	o	o	o	o	o	o	o	o	o	Boron
o	o	o	o	+	+	+	+	o	o	o	o	o	o	o	o	o	o	+	o	o	+	+	+	o	o	o	o	o	o	Calcium
o	o	o	o	o	o	o	o	o	o	o	o	o	o	o	o	o	o	+	o	o	o	o	o	o	o	o	o	o	o	Chondrointin
o	o	o	o	+	o	o	o	o	o	o	o	o	o	o	o	o	o	o	o	o	+	+	+	o	o	o	o	o	o	Copper
o	o	o	+	o	+	+	+	o	o	o	o	o	o	o	o	o	o	+	o	o	o	o	o	o	o	o	o	o	o	CO Q 10
o	o	o	o	+	+	+	+	o	o	o	o	o	o	o	o	+	o	o	o	o	+	+	+	+	o	o	o	o	o	Folate
o	o	o	o	o	o	o	o	o	o	o	o	o	o	o	o	o	o	+	o	o	o	o	o	o	o	o	o	o	o	Glucosamine
o	o	o	o	-	-	-	-	o	o	o	o	o	o	o	o	o	o	o	o	o	o	o	o	o	o	o	o	o	o	Homocysteine
o	o	o	o	o	o	o	o	o	o	o	o	o	o	o	o	o	o	o	o	o	+	+	+	o	o	+	o	o	o	5HTP
o	o	o	o	o	o	o	o	o	o	o	o	o	o	o	o	o	o	o	o	o	+	+	+	o	o	o	o	o	o	Inositol
+	o	o	o	o	o	o	o	o	o	o	o	o	o	o	o	o	o	o	o	o	o	o	o	o	o	o	o	o	o	Lecithin
o	o	o	o	o	o	o	o	o	o	o	o	o	o	o	o	o	+	o	o	o	o	o	o	o	o	o	o	o	o	Lipoic Acid
o	o	o	o	o	+	+	+	o	o	o	o	o	o	o	o	o	o	o	o	o	o	o	o	o	o	o	o	o	o	L-Carnitine
+	o	o	o	+	+	+	+	o	o	o	o	o	o	o	o	o	o	o	o	o	+	+	+	o	o	o	o	o	o	Magnesium
o	o	o	o	+	o	o	o	o	o	o	o	o	o	o	o	o	o	o	o	o	o	o	o	o	o	o	o	o	o	Manganese
o	o	o	o	o	o	o	o	o	o	o	o	o	o	o	o	o	o	o	o	o	o	+	+	o	o	o	o	o	o	Melatonin
o	o	o	+	o	+/o	+/o	+/o	o	o	o	o	o	o	o	o	o	o	+	+	o	o	+	+	+	o	o	o	o	o	Omega 3 FA
o	o	o	o	o	o	o	o	o	o	o	o	o	o	o	o	o	o	o	o	o	+	+	+	o	o	o	o	o	o	Omega 6 FA
o	o	o	o	o	+	+	+	o	o	o	o	o	o	o	o	o	o	o	o	o	o	o	o	o	o	o	o	o	o	Potassium
o	o	o	o	o	o	o	o	o	o	o	o	o	o	o	o	o	+	o	o	o	o	o	o	o	o	o	o	o	o	Proanthocyanidins
o	o	o	o	o	o	o	o	o	o	o	o	o	o	o	o	o	o	+	o	o	+	+	+	o	o	-	o	o	o	SAMe
o	o	o	o	o	o	o	o	o	o	o	o	o	o	o	o	o	o	o	o	o	o	o	o	+	o	o	o	o	o	Selenium
o	o	o	o	+	o	o	o	o	o	o	o	o	o	o	o	o	o	o	o	o	o	o	o	o	o	o	o	o	o	Silicon
o	o	o	o	o	-	-	-	o	o	o	o	o	o	o	o	o	o	o	o	o	o	o	o	o	o	o	o	o	o	Sodium
o	o	o	o	o	o	o	o	o	+/o	o	o	o	o	o	o	o	+	o	o	o	o	o	o	o	o	o	o	o	o	Vitamin A
+	o	o	o	o	o	o	o	o	+	o	o	o	o	o	o	+	o	o	o	o	o	o	o	+	o	o	o	o	o	Vitamin B1
+	o	o	o	o	+	+	+	o	o	o	o	o	o	o	o	o	o	o	o	o	o	o	o	o	o	o	o	o	o	Vitamin B3
+	o	o	o	+	+	+	+	o	o	o	o	o	o	o	o	o	o	o	o	o	+	+	+	o	o	o	o	o	o	Vitamin B6
o	o	o	o	o	+	+	+	o	o	o	o	o	o	+	o	o	o	o	o	o	+	+	+	o	o	o	o	o	o	Vitamin B12
+	o	o	o	+	+	+	+	o	+	o	o	+	o	o	o	+	+	o	o	o	+	+	+	+	o	o	o	o	o	Vitamin C
o	o	o	o	+	o	o	o	o	o	o	o	o	o	o	o	+	o	o	o	o	o	o	o	o	o	o	o	o	o	Vitamin D
+	o	o	o	o	+	+	+	o	o	o	o	o	o	+	o	o	+	+/o	o	o	o	o	o	+	o	o	o	o	o	Vitamin E
o	o	o	o	+	o	o	o	o	o	o	o	o	o	o	o	o	o	o	o	o	o	o	o	o	o	o	o	o	o	Vitamin K
+	o	o	o	+	o	o	o	o	+	o	o	+	o	o	o	o	o	+	o	o	o	o	o	+	o	o	o	o	o	Zinc

Legend

- **+**   Means: Improves the Situation, Prevents the Situation, or Produces a Desirable Effect.
- **-**   Means: Worsens the Situation, Causes the Situation, or Produces an Undesirable Effect.
- **o**   Means: Has No Effect on the Situation.
- **n/a**   Means: Not Applicable.
- **?**   Means: Unknown Effect.
- **@**   Means that any result (+,-,0) is possible

Botanical and Herbal Options

Alzheimer's Disease	Ovarian Cancer	Uterine Cancer	Breast Cancer	Osteoporosis	Stroke	Blood Clots	Heart Attack	Headaches	Acne	Decreased Sex Drive	Weight Gain	Incontinence	Urinary Tract Infection	Vaginal Dryness	Hair Growth	Hair Loss	Dry Skin	Joint Pain	Breast Pain	Cravings	Depression	Irritability	Mood Swings	Forgetfulness	Fatigue	Insomnia	Night Sweats	Hot Flashes	Irregular Periods	
o	o	o	o	o	o	o	o	o	o	o	o	o	o	o	o	o	o	+	o	o	o	o	o	o	o	o	o	o	o	Aloe Vera
o	o	o	o	o	o	o	o	-	o	o	-	o	o	+	+	o	o	o	o	o	+	+/o	+	o	o	+	+	+	o	Black Cohosh
o	o	o	o	o	o	o	o	o	o	o	o	o	o	o	o	o	o	o	o	o	+	+	+	o	o	o	o	o	o	California Poppy
o	o	o	o	o	o	o	o	o	o	+	o	o	o	o	o	o	o	o	o	o	o	o	o	o	o	o	o	o	o	Cayenne
o	o	o	o	o	o	o	o	o	o	o	o	o	o	o	o	o	o	o	o	o	+	+	o	o	+	o	o	o	o	Chai Hu Long Gu Muli Wang
o	o	+	o	o	o	o	o	+/o	o	+	o	o	o	+	o	o	o	o	o	o	+	o	o	o	o	+	o	o	+	Chasteberry
o	o	o	o	o	o	o	o	o	o	+/o	o	o	o	o	o	o	o	o	o	o	o	o	o	o	o	o	o	o	o	Cubeb
o	o	o	o	o	o	o	o	o	o	+	o	o	o	o	o	o	o	o	o	o	o	o	o	o	+	+	+	+	o	Damana
o	o	o	o	o	o	o	o	o	o	o	o	o	o	+	o	o	o	o	o	o	o	o	o	o	o	o	o	o	o	Dong Quai
o	o	o	+/o	o	o	o	o	o	o	o	+	o	o	o	o	o	o	o	+	o	+/o	+	+	o	o	o	o	o	o	Evening Primrose
o	o	o	o	o	+	+	o	+	o	o	o	o	o	o	o	o	o	+	o	o	o	o	o	o	o	o	o	o	o	Feverfew
+	o	o	o	o	+	+	o	o	o	o	o	o	o	o	o	o	o	o	o	o	o	o	o	+	o	o	o	o	o	Ginkgo Biloba
o	o	o	o	o	o	o	o	o	o	o	o	o	o	o	o	o	o	o	o	o	o	o	o	+	o	-	o	o	o	Gotu Kola
o	o	o	o	+	o	+	+	o	o	o	o	o	o	o	o	o	+	o	o	o	o	o	o	o	o	o	o	o	o	Green Tea
o	o	o	o	o	+	+	+	o	o	o	o	o	o	o	o	o	o	o	o	o	o	o	o	o	o	o	o	o	o	Hawthorne
o	o	o	o	+	+	+	+	o	o	o	o	o	o	o	o	o	o	o	o	o	o	o	o	o	+	+	o	o	o	Hops
o	o	o	o	o	o	o	o	o	o	o	o	+	o	o	o	o	o	o	o	o	o	o	+	+	+	+	+	+	o	Joyful Change
o	o	o	o	o	o	o	o	o	o	o	o	o	o	o	o	o	o	o	o	o	o	o	o	o	+	+	o	o	o	Kava Kava
o	+	+	+	o	o	o	o	o	o	o	o	o	o	o	o	o	o	o	o	o	o	o	o	o	+	o	o	o	o	Licorice root
o	o	o	o	o	o	o	o	+/o	o	o	o	o	o	o	o	o	o	o	o	o	o	o	o	o	+	+	o	o	o	Passion Flower
+/o	+/o	+	+	+	+	+	+	+	+/o	+/o	+/o	+/o	+/o	+	+/o	+/o	+/o	+/o	+/o	+/o	+/o	+/o	+/o	+	+/o	+/o	+	+	+/-	Phytoestrogen
o	o	o	o	o	o	o	o	o	o	o	o	o	o	o	o	o	o	o	o	o	+	+	+	o	o	o	o	o	o	St. John's Wort
o	o	o	o	o	o	o	o	o	+	o	o	o	o	o	o	o	o	o	o	o	o	o	o	o	o	o	o	o	o	Tea Tree Oil
o	o	o	o	o	o	o	o	o	o	o	o	o	o	o	o	o	o	o	o	o	+	+	+	o	+	+	o	o	o	Valerian
o	o	+	o	o	o	o	o	o	o	o	o	o	o	+	o	o	o	o	o	o	o	o	o	o	o	o	o	o	o	Wild Yam
o	o	o	o	o	o	o	o	o	o	o	o	o	o	+	+	o	o	o	o	o	o	o	o	o	o	o	o	o	o	Wu Pian

Legend

- **+** Means: Improves the Situation, Prevents the Situation, or Produces a Desirable Effect.
- **-** Means: Worsens the Situation, Causes the Situation, or Produces an Undesirable Effect.
- **o** Means: Has No Effect on the Situation.
- **n/a** Means: Not Applicable.
- **?** Means: Unknown Effect.
- **@** Means that any result (+,-,0) is possible

Hormonal Medication Options

Category	Alzheimer's Disease	Ovarian Cancer	Uterine Cancer	Breast Cancer	Osteoporosis	Stroke	Blood Clots	Heart Attack	Headaches	Acne	Decreased Sex Drive	Weight Gain	Incontinence	Urinary Tract Infection	Vaginal Dryness	Hair Growth	Hair Loss	Dry Skin	Joint Pain	Breast Pain	Cravings	Depression	Irritability	Mood Swings	Forgetfulness	Fatigue	Insomnia	Night Sweats	Hot Flashes	Irregular Periods	Medication
Estrogen	+	o/-	-	o/-	+	@	@	@	o/-	+	+/-	+	+	+	+	+	+	+	+	+	+	+	+	+	+	+	+	+	+	+/-	Bioidentical Estrogen
	+	o/-	-	o/-	+	-	-	@	o/-	+	+/-	+	+	+	+	+	+	+	+	+	+	+	+	+	+	+	+	+	+	+/-	Estrogen Gel
	+	o/-	-	o/-	+	+	+	@	o/-	+	+/-	+	+	+	+	+	+	+	+	+	+	+	+	+	+	+	+	+	+	+/-	Estrogen Patch
	+	o/-	-	o/-	+	@	@	@	o/-	+	+/-	+	+	+	+	+	+	+	+	+	+	+	+	+	+	+	+	+	+	+/-	Estrogen Pellets
	+	o/-	-	o/-	+	@	@	@	o/-	+	+/-	+	+	+	+	+	+	+	+	+	+	+	+	+	+	+	+	+	+	+/-	Estrogen Pills
	+	o/-	-	o/-	+	@	@	@	o/-	+	+/-	+	+	+	+	+	+	+	+	+	+	+	+	+	+	+	+	+	+	+/-	Estrogen Shots
	+	?	-	o	+	-	-	@	o/-	+	+/-	+	+	+	+	+	+	+	+	+	+	+	+	+	+	+	+	+	+	+/-	Estrogen Vaginal Cream
	+	o/-	-	o/-	+	+	+	@	o/-	+	+/-	+	+	+	+	+	+	+	+	+	+	+	+	+	+	+	+	+	+	+/-	Estrogen Vaginal Ring
	+	o/-	-	o/-	+	@	@	@	o/-	+	+/-	+	+	+	+	+	+	+	+	+	+	+	+	+	+	+	+	+	+	+/-	Estrogen Vaginal Tablets
	o	o	o	o	+	o	o	o	o	o	o	o	o	o	+	o	o	o	o	-	o	o	o	o	+	+	+	o	+	-	Tibolone
Progesterone	o	o	+	o	+/o	o	o	o/-	+	o	o	-	o	o	o	o	o	o	o	o	o	o	o	o	o	+	+	+	o	o	+	Progesterone Birth Control Pills
	o	o	+/o	+/o	+	+	+	+	+	+	+	o	o	o	o	o	+	o	-	o	@	o	-	+	o/+	+	+/-	+/-	-	Progesterone Cream
	n/a	n/a	n/a	n/a	n/a	n/a	n/a	n/a	n/a	n/a	n/a	n/a	n/a	n/a	n/a	n/a	n/a	n/a	n/a	n/a	n/a	n/a	n/a	n/a	n/a	n/a	n/a	n/a	n/a	n/a	Progesterone Gel
	n/a	n/a	n/a	n/a	n/a	n/a	n/a	n/a	n/a	n/a	n/a	n/a	n/a	n/a	n/a	n/a	n/a	n/a	n/a	n/a	n/a	n/a	n/a	n/a	n/a	n/a	n/a	n/a	n/a	n/a	Progesterone IUD
	o	o	+/o	o	+	-	-	+	+	+	-	o	o	o	o	o	-	o	o	o	-	+	+	+	+	+	-	Progesterone Pills
	o	o	+/o	o	+	-	-	+	+	+	-	o	o	o	o	o	-	o	o	o	+	+	o	+	+	-	Progesterone Shots
	o	o	+/o	+/o	+	+	+	+	+	+	-	o	o	o	o	o	-	o	o	o	-	+	+	o	o	o	-	USP Progesterone
Estrogen Plus Progesterone	+/o	o/-	+	-	+	-	-	o/-	+	+	+	+	+	+	+	+	+	+	+	+	+	+	+	+	+	+	+	+	+	o	Continuous HRT Pills
	+/o	o/-	+	-	+	-	-	o/-	+	+	+	+	+	+	+	+	+	+	+	+	+	+	+	+	+	+	+	+	+	+	Cyclic HRT Pills
	+/o	+	+	o/-	+	-	-	+	+	+	+	+	+	+	+	+	+	+	+	+	+	+	+	+	+	+	+	+	+	+	Estrogen + Progesterone Birth Control Pills
	+/o	+	+	o/-	+	o	o	+	+	+	+	+	+	+	+	+	+	+	+	+	+	+	+	+	+	+	+	+	+	+	Estrogen + Progesterone Birth Control Patch
	+/o	o/-	+	-	+	o	o	o/-	+	+	+	+	+	+	+	+	+	+	+	+	+	+	+	+	+	+	+	+	+	o	HRT Patches
Testosterone	+	o	o	-	+	+	+	+	o	-	+	o/-	o	o	+/o	-	-	o/-	o	o	o/-	o	o	o	+	o	o	o	o	o	Bioidentical DHEA
	o	o	o	-	+	+	+	+	o	o/-	+	o	o	o	+	-	o/-	o	o	o	o	o	o	o	o	o	o	o	+	o	Testosterone Cream
	o	o	o	o/-	+	+	+	+	o	o/-	+	o	o	o	+/o	-	o/-	-	o	o	o/-	o	+	+/-	+/-	o	o	o	o	o	Testosterone Pills
	+/o	o/-	o/-	o/-	+	-	-	-	o/-	-	+	-	+	-	+	-	+	+	+	+	+	+	+	+	+	+	+	-	Estrogen + Testosterone Pills
Other Hormones	o	o	o	o	+	o	o	o	o	o	o	o	o	o	o	o	o	o	o	o	o	o	o	o	o	o	o	o	o	o	Calcitonin
	o	o	o	o	o	o	o	o	o	o	o	o/-	o	o	o/-	o	o	o	o	o	o	o	o	o	o	o	o	o	@	o	Infertility Meds
	o	o	o	o	+	o	o	o	o	o	o	o	o	o	o	o	o	o	o	o	o	o	o	o	o	o	o	o	o	o	Teriparatide

Legend

- **+** Means: Improves the Situation, Prevents the Situation, or Produces a Desirable Effect.
- **-** Means: Worsens the Situation, Causes the Situation, or Produces an Undesirable Effect.
- **o** Means: Has No Effect on the Situation.
- **n/a** Means: Not Applicable.
- **?** Means: Unknown Effect.
- **@** Means that any result (+,-,0) is possible

Non-Hormonal Medication Options

Alzheimer's Disease	Ovarian Cancer	Uterine Cancer	Breast Cancer	Osteoporosis	Stroke	Blood Clots	Heart Attack	Headaches	Acne	Decreased Sex Drive	Weight Gain	Incontinence	Urinary Tract Infection	Vaginal Dryness	Hair Growth	Hair Loss	Dry Skin	Joint Pain	Breast Pain	Cravings	Depression	Irritability	Mood Swings	Forgetfulness	Fatigue	Insomnia	Night Sweats	Hot Flashes	Irregular Periods	
o	o	o	o	o	o	o	o	o	+	o	o	o	o	o	o	o	o	+	o	o	o	o	o	o	o	o	o	o	o	Acetaminophen
o	o	o	o	+	o	o	o	o	o	o	o	o	o	o	o	o	o	o	o	o	o	o	o	o	o	o	o	o	o	Alendronate (Fosamax)
o	o	o/-	+	-	o	o/-	o	o	o	-	o	o	o	o	o	o	o	-	o	o	o	o	o	o	o	o	o	-	o	Anastrozale (Armidex)
o	o	o	o	o	o	o	o	o	o	o	o	+	o	o	o	o	o	o	o	o	o	o	o	o	o	o	o	o	o	Anticholinergics
o	o	o	o	o	o	o	o	o	o	o	o	o	o	o	o	o	o	o	o	o	o	o	o	-	o	+	+	o	o	Antihistamines
o	o	o	o	o	o	o	o	+	o	o	o	o	o	o	o	o	o	o	o	o	o	o	o	-	o	+	+	o	o	Antihypertensives
o	o	o	o	o	o	o	o	o	o	o	o	+	o	o	o	o	o	o	o	o	o	o	o	o	o	o	o	o	o	Antispasmodics
o	o	o	o	o	+	+	+	+	o	o	o	o	o	o	o	o	o	o	o	o	o	o	o	o	o	o	o	o	o	Aspirin
o	o	o	o	-	o	o	o	o	o	o	o	o	o	o	o	o	o	o	o	o	-	-	o	+	o	o	o	o	o	Benzodiazepines
o	o	o	o	o	o	o	o	o	+	o	o	o	o	o	o	o	o	o	o	o	o	o	o	o	o	o	o	o	o	Benzoyl Peroxide
o	o	o	o	-	o	o	o	o	o	+/o	o/-	o	o/-	o	+	+	o	o	o/-	o	o	o	o	o	o	o	o	o	o/-	Deamethasone
o	o	o/-	+	-	o	o/-	o	o	o	-	o	o	o	o	o	-	o	o	o	o	o	o	o	o	o	o	o	-	o	Exemestane (Aromasin)
o	o	o	o	+	o	o	o	o	o	o	o	o	o	o	o	o	o	o	o	o	o	o	o	o	o	o	o	o	o	Ibandronate (Boniva)
o	o	o	o	o	o	o	o	o	o	o	o	o	o	o	o	o	o	o	o	o	o	o	o	+	+	o	o	o	o	Imidazopyridines
o	o	o	o	o	o	o	o	o	o	o	o	+	o	o	o	o	o	o	o	o	o	o	o	o	o	o	o	o	o	Incontinence Surgery
o	o	o	o	o	o	o	o	o	o	o	o	+	o	o	o	o	o	o	o	o	o	o	o	o	o	o	o	o	o	Injectable Substances into Bladder (Collagen)
o	o	o/-	+	-	o	o/-	o	o	o	o	-	o	o	o	o	o	-	o	o	o	o	o	o	o	o	o	o	-	o	Letrozole (Femara)
o	o	o	o	o	+/o	o	o	o	o	o	o	o	o	o	+	o	o	o	o	o	o	o	o	o	o	o	o	o	o	Minoxidil
o	o	o	o	o	o	o	o	o	o	o	o	o	o	o	o	o	o	o	o	o	o	o	o	o	o	o	+	+	o	Neurottin (Gabapenin)
o	o	o	o	o	o	o	o	+	o	o	o	o	o	o	o	o	o	+	o	o	o	o	o	o	o	o	o	o	o	NSAIDs
o	o	o	o	+	-	-	+	o	+/o	+/o	+/o	+/o	o	-	+/o	+/o	+/o	+/o	+/o	+/o	+/o	+/o	+/o	+/o	+/o	+/o	+/o	-	o	Raloxifene (Evista)
o	o	o	o	+	o	o	o	o	o	o	o	o	o	o	o	o	o	o	o	o	o	o	o	o	o	o	o	o	o	Risedronate (Actonel)
o	o	o	o	o	o	o	o	o	o	o	o	o	o	+	+	o	o	o	o	o	o	o	o	o	o	o	o	o	o	Spironolactone
o	o	o	o	o	o	o	o	o	-	+	+	o	o	o	o	o	o	o	o	+/o	+	+	+	-	o	+	+	+	o	SSRI Antidepressants
o	o	o	o	o	o	o	o	+	o	o	o	o	o	o	o	o	o	o	o	o	o	o	o	o	o	o	o	o	o	Statins
o	o	o	o	-	o	o	o	o	o	+/o	-	o	o/-	o	+	o	o	+	o	o/-	o	o	o	o	o	o	o	o	o/-	Steroids
o	o	-	+	+	-	-	+	o	o	-	o	o	o	-	o	o	o	o	-	o	o	-	o	o	-	o	-	-	-	Tamoxifen (Nolvadex)
o	o	o	o	o	o	o	o	o	o	o	o	+	o	o	o	o	o	o	o	o	o	o	o	o	o	o	o	o	o	Tolteridine
o	o	o	o	o	o	o	-	o	o	-	o	+	o	o	o	o	o	o	o	o	+	+	+	-	-	+	o	o	o	Tricyclic Antidepressants
o	o	o	o	o	o	o	o	o	o	o	o	o	o	o	+	o	o	o	o	o	o	o	o	o	o	o	o	o	o	Vaniqa Cream
o	o	o	o	o	o	o	o	+	o	o	o	o	o	o	o	o	o	o	o	o	o	o	o	o	o	o	o	o	o	Vasoconstrictors
o	o	o	o	o	o	o	o	o	o	+/o	o	o	o	o	o	o	o	o	o	o	o	o	o	o	o	o	o	o	o	Viagra/Cialis/Levitra
o	o	o	o	o	o	o	o	o	+	o	o	o	o	o	+	+/o	o	o	o	o	o	o	o	o	o	o	o	o	o	Vitamin A Meds

Legend

+   Means: Improves the Situation, Prevents the Situation, or Produces a Desirable Effect.

-     Means: Worsens the Situation, Causes the Situation, or Produces an Undesirable Effect.

o   Means: Has No Effect on the Situation.

n/a   Means: Not Applicable.

?   Means: Unknown Effect.

@   Means that any result (+,-,0) is possible

Section I:

Introduction

It Doesn't Have To Be This Way

You're a woman, and you wonder:

What's happening? You begin noticing that you have episodes of sudden increases in body temperature during the day and at night. You have difficulty sleeping because you awaken throughout the night in sweat-soaked sheets. You begin to exhibit mood swings, irritability, and depression. Your partner accuses you of being argumentative. Your kids and friends say you're no fun anymore. Because of this situation, you feel fatigued just about all the time. As if that weren't enough, you find that you're incredibly forgetful, and unable to focus on anything long enough to function in your normal, productive manner. To top it all off, you have dryness of your vagina which results in itching and painful intercourse. You want to do something to relieve yourself of your misery, but you just don't know where to begin.

You're a man, and you wonder:

What's going on with that special woman in your life? Is she going crazy? She could be your mother, your wife, your girlfriend, or your sister. You've always enjoyed a close, comfortable relationship with her, and you feel as though you know her quite well. But as she enters middle age, her behavior becomes bizarre. She acts like a completely different person! She's fragile in her mood to the point of making you feel like you're walking on eggshells. She isn't fun to be with anymore. And if she's your partner, her previous sexual interest in you is a distant memory. She complains of sweating a lot, and you just don't see what the big deal is. It may be that you live in a household with adolescents, too, and you just can't seem to make anyone happy these days. You're desperate for some guidance.

***

Just imagine dealing with menopause without adequate forewarning or preparation. Whether you're male or female, you are vaguely aware of the possibility that this may be menopause, but you really aren't sure because "menopause" is one of those taboo subjects. Coincidentally, it occurs at a time when things are already difficult for most people. Elderly parents need your help. Children are stumbling through adolescence, requiring you to stay focused and involved. You have college tuitions and retirement funds to think about. The last thing you need to contend with is a body full of confused hormones, or an adult partner behaving as erratically as the adolescents are.

If you're a woman, your mother probably didn't prepare you for this the way she did for the onset of your periods during puberty. That's ironic since puberty was temporary, while menopause is permanent. Your girlfriends make fleeting comments about menopause, but seem to know little about it. In your conversations with older women, you find that most of them either just endured menopause misery or consulted a physician who gave them a medication. These women didn't really understand the exact nature of the therapy.

So, you decide to do some research. As you scour the bookshelves for reading material, you encounter a number of books on menopause. It's bewildering! There's definitely more than one school of thought in the world of menopause. The books range from medical books to anti-medical books, from traditional to modern, from empowering to submissive, from humorous to angry. Most of them, however, promote one alternative for managing menopause over all other alternatives. One is dedicated solely to the use of progesterone cream. Another recommends herbal therapy. There's one that supports no therapy or intervention at all, and suggests that lifestyle changes alone are the answer. There's even one that promotes yoga as the only way to manage the change successfully. Another advertises a special menopause diet. A medical book presents hormones as the "one size fits all" answer for menopause. What's a woman to do?

It Doesn't Have To Be This Way

You notice a couple of books which cover the topic of menopause more broadly and offer a variety of options for management, but they are highly technical, detailed, and riddled with scientific terminology. You'd need a medical dictionary to make sense of them.

Many of the authors recommend that you do what they themselves have done for their own menopause. Some present various "types" of menopause and expect you to fit into one category or another. Inevitably, they seem to treat all women as carbon copies of one another. They assume that there is *one* option that's best for the entire female population, or that each woman falls into one of only a few categorical types. You think that surely the menopausal experience must vary from woman to woman. You wonder why these books advocate treating all women similarly at such an important time in their lives ... a time when they're all so different. Most books seem more like persuasive campaigns than unbiased guidance on options for management of a normal phase of life.

You find yourself thinking:

"If I already *knew* how I wanted to manage menopause, I might choose one of these books which focuses on that particular approach. What *I* want is a book that explains *all* that I need to know, lays out all the options *without* bias, and helps me decide for *myself* what's best for me. I'm not looking for someone else's opinion here. I don't fit into an artificial category that determines what I should do for menopause. I'm unique. I want to do things *my* way!"

You then notice that menopause authors have credentials ranging from fitness instructors, to naturopathic doctors, to medical doctors, to women who have experienced menopause personally, but have no credentials at all. Some are published authors on other topics who also wrote a book on menopause.

If you're male, you feel defeated in your effort to understand what's going on with your special woman and play a supportive role for her. It sure seems odd that there is so little information written for the male perspective. The books for men are mostly personal stories by guys commiserating about their roles as bystanders. Most advise you to just keep your distance while your special woman deals with menopause alone. The number of choices for men pales in comparison to the books about menopause written for women. You find that odd since this is a couples' issue for menopausal women with a male partner. You don't need to understand everything as thoroughly as a woman does, but you *do* want to have a basic understanding of what menopause is, and you want advice on how to be most empathetic. There seems to be plenty of material for males on dealing with puberty and adolescence. Why is it so different for menopause?

If you're female, you realize that you'll have to invest enough energy to read all of these books in their entirety. Then you'll have to compare each one's biases. Only then will you have the knowledge you need to make any decisions as to how you wish to manage your own menopause. How unrealistic! Since time is of the essence, and since you need help now, you decide to go to your doctor to address menopause on a personal level.

After having waited the frustratingly long time it took to get an appointment with your physician, you finally find yourself face-to-face with your healthcare provider. You list your symptoms:

- hot flashes
- night sweats
- insomnia
- mood swings
- irritability
- depression
- forgetfulness
- fatigue
- vaginal dryness
- diminished sex drive, and
- weight gain.

Recollection of these complaints required no written list. Your days are so continually plagued with these symptoms that your life is in complete turmoil. You're ineffective at work; you aren't loving towards your partner; you don't feel happy anymore; and your family and colleagues claim that you're unpleasant to be with. You've prepared yourself for a lengthy discussion with your physician about your symptoms and your preferences for managing them. You even requested extra time when you scheduled the appointment. You have the reasonable expectation that your healthcare provider will help you apply the basic information about menopause to your own physical, mental, and emotional situation. You expect help in balancing the pros and cons of various options. You've waited a long time for this appointment and you've suffered all the while.

But before you even finish your first sentence, your physician has summarily diagnosed your list of concerns as *"just menopause."* In a dismissive, perfunctory gesture, he/she has handed you a prescription, patted you on the hand, and said, "Take this. It's what I give all my menopausal patients."

You counter with:

"Is this my *only* option? What about lifestyle changes, herbal therapy, and other non-pharmaceutical options? I'm not opposed to taking hormones, but how can I be sure that this is the best choice *for me*? I just want to find what works best for me, and I want to discuss the benefits and risks of various options."

Your physician responds:

"Well, go right ahead and try other things if you wish, but you're on your own with those voodoo medicines. Physicians have nothing to do with any of those alternative methods."

As you leave that six minute office visit, you realize that you have the choice of accepting your physician's recommendation and taking a drug you know nothing about, or forging into the world of botanical/herbal therapy with no guidance from the medical profession. You've heard pros and cons about both medical and non-medical options. You feel unsure of yourself, insecure about your knowledge and choices, and victimized by the limited resources available to you.

The fact that all women go through menopause doesn't make it a minor event. Actually, it's one of life's most major events for women and men. It's a hormonal rollercoaster that disrupts your quality of life and ability to function normally. And there's nothing "routine" about it. Sure, it's a common aspect of female existence, but you've never gone through it before, and you'll never go back to your pre-menopausal state. So, for you as an individual, it's your one and only, one-of-a-kind event that isn't like anyone else's. You're an adult. You know yourself better than anyone else does. If your healthcare professional simply took the time to explain the process of menopause, the pertinent health issues, and the management options, you could make a wise, rational decision. Why is it so difficult to accomplish this? If menopause is a normal, natural process, then why is unbiased, comprehensible information so elusive?

STOP!

You can wake up now. You've been having a nightmare. Fortunately, it's over. The scenario you've just read doesn't have to happen to you. And hopefully, it hasn't *already* happened to you. Whether you're reading this before, during, or well beyond your menopausal transition, this book will serve you well. It will allow you to manage **your** menopause **your** way, before, during, and after the transition.

Chapter 1:
An Introduction to the Mystery of "Menopause"

The Longest Female Phase

Menopause is a natural process which all women experience if they're fortunate enough to live that long. It's as natural as infancy, childhood, adolescence, pregnancy, and death. And the time that you'll spend experiencing menopause ranges from one third to one half of your entire life. That's right. Think about it. Menopause occurs at about age 51, and we're living into our 80s, 90s, and even past 100. Menopause marks the last hormonal phase of a woman's life. Once you become menopausal, you'll remain menopausal for the *rest of your life*! This long duration of life after the reproductive phase is most profound for humans. Most mammals live long enough to reproduce, but may not live long after that.

Yet, the level of familiarity on the subject of menopause pales in comparison with that on the other phases of life. How can this be? Everyone, whether female or male, young or old, will either experience menopause personally or interact with a woman who is menopausal. Because menopause is more than just a subtle, minor event, it deserves special attention. It isn't fair to you or your family and friends to gloss over this important part of the female life cycle.

Menopause isn't just a phase. It's actually a population explosion. If you look at the numbers of menopausal women, they will astound you. Get this:

- In the year 2000, the United States alone had almost 42 million women over the age of 50. That amounted to nearly one out of every three women.[1]
- Every year, approximately 2 million women in the U.S. reach the age of 50.[1]
- Worldwide, the number of postmenopausal women was 569 million in the year 2000.[1]
- By the year 2020, there will be 967 million postmenopausal women.[1]
- By the year 2030, there will be 1.2 billion postmenopausal women.[1]
- These figures don't even include the 600,000 women who become menopausal by surgical means each year.[1]

Surprisingly, it seems that mere acceptance of menopause is lacking. The majority of women are not prepared for it in advance. Stories abound of women who had no idea what was happening when they began to experience the signs and symptoms of menopause. These are mature adults who feel clueless about their own bodies. I don't want you to be one of them. Just as mothers prepare their daughters for the onset of their menstrual cycles so that they will accept them as a part of normal female existence, medical professionals should prepare women for the onset of menopause. Historically, though, such preparation has been neglected.

You shouldn't have to settle for confusion and lack of preparation for the longest phase of your life.

Information Sources

Practical, impartial, simple information on menopause is sparse. Yet, there are more books on menopause than on any other subject in women's health.[2] Most of the available literature on menopause is biased, favoring certain options over all others, and promoting those particular biased options to all women. Such an approach is absurd! The simple fact is that *no two women are alike.* We all differ with regard to our genetic backgrounds, health statuses, body types and shapes, personal preferences, perceptions, and attitudes about menopause itself. You are unique. *You know yourself better than anyone else does.* As long as you have complete and accurate information, you will make the best decisions with regard to management of your own menopausal experience.

I think the best way to approach the question of whether and how to manage menopause is to gain as much knowledge as possible about all the issues. This book will give you exactly what you need to meet that goal. Once you have complete and accurate information about menopause, ask yourself whether or not you prefer to manage menopause at all. If your answer is, "No," you've made your decision as an informed adult. If your answer is, "Yes," you then need to decide which option(s) you prefer to pursue. This book will help you navigate the choices without having to go to a multitude of individual biased sources.

You shouldn't have to rely on mass media to learn about menopause. Nor should you assume that your mother has told you all that you need to know. As with most medical and health choices, friends and colleagues don't have adequate knowledge or experience to advise one another. It's no secret that the medical profession has devoted too little time to counseling on menopause. Most women are starved for information, but the only information available to them is scanty, biased, or distorted. In many cases, these women are the victims of medical professionals who are limited in *their* knowledge about menopause. Rather than offering choices, physicians substitute their own judgments and preferences for those of their patients, leaving patients with little knowledge and plenty of uncertainty about their options. Many physicians distribute the same medication to all their menopausal patients, even those who don't want any form of medical therapy at all. Some women who are taking hormones have no idea as to why they are doing so.

There is a vast array of information available on menopause. However, because of the overwhelming quantity of contradictory information, most women feel confused. With the barrage of media information, marketing, hype, and scare tactics that abound, most women have a difficult time assessing what's accurate.

This book is my attempt to communicate with you in a manner which dispels the confusion. I plan to communicate with you so clearly that you not only understand what menopause is and what to expect when you encounter it, but also how to apply all aspects of that information to yourself as a unique individual. I want you to be able to form preferences about the best way to manage your own menopause based on accurate, unbiased information. I want you to feel empowered to trust yourself. I want you to feel free to change your mind and your management as you evolve over the years. That's a lofty goal, and one which I embrace with great enthusiasm and care.

Don't settle for anything less than a full understanding of menopause. You'll spend almost half of your life as a menopausal woman. You owe it to yourself to make them very good years.

More Than Just The Golden Rule

As an obstetrician/gynecologist, I believe that my most important role is that of an educator. To be a good educator requires attention to some basic principles. But, it requires something else far beyond that. I'm sure you're familiar with "The Golden Rule." It's the simple principle of treating each patient just as I would want my caretaker to treat me. That's a good start. But wait a minute! What if your desires are *different* from mine? Should I simply impose my own desires on you anyway? Should I tell you that I can't help you? Of course not! It means that I need to go *beyond* The Golden Rule to give you what *you* want.

I love learning, so I tend to go to school again and again. One of my educational endeavors was law school. (Yes, I'm sort of a nerd!) When I was in law school, I concentrated heavily on health law. One of the most basic concepts in health law is something called "the standard of care." It's a term which refers to the appropriate duty a physician has to a patient in terms of informed consent and medical care. As with most things in the legal profession, there are many ways to define "standard of care." Here's a list of some of the definitions for that term:

1. The care which a reasonable physician in the same circumstance would deliver to an average patient
2. The care which the reasonable patient would expect in a similar circumstance
3. The care which *this particular patient* would expect in *her actual* circumstance

An Introduction to the Mystery of "Menopause"

As you compare those definitions, what do you notice about them? The first one is all about the *physician's* point of view, without regard for the patient's wishes at all. It's the professional-community standard. It requires that your doctor provide information and care equal to that of another professional with similar training. It assumes that all patients are the same, defined as "the average patient." I'm sure you don't consider yourself an "average patient" under any circumstance. And even if your physician is reasonable in terms of the same circumstance for another patient, do you really think that all you deserve is the standard treatment for the average patient?

The second definition takes into account the wishes of the "reasonable patient," which is just another way of implying "average patient." But it doesn't take into account the fact that your personal desires or needs may be completely different from those of the "average patient." It's the reasonable-person standard. It requires that your doctor provide information and care which a reasonable person with the same diagnosis or situation would need. *Your* needs may be entirely unique. If they are, and your physician meets this standard of care, you won't feel as though your needs have been met at all. Whose definition of "reasonable" counts here, anyway, yours or your physician's?

The third definition is the one I like the best. In fact, it's the only one I like at all. It's the particular patient in her unique circumstance standard. It makes the most sense, doesn't it? It's all about **you**, as an individual with unique needs and desires. It requires your physician to interact with you sufficiently to get to know you. It means that you would probably want to know *everything* about your situation, and you'd want to know *all* your options. You would want your physician to *tailor* everything to your particular needs. That's what any reasonable patient expects. Simply put, that's what you deserve.

You Decide

Your decision is what this book is all about. You're not interested in knowing what I do for my menopause. You're not interested in what I would do if I were you. You want complete information to apply to your unique circumstance, and you want to have the freedom to choose your **own** options.

That doesn't mean that you're on your own. You certainly may request some guidance. But you'll have the fundamental knowledge so that you can participate to whatever extent you desire. You'll be empowered to manage *your* menopause in the way that's best for *you*.

My interaction with each patient is a partnership. There is mutual respect for the elements we each contribute to the process of managing her unique situation. I offer knowledge, experience, and scientific evidence. She offers self awareness, personal preferences, family history, and the final decision as to which option she prefers. In this book, I vow to do my best to deliver information to you based on my knowledge and experience. I will respect your right to honor your own preferences. I hope you do, too.

Any time you make your own decision about management or treatment of a problem, you always have more peace of mind and motivation to create a positive outcome than someone who has no personal stake in the matter. In all my years of practicing obstetrics and gynecology, I have never made a decision *for* a patient. What I have done is empower her to make the best decision for herself. This takes time. Some patients make decisions quite readily. Others require more consideration of the benefits and risks of their options. I do whatever it takes to ensure that my patient has all the information she needs to feel secure with her fund of knowledge and her final decision.

Now, not everyone makes a decision with which I agree. But everyone has the right to make her own decision. The key is to ensure that you are not overlooking data which would cause you to alter that decision. I have never had a patient choose an option that was intentionally harmful to herself once she fully understood all of the ramifications of her choices.

Years ago, it was common for a patient to avoid any part in the decision-making process for medical issues. The common response from the patient was, "Whatever you recommend, Doctor," or "I'll do whatever you think is best." This response is neither healthy nor appropriate. It relinquishes both the consideration of alternatives and the final decision to the physician. Rather than accepting such a responsibility, the physician should discuss all of the options anyway.

An Introduction to the Mystery of "Menopause"

The patient's delegation of the final decision to the physician is just the *beginning* of the decision-making process rather than the end.

Likewise, asking a physician what they would do in a similar situation or what they would want for their wife or daughter is simply an expression of uncertainty. It indicates that you need more information. Why in the world would you care what someone's wife or daughter would choose in a similar situation? Why would you assume that your physician has the same value system and personal preferences that you have? In reality, it doesn't matter what anyone else would do. It is the job of your healthcare provider to present information in a factual, statistical, unbiased manner, and to tailor that information to your personal situation in a way that allows you to easily feel at least a slight preference for one or two options. It may take time to narrow down your choice to one final decision. But, once you understand the scientific aspects of your situation, you know yourself well enough to find a match between the facts and your preferences.

The American medical community is encountering the largest number of menopausal women ever.[3] Approximately 45 million women will enter their menopausal years over the next two decades.[4] With the huge numbers of women from the baby boom generation entering their menopausal years, simple, useful, nonbiased information on menopause is long overdue. My goal is to provide this information in a manner that allows you to make choices which best suit your needs and desires.

In writing this book, it is *not* my purpose to recommend only the "best course of action" with regard to management of your menopause. It would be quite presumptuous of me to assume that I know what is best or most desirable for you. This is a book, for heaven's sake. As such, you and I don't have the luxury of interacting. I would hope that you would find it offensive for me to assume that I know your needs better than you do.

There are no anecdotes in this book. I don't think that giving you a variety of other women's experiences with menopause makes much sense. You're not going to be a clone of any of them. You may have similarities to one or more of them, and your *differences* may be more important than the similarities. You shouldn't have to decipher which similarities or differences are most pertinent for choosing your own course of action. You shouldn't feel pressure to follow a course of action similar to the one that the "anecdotal model" chose. *You* are an original. So, I'll give you the information you need, and you can apply it to the one and only *you*. You get to create your own style of managing *your* unique menopause.

Likewise, I won't waste your time by telling you what I would do in various circumstances. It's not that I don't have personal experience with this stuff. I became menopausal in 1994, at the age of 34. So, I've lived through many wonderful years as a menopausal woman. I intend to live through many decades more. I've tried the majority of the available options. I've done so because I'm a curious person who believes in trying things out to find what works best for me. But more than that, I've tried a variety of things because I wanted to know first hand about menopausal options for the sake of my patients. I know that I can give you more information and relate better to your experience if I've tried a lot of these things personally. I've gone to a health store or vitamin shop on a number of occasions and purchased one of everything they have in stock for menopause. You can imagine the looks and comments I've gotten at the check-out counter. Nevertheless, these shopping sprees have enabled me to do a better job in helping other women with managing their own menopause. I've tried a variety of the pharmaceutical options, too. I guess you could say that I've used myself as a lab animal.

There are two reasons that I won't be giving you testimonials about my own menopause. First, you probably don't care what my own personal choices are; and second, I would not want my own choices to sway the decisions you make for yourself. I wouldn't want you to forfeit your opportunity to exercise your own opinion or substitute my judgment for your own.

On the other hand, I don't want you to consider this a do-it-yourself book for managing menopause. It *is* a self help book to the extent that it will serve as an educational reference which gives you a comprehensive fund of knowledge about menopause. You *will* be prepared for menopause; you *will* be an informed patient in your dealings with healthcare providers; and you *will* be a smart consumer in assessing products for management of your menopause. You'll know the correct terminology to request exactly what you want, and you'll know what your options are. In other words, you won't have to settle for anything less than *your* menopause *your* way.

Empowerment

The only opinion that matters is *yours*. That is, of course, as long as you aren't in denial about your circumstances. You must be careful to avoid belittling any risk factor that exists for you. Be honest with yourself about the need to weigh a factor heavily with regard to the attention it deserves. For example, even if you smoke only occasionally, you're still a smoker, and all the risk factors related to smoking apply to you. When in doubt, err on the side of being extra careful rather than adopting a cavalier attitude of being invincible. By utilizing a conservative approach, you can rest assured that you'll make safe choices.

If I succeed in accomplishing the goals I've set for myself in writing this book, it will provide you with all you need to make excellent choices. I have no intention of letting you down.

In law, the answer to almost any question is, "It depends." The same can be said about answering questions as to your best options for menopause. Addressing options for management of menopause involves considering many variables. Here's a list of the factors you must consider in choosing how to manage your own menopause:

1. Your age
2. Whether you're approaching, experiencing, or beyond the transition into menopause
3. Presence or absence of symptoms of menopause
4. Presence or absence of vaginal bleeding (periods)
5. Personal history of medical problems
6. Risks for medical problems
7. Family history of medical problems
8. Personal history of surgical procedures
9. Body habitus (shape, height, weight, and where you accumulate fat)
10. Dietary habits

11. Exercise habits
12. Tobacco use
13. Personal preferences with regard to medical versus non-medical choices
14. Past experiences with menopausal management options
15. Geographic residence and proximity to available resources
16. Short-term and long-term goals

Now, although this is quite a lengthy list, you know the intricacies of all these variables as they pertain to you personally. We aren't dealing with a monumental mental exercise here. However, it's ludicrous to think that someone other than yourself would be able to adequately consider and balance all of these factors and make a proper decision for you. I resent books that promote a particular menopause management option for all women. I hope you do, too. Menopause is about empowerment. You have the power and the wisdom to consider your choices and to make wise decisions. When it comes to menopause, *it's all about YOU*!

This information is very straight-forward, complete, and nonbiased. I think you'll find it surprisingly easy to use the information in this book to manage your menopausal transition in a manner which suits you best. The information here will serve as a safety net to ensure that you don't overlook the health issues you need to acknowledge in making choices. Honor your preferences and take control.

Chapter 2:
An Orientation to the Parts and Processes of Menopause

We'll start with the basics to lay the foundation for a full discussion on menopause. While some of this may seem elementary to you, I want anyone reading this book to understand it. So, I'd rather give you a review than omit something fundamental. The first thing you need is a definition for menopause, so we'll start there.

<u>**Menopause**</u> is the process during which you transition from the reproductive to the non-reproductive phase of your life. You were born with over a million immature eggs in your ovaries. With each menstrual cycle, you've ovulated an egg (or maybe two in certain instances of twinning). During your reproductive years, you've only had approximately 450 menstrual cycles, and many of your eggs have just shriveled up. With all this ovulating and shriveling up of your eggs, the more than one million that you were born with dwindle. When you have only about 1000 left, you reach a critically low number of eggs and your fertility begins to wane. Menopause signifies the end of the reproductive portion of your life. It's the time when menstrual periods stop. "Meno" means menstruation, and "pause" means stop. Menopause results when the ovaries stop producing eggs.

Traditionally, the primary focus with regard to menopause is on the hormone estrogen, because menopause constitutes a time when estrogen production from the ovaries ceases. However, as I will explain later, this is a simplified version of a much more elaborate series of changes in the levels of numerous hormones over time.

Puberty in Reverse

The best way to understand menopause is to use puberty as an analogy. Remember those wonderful early adolescent years when your body began changing into its adult form? We call those collective physical changes "puberty." While many events occur during puberty, one of the most significant occurrences for females is the onset of menstrual periods. The medical term for the first period is "menarche." Because of menarche, puberty is the process that defines the beginning of a woman's reproductive years.

There is a tendency to use the terms "puberty" and "adolescence" interchangeably. While they are closely related, they don't really refer to the same thing, so let's make a distinction between them. <u>Puberty</u> is the time when the potential for reproduction begins. It includes breast development, appearance of pubic hair, growth of hair in the arm pits, and the first period ("menarche"). So, the word puberty refers to the physical changes which make your body capable of reproduction.

It would be grand if that's all there were to our transition into adulthood. We'd reach full maturity in our early teens and reflect on it as a fairly simple transition. But Mother Nature has made sure that we have more than just fleeting memories of that special time in our lives. She's added adolescence to the process of becoming an adult. <u>Adolescence</u> is the time between puberty and full maturity. During adolescence, you have predictable monthly cycles which end in a period. The medical term for this is "menstrual cycles." It's also the time when you have emotional changes, acne, weight gain, and relationship conflicts (especially with your parents). Most adolescents want a lot of sleep, and have cravings for carbohydrates. It's a time of confusion for the body and the mind.

For most people, it's not the actual bodily changes of puberty that make adolescence difficult. It's all the stuff that goes along with it. Reflect back on your adolescent years. If you're like most women, you

An Orientation to the Parts and Processes of Menopause

probably think that starting your periods would have been a breeze if you hadn't had to deal with all the emotional and physical aspects that accompanied adolescence, also. And it would have been much nicer if it hadn't gone on for so many years!

Well, now you're at the other end of the reproductive spectrum. Menopause is the time when your menstrual cycles (periods) cease. It's that time when you can declare yourself as belonging to the non-reproductive population. As you'll see later in this book, menopause is like puberty in that it involves a lot more than just putting your periods in the past. There are a variety of physical, emotional, and behavioral changes which make it much more interesting than that. And it takes time to make the full transition.

As you can see, menopause and puberty are at opposite ends of the reproductive spectrum. Puberty defines the beginning of reproductive capacity while menopause defines the end of reproductive capacity. The two processes are, in essence, mirrors or opposites of one another. Because they mark the beginning and the end of the same physiologic state, it's only natural that they resemble one another in terms of what you'll notice when you are experiencing either one.

Think back on your own experience during puberty. Wasn't it wonderful? Didn't you just love it? I'll bet it was a breeze for you and a joy for your parents, right? At this point, you're probably thinking, "Wait a minute. You must be kidding!" If so, you get my drift. The point is that puberty and menopause are both a little rough.

Here are some of the ways in which menopause and puberty mimic one another: Both are a result of hormonal changes occurring over a period of months or years. In both instances, these hormonal changes affect physical, emotional, and social aspects of your life. Think back on how difficult it is for adolescents to adjust to the process of puberty. They experience mood swings, irritability, desirable and undesirable bodily changes, acne, new behaviors, and new sexual issues. Likewise, a menopausal woman may have any or all of these same occurrences. Just as it may be difficult for family members to understand and relate to an adolescent experiencing puberty, they may have the same difficulty understanding or relating to a menopausal woman.

Menopause = Puberty in reverse:

Puberty	Menopause
Begin reproductive years	End reproductive years
Periods begin	Periods end
Physical changes	Physical changes
Emotional changes	Emotional changes
Behavioral changes	Behavioral changes
Difficult for family members	Difficult for family members
Some aspects are temporary; others are permanent	Some aspects are temporary; others are permanent

Fortunately, menopause offers much more in the way of options for management than puberty does. This book gives you complete and accurate information in a simple format. It helps you understand menopause and all of its various manifestations. Once you have this understanding, you'll readily see that menopause is a process for which there are many management options. It's not a disease any more than puberty is. However, there are many opportunities to make menopause much more enjoyable and tolerable than puberty. Hopefully, this book will assist you in making both your transition into menopause and the ensuing menopausal years as simple and pleasant as possible.

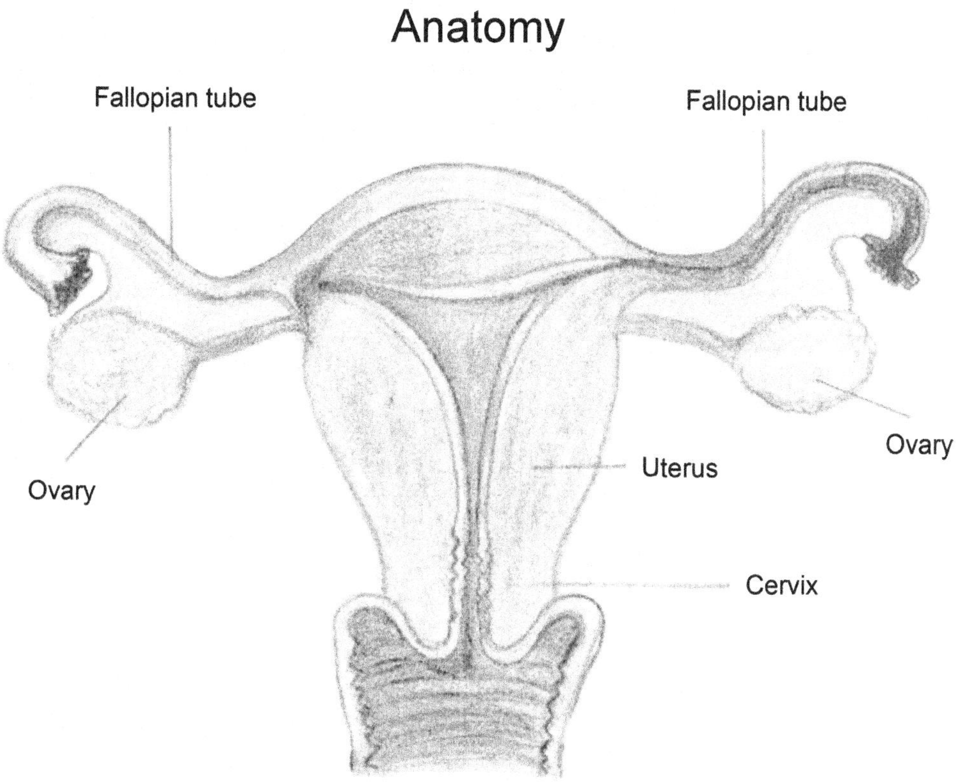

An Orientation to the Parts and Processes of Menopause

Anatomy

Figure 1: Female reproductive organs

Here's a picture of the female reproductive organs. There are four basic body parts, but only one of them has a direct role in bringing about the process of menopause. We'll address each anatomical structure separately. This may seem incredibly basic to you, and it is. However, I'd rather bore you with some things you already know than skip something you don't know. Who knows, you may be surprised. It's not uncommon for people to realize that they had a misunderstanding about some of the basics. So, read on.

The **cervix** is the doorway, or gateway, to the uterus. It's actually part of the uterus, but it protrudes into the vagina. Your doctor can actually see it if he/she looks into the vagina, and it's the site where a pap smear is taken. It consists of muscular and fibrous tissue, and it has a tough, firm consistency.

Menopause

If you were to view your cervix by looking into your own vagina, you would say it looks just like a donut. Yes, a donut! It's round with a hole in the middle of it. The central hole can open to varying degrees to let things pass in and out of the uterus.

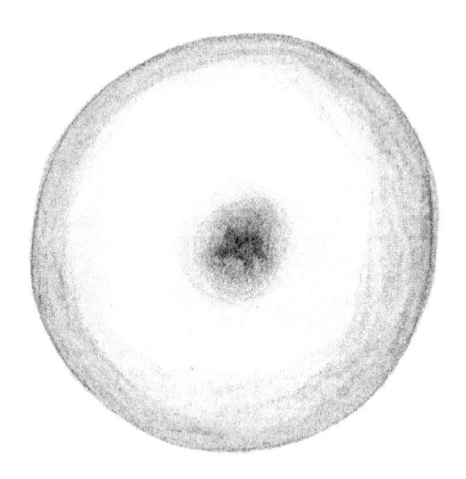

Figure 2: Cervix

The cervix has varying roles depending on what's going on in the reproductive tract at the time. During menstruation, it is the orifice through which blood exits the uterus in the form of a period. Its reproductive functions include allowing sperm to swim through the orifice, up the uterus, and into the fallopian tube to fertilize an egg. Then it serves the function of staying closed to hold the growing baby in the uterus. When it's time for delivery, it dilates to let the baby out. The cervix has no role in the process of menopause. Think of it as nothing more than a doorway or gateway. All it does is allow things to pass into and out of the uterus. It allows sperm to enter the uterus, and it allows your menstrual flow and babies to exit the uterus. It has nothing to do with hormones.

The **uterus** is directly attached to the cervix. In fact, the cervix and the uterus are actually one continuous structure. Taken together, they look like an upside down pear. The uterus and cervix together are actually just about the size of a small pear, also.

An Orientation to the Parts and Processes of Menopause

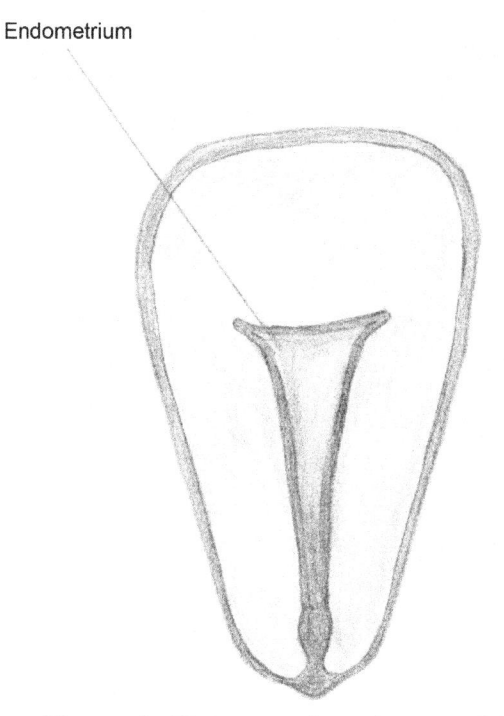

Figure 3: Uterus with endometrial lining

The uterus, like the cervix, has different functions depending on what's going on in the neighborhood. The best way to appreciate the functions of the uterus is to separate the uterus into two layers. The inner layer is the uterine lining, which lines the hollow cavity of the uterus. The outer layer is a thick, muscular layer with a consistency similar to that of the cervix. Let's address the functions of each of these layers, one at a time.

First, we'll focus on the inner lining of the uterus, which is called the "*endometrium*." This is the part of the uterus that is most sensitive to hormones. It doesn't produce hormones; it only *responds* to them. So, it changes according to changes in hormone levels. Over the course of a month, the inner lining of the uterus thickens as the level of estrogen gradually rises. At the end of the monthly cycle, when the lining is thick, the uterine lining does one of two things. If pregnancy has occurred (from the union of egg and sperm), the uterine lining functions as a nice, thick cushion into which the fertilized egg can bury. It serves as a burrow for the developing baby. Progesterone is the hormone which allows the lining to remain thick enough to support a pregnancy. On the other hand, if no pregnancy has occurred, there is no reason for the lining to remain thick. In that case, the progesterone level drops drastically, allowing the lining to shed. The process of shedding the uterine lining is what constitutes a period. Then the cycle begins again.

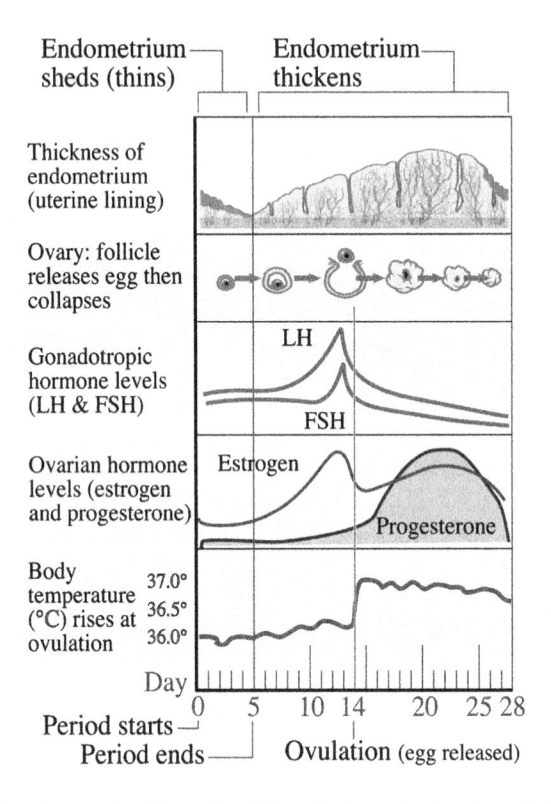

Figure 4: Hormone cycle and effect on endometrial lining and ovulation

The outer layer of the uterus is nothing more than a thick muscle, similar in consistency to the cervix. The uterus really functions like any other muscle in your body. All it knows how to do is contract, relax, or stretch. During pregnancy, it stretches to house a baby. As the pregnancy progresses, the muscular layer becomes thinner, stretching to accommodate the growing baby. When it's time for delivery, it contracts to expel the baby. So, the contractions of labor are nothing more than muscular contractions of the uterine muscle. When there is no pregnancy, the uterine muscle stays relaxed most of the time. Then, at the end of your menstrual cycle each month, it contracts to expel the menstrual blood in the form of a period. Contractions enable the uterus to expel its contents. Both menstrual cramps and labor pains are contractions of the uterine muscle.

An Orientation to the Parts and Processes of Menopause

The **fallopian tubes** extend outward from both sides of the uterus. There are two fallopian tubes. They are soft, thin, frail structures. The fallopian tubes serve as a bridge, or connection, between the uterus and the ovaries. As the picture illustrates, each fallopian tube comes in contact with one of the two ovaries, so that there is a fallopian tube – ovary unit on each side of the uterus.

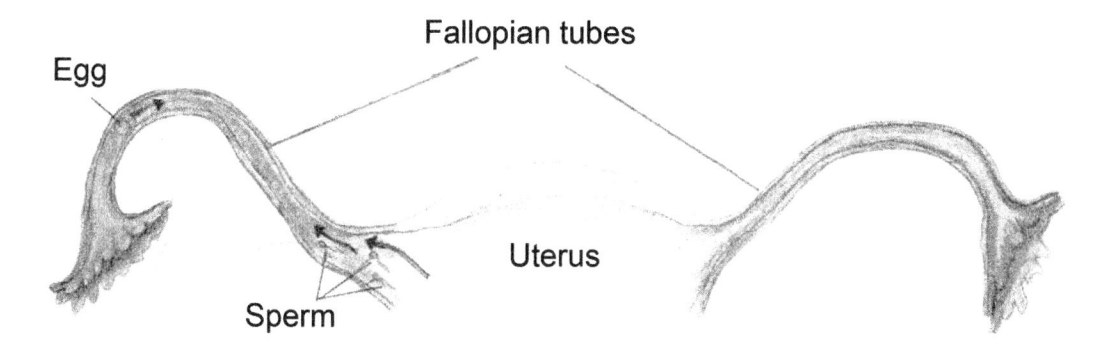

Figure 5: Fallopian tubes

Think of the fallopian tubes as highways along which the egg and sperm travel in order to unite with one another. The egg travels from the ovary and into the fallopian tube toward the uterus. The sperm travels up from the vagina, through the cervix, through the uterus, and into the fallopian tube. The egg and sperm have a head-on collision in the fallopian tube, and that constitutes fertilization of the egg.

The end of the fallopian tube that is in contact with the ovary has finger-like extensions which drape over the ovary. These fingers are able to grasp an egg as it is extruded from the ovary. That's how the egg gets into the fallopian tube. Once in the fallopian tube, the egg travels to the uterus, regardless of whether or not it gets fertilized along the way.

If a sperm unites with the egg in the fallopian tube, and fertilization occurs, it results in the beginning of a pregnancy. That fertilized egg travels to the uterus, where it buries into the thick, cushioned uterine lining. If the egg doesn't get fertilized, it simply travels down the fallopian tube to the uterus and gets flushed out of the body with the menstrual period.

Menopause

The **ovaries** are two glistening, round, structures that dangle just below the finger-like projections of the fallopian tubes. They have the greatest responsibility of all the reproductive organs. They are active during the reproductive phase of your life. Their size and appearance change depending on whether or not you are pre- (before) or post- (after) menopausal.

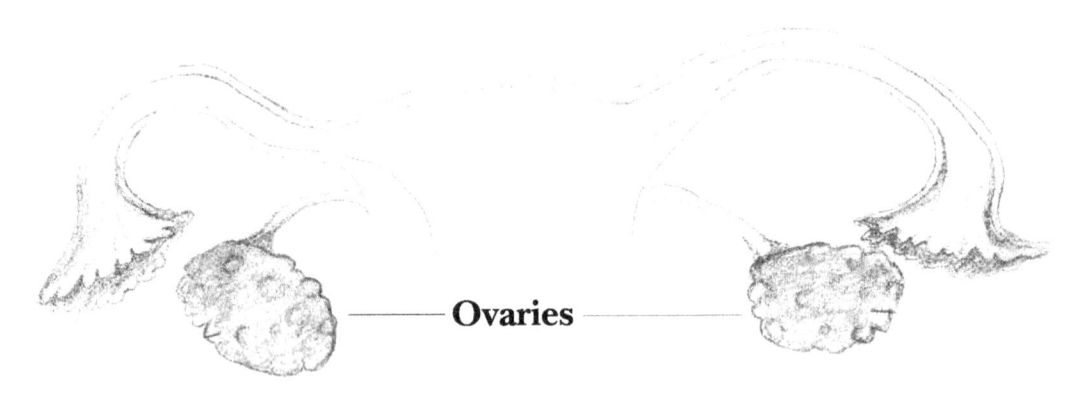

Figure 6: Ovaries

Before menopause, the ovaries are plump, walnut-sized, smooth, and extremely active. They are soft and full. They contain hundreds of thousands of eggs, all of which are already present at the time of birth. Over the years between menarche and post-menopause, one egg matures each month and leaves the ovary through a process called ovulation. When you think about it, a very small percentage of the available eggs are actually used during your lifetime. Usually, the ovaries alternate each month in preparing an egg for ovulation. But if you only had one ovary, that one ovary would take over the job full time and ovulate every month. Now that's an example of how creative and smart Mother Nature is. Having two ovaries instead of only one is just brilliant.

The ovaries are also hormone factories. They produce the vast majority of estrogen in the human female body. The production of estrogen and the preparation of eggs for ovulation are linked. The level of estrogen determines the ovary's ability to make an egg mature enough for ovulation.

An Orientation to the Parts and Processes of Menopause

After menopause, the ovaries are shriveled, grape-sized, wrinkled, and dormant. Instead of the soft, full consistency that they once had, they are now very hard, firm, and nodular. They have discontinued the process of preparing eggs for ovulation. They have drained themselves of all hormone production. You could say they've retired and gone out of business. They have served their purpose and have no significant function any longer.

Now, if you had to designate which anatomical structures have the largest role in the process of menopause, I'll bet you would have no hesitation in choosing the *ovaries*. As you can gather from this basic description of the parts and their functions, it's quite obvious that the ovaries literally govern the process of menopause. In fact, menopause is all about your ovaries, your eggs, and the hormone estrogen. So, in any discussion concerning menopause, narrow your focus to the ovaries.

Forget about the uterus in terms of what *causes* menopause. It plays no part in bringing about menopause. Many people mistakenly believe that the uterus is pertinent in producing hormones and causing menopause. That's not correct. Don't make the same mistake. Think ovaries!

"I'm Not Sure Which Surgical Procedure I've Had."

The title of this section isn't an exaggeration. It's quite common for a woman who has had surgery to admit that she is unsure as to the surgical procedure she's had. It's also common for a woman to assume she knows which anatomical parts were removed during surgery, but to be incorrect in her assumption. There are many misconceptions and misunderstandings about what was removed, what remains, why surgery was necessary in the first place, and a host of other particulars. One of the most significant problems is that people tend to mislabel procedures. Thus, they use the name of a common surgical procedure to describe something other than that particular procedure. The result is total confusion for the woman, her healthcare provider, and everyone with whom she communicates about her surgery. In some cases, the incorrect term for a surgical procedure is *so* rampant that it's very difficult to erase the misconceptions that seem to be shared by so many people.

So, let's get the terms right and match them with the proper procedures. Then let's designate which ones result in menopause and which ones don't. Once again, this is an area in which you may presume that you already know what's what, but don't bet on it. You may be surprised. The misconceptions are so common that most people are amazed once they learn the truth.

Total Hysterectomy is the term for surgical removal of the *uterus and cervix* **only** (Total = with the cervix, Hyster = uterus, Ectomy = removal of). Realize that the word "total" does *not* mean that the ovaries were removed. Total Hysterectomy does **not** cause menopause.

If you'll reflect back on what you learned when I described the uterus and the cervix, I told you that the uterus and the cervix are actually *one* structure. (It looks just like an upside down pear.) There's no true demarcation as to where the uterus ends and the cervix begins. So, the "total uterus" consists of both the uterus **and the cervix.** They're naturally attached. If you think of it this way, it will make sense to refer to removal of the uterus and cervix as a "Total Hysterectomy."

This is one of the most common areas of misconception. Very few people can correctly define "Total Hysterectomy." Most of them think it means all the female reproductive organs were removed. They'll say it means "total clean-out" or that "nothing is left." Almost everyone thinks it means removal of the ovaries. Test this yourself. Go around and ask a few people what the term means. I'll be surprised if you get a single correct answer. I'll bet that some of them are so sure of themselves (wrongly), that they'll actually fight with you about it. Even women who've had hysterectomies themselves will get it wrong. (Thus the title of this section!)

If your uterus and cervix are absent, but you still have your ovaries, you will still produce the hormone estrogen. You'll still have cycles, also. You just won't have a uterus to respond to the hormone cycles or to shed its lining in the form of a period. So, you will experience natural menopause at the average age of menopause (approximately 51), marked by the usual signs and symptoms of menopause, minus the dwindling of periods. This makes sense, doesn't it? Simply put, as long as you have ovaries that function properly, you haven't encountered menopause.

Subtotal or Partial Hysterectomy is the term for surgical removal of the uterus *without* removal of the cervix (Subtotal/Partial = without the cervix, Hyster = uterus, Ectomy = removal of). This does **not** cause menopause.

Once again, think about the uterus and the cervix as one structure (the upside down pear). If your surgeon doesn't remove the "total" structure, but instead leaves a portion of it in place (the cervix), she's performed a "Subtotal Hysterectomy." Here's another way of saying this: If your surgeon removes only "part" of that structure, it makes sense to call it a "Partial Hysterectomy." The key is to think of the uterus and the cervix as one structure with two parts.

Notice that the words "subtotal" or "partial" do *not* refer to the ovaries in any manner! They do *not* mean the ovaries were left in place. Rather, they mean that the **cervix** was left in place. This is another area of extreme confusion. Go ahead and conduct another experiment. Ask some people what "Partial Hysterectomy" means. Most of them will tell you it means removal of the uterus without the ovaries. Wrong!

With a Subtotal Hysterectomy or Partial Hysterectomy, you'll have the same results as with a Total Hysterectomy. You'll have hormone cycles until natural menopause occurs. You'll have no periods because there is no uterus in which to build up a lining that can shed. Remember, other than serving as a passageway for sperm, menstrual blood, or a baby, the cervix has no purpose. Since the uterus is absent, there is no build-up of its lining, no periods, and no possibility of pregnancy. The cervix just plugs the top of your vagina.

Unilateral Salpingectomy is the term for surgical removal of one fallopian tube (Uni = one, Lateral = side, Salpinx/Salpingo = fallopian tube, Ectomy = removal of)). This has no effect on menopause, and does **not** cause menopause. The result is that an egg and sperm have no meeting place on that side of the uterus. If pregnancy occurs, it will originate on the opposite side, using the other fallopian tube as the meeting place for the egg and sperm.

MENOPAUSE

With a salpingectomy, there are no noticeable changes in periods, hormone cycles, or menopause. The body knows that one fallopian tube is gone, so it uses the opposite fallopian tube and ovary for all its functions. Even though one fallopian tube is gone, you won't even be aware of it.

Bilateral Salpingectomy is the term for removal of both fallopian tubes (Bi = two, Lateral = sides, Salpinx/Salpingo = fallopian tube, Ectomy = removal of). This does **not** cause menopause. However, it may decrease the blood supply to the ovaries, resulting in lower levels of estrogen production by the ovaries. While such an effect is not common, it is possible.

The obvious result of Bilateral Salpingectomy is that eggs and sperm cannot travel to a meeting place and unite. That's why "tying the tubes" (tubal ligation) is a very reliable means of permanent pregnancy prevention.

After Bilateral Salpingectomy, the ovaries continue to produce eggs and hormones. Since there's no place for the egg to travel, it simply tumbles out of the ovary and falls into the surrounding area, where it dissolves.

The uterus functions in its usual fashion, responding to hormones and shedding its lining according to hormone cycles.

Unilateral Oophorectomy is the term for surgical removal of a single ovary (Uni = one, Lateral = side, Ooph/Oophor = ovary, Ectomy = removal of). As long as the other ovary is still present and functional, this does **not** cause menopause.

Remember, with just one ovary, you still have monthly ovulation, hormone cycles, monthly periods, the same pregnancy potential, and natural menopause at approximately age 51.

Here's another situation in which your body accommodates the absence of one ovary by using the other ovary for all its functions. You would perceive that everything is running normally, with no difference in your cycles. You could still get pregnant with no problem.

An Orientation to the Parts and Processes of Menopause

Bilateral Oophorectomy is the term for surgical removal of both ovaries (Bi = two, Lateral = sides, Ooph/Oophor = ovaries, Ectomy = removal of). **This causes immediate menopause.**

This is logical, right? Without your ovaries, you have no eggs and no estrogen, which matches the definition for menopause. Rather than experiencing the gradual, prolonged onset of menopause over months or years as with natural menopause, you would have sudden onset of menopause on the day of the surgery. Thereafter you would notice the signs and symptoms of menopause, and they would probably be more significant than with natural menopause. In other words, you would transition directly from pre-menopause to post-menopause, omitting the transition process, which we call peri-menopause (unless you had already begun peri-menopause before your surgery). We'll discuss these three phases of menopause in detail in the next chapter.

In fact, you should think of menopause as ovaries that are absent in either the physical sense or the functional sense. Menopause is all about the ovaries. The only surgical procedures which result in menopause are those that involve removal of the ovaries.

If your uterus were still present after a Bilateral Oophorectomy, it would have no functional purpose. The ovaries would not be present to produce hormones, so the uterus would not thicken and shed its lining. Of course, if you took hormones in the form of a medication or an herb, your uterus would still respond.

Unilateral Salpingo-oophorectomy is the term for surgical removal of one fallopian tube and ovary, on one side of the uterus (Uni = one, Lateral = side, Salpinx/Salpingo = Fallopian tube, Ooph/Oophor = ovary, Ectomy = removal of). The uterus is still there, and there is still one ovary. This does **not** cause menopause if the other ovary is left in place and functions normally.

The result is that life goes on as usual on the other side with the remaining fallopian tube and ovary. So, you have hormone cycles, eggs and sperm meeting, pregnancy occurring, and periods. Natural menopause occurs at about age 51.

Menopause

Bilateral Salpingo-oophorectomy is the term for surgical removal of both fallopian tubes and both ovaries (Bi = two, Lateral = sides, Salpinx/Salpingo = fallopian tubes, Ooph/Oophor = ovaries, Ectomy = removal of). **This causes immediate menopause.**

In this case, the uterus and cervix are present, but the ovaries and the fallopian tubes are absent. There is no hormone production and there are no eggs. The uterus just sits there doing nothing. It has no hormones to build up its lining. Once again, if you took hormones in the form of a medication or an herb, the uterus would respond to them.

Total Hysterectomy, Bilateral Salpingo-oophorectomy is the term for removal of the uterus, cervix, both fallopian tubes, and both ovaries (Total = with the cervix, Hyster = uterus, Ectomy = removal of, Bi = two, Lateral = sides, Salpinx/Salpingo = fallopian tubes, Ooph/Oophor = ovaries, Ectomy = removal of). This is what some call a "clean out." Obviously, all reproductive potential is lost, and there is no more hormone production. **So, this causes immediate menopause.**

In this case, you would immediately cease having periods and hormone cycles. Rather than natural menopause which is gradual, you would have sudden onset of the signs and symptoms of menopause at the time of the surgery. If you were pre-menopausal, you would become post-menopausal, skipping peri-menopause.

Note that this is what most people misconstrue as a "Total Hysterectomy." Now do you understand why they're all wrong? Most of them have never heard the term "Total Hysterectomy, Bilateral Salpingo-oophorectomy."

Subtotal (or Partial) Hysterectomy, Bilateral Salpingo-oophorectomy is the term for removal of the uterus **without** the cervix, plus removal of both fallopian tubes and both ovaries (Subtotal/Partial = without the cervix, Hyster = uterus, Ectomy = removal of, Bi = two, Lateral = sides, Salpinx/Salpingo = Fallopian tubes, Ooph/Oophor = ovaries, Ectomy = removal of). With this procedure, you're left with your cervix at the top of your vagina, but it's attached to nothing. There's no uterus to shed its lining, no ovaries to produce hormones or eggs, and no fallopian tubes. You have no periods. The cervix serves no purpose. **This causes immediate menopause**.

Do you see the additive nature of the terms? All we're doing here is designating each part that is removed in the name of the surgical procedure. It's that simple. If you want to break it down into the root words, it goes like this:

Hyster = uterus
Total = uterus and cervix
Subtotal or partial = uterus without cervix
Salpinx or salpingo = fallopian tube
Ooph or oophor = ovary
Uni = one
Bi = two
Lateral = side
Ectomy = removal of

By combining these root words and adding them together, you can have any combination of procedures.

Now, I'm sure you've heard many people refer to a clean out of the uterus, cervix, both fallopian tubes, and both ovaries as a "Total or Complete Hysterectomy." Well, they are totally and completely incorrect. Now you see why. Misuse of the term "Total Hysterectomy" along with misunderstanding of its true meaning have become so commonplace that the vast majority of people have no idea that they are way off in their definition. Please use this guide to figure out exactly which surgical procedure(s), if any, you've had before trying to decide how to manage menopause. It really makes a difference in shaping your preferences. If you make decisions based on incorrect information, you may do more harm than good.

One final note: Some surgeries are done through an incision in the abdomen. Some are done through a telescope (called a laparoscope). Others are done through the vagina. You *cannot* determine the procedure you have had based on the approach or the incisions. So, don't let that misguide you, either. It's all about which anatomical parts were removed. Leave it at that and you'll be well informed.

Surgical and Premature Menopause

There are two special categories of menopause. They are special because they constitute an "unnatural" menopause. In other words, the timing or the means by which menopause comes about are abnormal or unnatural.

Premature menopause is menopause which occurs at an age earlier than the average age range of 45 to 55. The strict definition of premature menopause is menopause which occurs earlier than age 45. It usually refers to menopause occurring during the age range of 30 to mid 40s. Premature menopause occurs in fewer than one out of every 100 women. Sometimes, the average age of menopause is similar from one generation to the next within families. However, this isn't always true. In any case, it is good to know the age at which your mother and grandmother transitioned into menopause. This is only pertinent if they had natural menopause (as opposed to surgical menopause).

Surgical menopause is menopause which results from surgical, medical, or x-ray therapy that disrupts or destroys the blood supply to the ovaries. Chemotherapy is a common cause of "surgical menopause." Intense radiation therapy for cancer treatment is another common cause of "surgical menopause." And, obviously, surgery is a common cause of "surgical menopause" (on which you're now practically an expert). Of course, you could be specific and refer to these as chemotherapy-induced or radiation-induced menopause if you wish. In any case, think of surgical menopause as *sudden, immediate* menopause. Before the surgery, chemotherapy, or radiation therapy, you're pre-menopausal. Afterwards, you're post-menopausal. This is in sharp contrast to natural menopause, in which it takes years to transition from pre- to post-menopause.

Both of these conditions are very different from natural menopause occurring in your early 50s. Thus, you must treat them differently. Together, surgical and premature menopause affect one out of every

An Orientation to the Parts and Processes of Menopause

12 women. The symptoms of menopause may be more sudden, more severe, and more debilitating for these women. They may be at much greater risk for some of the health risks of aging and menopause. It's important to exercise more intense management of menopause when it is premature or surgical.[1] While I apply the word "options" to the management of menopause, some of these things are not optional for women who experience surgical or premature menopause. For them, some of the aspects of menopause management are actually mandatory.

Some women experience menopause as a result of radiation (x-ray) therapy in the pelvic area to treat cancers. That's because radiation therapy really amounts to intense, heavy doses of radiation which damage the ovaries just as if they were burned. That's desirable if there is cancer nearby, so it's an acceptable side effect of radiation therapy if it will cure cancer. The result is that the ovaries stop working just as they do with menopause. You would handle this as a surgical menopause. If it occurs at an age younger than 45, you would also handle it as a premature menopause.

Chemotherapy can cause menopause. That's because some chemotherapy drugs are toxic to the ovaries. It really depends on which drugs are used. Once again, the benefits of curing cancer outweigh the risks of forgoing a cure for cancer just to avoid menopause. This constitutes a surgical form of menopause. If it occurs before age 45, it's also premature menopause.

Neither surgical nor premature menopause will ruin your life. You'll just experience the transition into the non-reproductive phase of your life earlier or by different means. Be glad that you're reading a book which gives you so many tools for improving your quality of life, both now and later.

Our focus will center on quality of life with regard to everything we discuss. The most important thing is to remember that "quality of life" is defined by each woman individually. Since no two women are alike, the information in this book will allow you to tailor all of your choices to your personal and particular needs. Not only that; you will also have the option of changing your mind and adjusting your choices to your new situation at any time. You are in total control. The goal is to give you the information with which to assess your options, make wise choices, and avoid any harm to yourself. So, let's get started!

Chapter 3:
Terminology: The Language of Menopause

Hormones

A discussion of menopause invariably involves a discussion of hormones. Each hormone has its own personality, and plays a role in your menopausal experience. Understanding the individual hormones and their actions will help you identify which hormone's presence or absence is contributing to your symptoms.

Estrogen is the major character in menopause. It's the primary female hormone. It's the hormone that makes your skin soft, your voice high in pitch, your features dainty, and your breasts more prominent than those of a male. While there are three different forms of estrogen in the human body, the major one is estradiol. The normal level of estradiol during your reproductive years is 50 – 150 pg/ml. The typical range during menopause is 0 – 45 pg/ml. (I'll be explaining all these strange terms which refer to quantities later.)

Progesterone is the partner hormone to estrogen. Estrogen and progesterone act in harmony with one another, fluctuating in a predictable and predetermined manner consistent with the reproductive state at hand (puberty, pregnancy, postpartum, menopause). Normal reproductive levels of progesterone are in the range of 0.1 – 0.5 pg/ml, whereas the menopausal range is less than 0.05 pg/ml. Progesterone has a calming, sedative effect on the body. The literal translation is Pro = for, Gest = gestation (or pregnancy), One = hormone. So, it is the hormone that supports pregnancy. It reduces anxiety and induces relaxation. A relaxed, anxiety-free environment is the best one for a healthy pregnancy.

Estrogen and progesterone have a predictable, coordinated pattern throughout your menstrual cycle. Just after your period ends, estrogen rises steadily over the first half of your cycle, peaking at mid-cycle, and then steadily declining. Progesterone doesn't begin to rise until mid-cycle, peaking about a week before the next period begins. Then it drops suddenly to very low levels. What does all this accomplish? Well, simply put, the estrogen thickens the lining of your uterus. Progesterone stabilizes the thick lining, maintaining it in its thickened state. The rapid *drop* in progesterone allows the thick uterine lining to shed in the form of a period. So, think of progesterone as the hormone that does two critical things: it controls how thick the uterine lining gets, and it allows the uterine lining to shed. You may wish to review Figure 4 again to recognize this. Be sure you really understand this dynamic between estrogen and progesterone. It's critical to many aspects of menopause and menopause management.

Testosterone is the male counterpart to estrogen. It's the primary male hormone that makes hair thick and coarse, skin rough, acne more prominent, and sex drive stronger. Females produce testosterone in the ovaries and adrenal glands, but the quantities are much smaller than in males. The normal level of testosterone during the reproductive years in a female is 0.4 – 1.0 ng/ml. During menopause it's 0.1 – 0.3 ng/dl. While the actual amount of testosterone decreases, it may be more concentrated than it was before.

In addition to natural menopause, anything that interferes with the blood supply to the ovaries can result in a decrease in testosterone levels. This includes surgical removal of the ovaries, chemotherapy, and radiation therapy. In general, testosterone levels decrease with menopause. However, it is the *relative* amount of estrogen to testosterone that matters in terms of your symptoms. In essence, you have more testosterone than estrogen during menopause. Testosterone levels decrease to a greater extent when menopause is surgical (Bilateral Oophorectomy, chemotherapy, radiation therapy). Testosterone falls by 40% to 60% with natural menopause and by 80% with surgical menopause.[1]

Terminology: The Language of Menopause

Follicle Stimulating Hormone (FSH) is the hormone that is produced in your brain and acts on your ovaries, causing your ovaries to produce *estrogen* (and eggs). FSH and estrogen have a special relationship, called "feedback." That means they respond to one another in a particular manner. In essence, the actions of one depend on the reactions of the other. It's the action-reaction phenomenon.

It goes like this: FSH tells the ovary to produce estrogen. If the ovary responds by increasing its estrogen production, the FSH level remains low. On the other hand, if the ovary doesn't increase its estrogen production, the FSH level rises. So, a low FSH is associated with a high estrogen level, and a high FSH is associated with a low estrogen level.

Think of your ovaries as a child, and FSH as their parent. If a parent tells her child to do something, he's supposed to mind, right? And if he doesn't, what's the parent going to do? Raise her voice! It's as if FSH speaks to the ovary, telling it to produce estrogen. FSH speaks softly, and, as long as the ovary responds by producing estrogen, the FSH has no reason to yell. If, on the other hand, the ovary were to ignore the soft voice of FSH, the FSH would raise its voice and scream at the ovary to produce estrogen.

It's a lot like the interaction you might have with your own child when you tell him to clean up his room. As long as he obeys, you have no reason to yell. But, if he doesn't, you raise your voice. Once he does respond, you stop yelling. A high FSH level represents the screaming voice of a dissatisfied parent. A low one represents the soft voice of a satisfied parent. A high estrogen level represents a child who obeys. A low estrogen level represents a child who doesn't.

Just think of "feedback" as a high-low relationship. When one is high, the other is low, and vice versa. Whenever I'm learning something, I love to take complicated information and boil it down to the simplest possible lesson. If I don't remember any of the details, I remember that simplistic, basic "bottom line." So, I'll do the same thing for you at times throughout this book.

The simplistic version of all this FSH and estrogen stuff is this: If your estrogen is low, your FSH is high. That's it.

The FSH level fluctuates throughout your menstrual cycle, ranging between 2 – 15 mIU/ml. At menopause, it skyrockets to greater than 30 mIU/ml.

FSH is also the hormone that causes the ovary to produce an egg which is primed for ovulation each month. The budding site for an egg is called a "follicle." The follicle is the nest for the egg. When FSH stimulates the follicle, the egg matures and eventually ovulates.

Luteinizing Hormone (LH) is the hormone that is produced in the brain and acts on the ovary to cause the ovary to produce *progesterone*. Just as FSH has a feedback relationship with estrogen, LH has the same kind of feedback relationship with progesterone.

In this case, LH tells the ovary to produce progesterone. The interaction between LH and progesterone is exactly like the one I described above using the parent/child analogy. When LH is high, progesterone is low, and vice versa.

As with FSH, the level of LH also fluctuates throughout your menstrual cycle, ranging between 2 – 20 mIU/ml. During menopause, it rises to greater than 40 mIU/ml.

It's Just a Phase

Because menopause is a process that takes place over time rather than being a sudden event, we use specific terms to distinguish the progressive phases of the process. The phases refer to the time frames before, during, and after the menopausal transition takes place. An understanding of these terms will help you in your understanding of menopause. Ultimately, it will assist you in your management of your own menopause.

Pre-menopause refers to the time before menopause begins (Pre = before, Meno = menstruation, Pause = stops). Premenopausal women are those who are not yet experiencing the signs or symptoms of menopause. This is the time *before* the transition begins.

Peri-menopause refers to the transition time between pre-menopause and post-menopause (Peri = time surrounding or near,

TERMINOLOGY: THE LANGUAGE OF MENOPAUSE

Meno = menstruation, Pause = stops). Just as puberty takes place over a period of many months or years, so does the process of menopause. Peri-menopause includes the time from the first sign or symptom of menopause until the time menopause is fully established. During this time, you may have some or all of the symptoms of menopause. They may be intermittent or continuous. For some women, this phase may persist for years. This is the time *during* the transition.

During peri-menopause, the levels of estrogen are erratic, changing frequently and unpredictably. That's because the levels of Follicle Stimulating Hormone (FSH) in the brain vary. FSH is the hormone that controls estrogen production. Therefore, if FSH production is irregular, so is the production of estrogen.

Earlier, you learned that focusing only on estrogen reduces an understanding of menopause to a more simplistic process than it actually is. Peri-menopause is the most significant phase to which this applies. When menopause occurs naturally (rather than surgically), the first hormone that begins to decline is progesterone. The lower than normal level of progesterone produces an imbalance in the ratio of estrogen to progesterone, resulting in a temporary excess of estrogen.[2] That's why periods can be so wacky in the early peri-menopausal years.

Think of peri-menopause as a time during which the ovaries are temperamental or confused. They function normally some of the time; they function partially some of the time; and sometimes they refuse to cooperate at all. This erratic behavior on the part of the ovaries produces a rollercoaster-like effect. The changes are unpredictable.

Because the levels of both FSH and estrogen are erratic during this phase, it's difficult to diagnose peri-menopause with a blood test for either of these hormones. The values will vary from day to day, depending on whether or not the ovaries are behaving normally or not on any given day. This explains why this phase can be so confusing to you, your partner, and your physician. The good news is that this erratic behavior is only temporary, similar to the temporary erratic behavior of any teenager during puberty. Understanding this and knowing that things will become more stable with time is the key.

MENOPAUSE

Unfortunately, there is a **_warning_** that I must issue about this phase: *Pregnancy* is still possible here. Remember, during this time, the ovaries produce eggs occasionally and unpredictably. Not only is pregnancy possible, but it is more difficult to determine which part of any cycle is likely to result in pregnancy. Additionally, the probability of *twins* increases at this time because the erratic behavior of estrogen results in crops of follicles undergoing maturation and releasing eggs. The result is ovulation of multiple eggs rather than just one. It just so happens that the decreasing level of progesterone which characterizes this phase results from the failed ovulations that occur for some of the eggs.

Just remember: You must exercise birth control during this time if you wish to avoid pregnancy. If pregnancy does occur, it's more difficult to diagnose due to the hormonal irregularity that existed to begin with. To make things even more interesting, pregnancy is much more likely to result in twins.

Because peri-menopause can last months or years, it's more difficult to define the average age of onset of peri-menopause. Some women actually begin to experience peri-menopause in their early 40s and continue the process for a decade. More commonly, peri-menopause begins in the late 40s or early 50s, with post-menopause occurring one or two years later.

Post-menopause refers to the time when menopause has been fully established (Post = after, Meno = menstruation, Pause = stops). In most cases, it is documented by the complete absence of menstrual periods for *12 consecutive months*. Thus, it takes a full year with no menstrual period before you can label yourself post-menopausal. This is the time *after* the transition.

Post-menopause designates the time when the estrogen level hits an all time low and remains low. It no longer fluctuates as it did during peri-menopause. It represents the time when the ovaries finally cease all production of eggs and estrogen once and for all. The ovaries actually "go out of business." This marks the time when pregnancy is no longer possible. In response to the low level of estrogen, the FSH level remains very high. (Remember, the FSH is screaming at the ovaries to produce estrogen, and when the ovaries fail to respond, the FSH level increases.)

Terminology: The Language of Menopause

The average age of completing peri-menopause and becoming post-menopausal is 51. Think back on our analogy to puberty. What is the average age of puberty? Well, it's approximately 12, but it varies. Some children begin puberty at age 10. Others don't show any signs of puberty until age 13. The same variance occurs in the age at which women end peri-menopause and become post-menopausal. Use age 51 as an average, but realize that you may be earlier or later than that in reaching post-menopause.

Regardless of the age at which you achieve post-menopause, *you'll remain post-menopausal for the remainder of your life,* which means that you'll spend a major portion of your life there. You'll spend one third to one half of your life as a post-menopausal woman, which is more time than you spent in infancy, childhood, adolescence, pregnancy, or menstruating. Of all your hormonal phases, menopause will occupy the most of your time. That's pretty significant, don't you think? Such a significant phase of life deserves a lot of attention and respect.

The fact that you reach the post-menopausal state and remain there for the rest of your life *doesn't* mean that everything will stay the same once you're post-menopausal. Think back on adolescence again. Once you made it through adolescence and reached early adulthood, you continued to change throughout your 20s, 30s, and 40s, right? And you continued to change in many different ways, too. Well, the same is true for post-menopause. You'll continue to evolve. Your health needs, emotional needs, personal preferences, knowledge, and choices will continue to change. Hopefully, you'll feel better about yourself than ever before. So, while post-menopause is the last phase, it's not a static one. It might even be the best one!

Because all these phases are not created equal, I'll be specific about which one I'm discussing. The term "menopause" is a general umbrella term, which includes both peri-and post-menopause. I'll use it to refer to both the transition into menopause and beyond.

WORKSHEET TIMEOUT:
Answer questions # 1, # 2, and # 3 on your worksheet.
Circle all that apply to you.

Chapter 4:
"How Will I Know When Menopause Comes a Knockin'?"

Signs and Symptoms of Menopause

There are many indicators that the process of menopause has begun. Even though it's a normal process, menopause is a shock to your body. It affects many parts of your body because they all have previously functioned in response to estrogen. Your brain, heart, bones, joints, skin, hair, vagina, bladder, and breasts all feel the crunch. So, there are symptoms of menopause that may involve many aspects of your body besides your ovaries and uterus. The order, extent, and inconvenience of these symptoms will vary greatly from one woman to another. First, simply view the list of signs and symptoms. Later we'll discuss each of them in detail. You may have only some of these symptoms or all of these symptoms. Some may occur for only a short time; others may remain indefinitely. Please note that certain unrelated medical conditions may also cause some of these symptoms. In general, it is the common occurrence of many of these symptoms at the appropriate time in your life that indicates the onset of menopause.

Here's the list of signs and symptoms which indicate the beginning of peri-menopause:

1. Menstrual periods that become farther apart
2. Hot flashes
3. Night sweats
4. Insomnia

5. Fatigue
6. Forgetfulness
7. Mood swings
8. Irritability
9. Depression
10. Cravings for sweets, carbohydrates, alcohol
11. Breast pain
12. Joint stiffness and joint pain
13. Dry skin
14. Hair loss on the scalp
15. Hair growth in undesirable locations
16. Vaginal dryness
17. Urinary problems (urinary tract infections [UTIs] and urinary incontinence)
18. Weight gain
19. Decreased or increased sex drive
20. Acne
21. Headaches

The severity of the symptoms of peri- and post-menopause varies from one woman to another. Some may be severe, while others are mild. They may appear in isolation or in conjunction with one another. Some may be apparent in the early stages of peri-menopause, while others may not be present until many years afterwards. These are the signs and symptoms to anticipate as an indication that the menopausal process may have begun.

Now, we've already established that menopause has many features similar to puberty and adolescence. But as you look at the list of signs and symptoms of menopause, you might also realize that menopause also has some features in common with some other aspects of being female. Some aspects of menopause actually resemble pregnancy. And some resemble aging. So, you might say that menopause is a combination of many hormonal and temporal events in your life. Let's review those signs and symptoms a little more closely, paying attention to some of these similarities.

First, let's list the signs and symptoms which resemble puberty and adolescence:

"How Will I Know When Menopause Comes a Knockin'?"

1. Mood swings
2. Irritability
3. Depression
4. Cravings for sweets and carbohydrates
5. Weight gain
6. Acne
7. Increased sex drive
8. Headaches

Now, let's list those which resemble pregnancy:

1. Hot flashes
2. Night sweats
3. Insomnia
4. Fatigue
5. Mood swings
6. Irritability
7. Cravings for various foods
8. Breast pain
9. Urinary problems (incontinence)
10. Weight gain

Finally, let's list those which resemble aging:

1. Less frequent periods
2. Insomnia
3. Fatigue
4. Forgetfulness
5. Joint stiffness and joint pain
6. Dry skin
7. Hair loss on the scalp
8. Hair growth in undesirable locations
9. Vaginal dryness
10. Urinary problems (UTIs and incontinence)
11. Weight gain
12. Decreased sex drive

And, voila! All accounted for. As you can see, some of these items fall into more than one category.

"Do I Need a Lab Test to Confirm Menopause?"

You might think that, with all of those significant and primarily bothersome signs and symptoms of menopause, we really don't need a laboratory test for the diagnosis of menopause. It may seem that any grown woman, taking note of her periods, emotions, and physical changes, would be capable of suspecting the onset of menopause. Like adolescence, you may think it possible (or inevitable) that friends and family members might even be able to diagnose menopause. If, indeed, your thinking is along these lines, you are absolutely correct. Just as we don't require a laboratory test to diagnose puberty or adolescence, we don't need one for menopause, either. Yes, once again, Mother Nature made it blatantly obvious. In fact, it is *so* obvious for most women that it's really difficult to overlook.

However, despite the clear signs and symptoms of menopause, it does differ from one woman to another. An important variable is the fact that not all women have all these signs and symptoms of menopause. Some women have very few of these attention-getting changes. So, there actually is a laboratory test to confirm menopause. The key thing to realize is that it isn't necessary in most cases. However, it's available for clarification.

A second reason that there's a test for menopause is because the signs and symptoms of menopause are not exclusive to menopause. In other words, there are medical diseases which exhibit some of the same signs and symptoms. Given the fact that some women only experience one or two of the signs and symptoms of menopause, it's important to ensure that we don't act too quickly and label something menopause when it's actually a disease. Thyroid problems, depression, dementia, and malnutrition are among the diseases which can mimic various aspects of menopause.

I'm a firm believer in peace of mind. If in doubt about whether you're experiencing menopause or some other medical phenomenon, get the test. Of course, if you're 50ish and you feel as though I'm describing *your* life as I list the signs and symptoms of menopause, you can be fairly safe in omitting the test. In short, if it *sounds* like menopause, and it *feels* like menopause, and others suggest that you *behave* as if it's menopause, then it probably *is* menopause.

Blood FSH Level

The most common laboratory test for menopause is a blood test for Follicle Stimulating Hormone (FSH). FSH is that hormone your brain produces to tell your ovaries to produce estrogen. When the ovaries respond appropriately and produce estrogen, FSH remains at a low level. If the ovaries fail to respond, and refuse to produce estrogen, the FSH level rises. Remember? It's as if the FSH is yelling at the ovaries to produce estrogen. The normal level of FSH before peri-menopause begins is 2 – 15 mIU/ml. The FSH level of a woman who is fully post-menopausal is greater than 30 mIU/ml.

Notice that I skipped any mention of the typical FSH range for peri-menopause. That's because this is where things get tricky. Reflect back to the definition and description of peri-menopause. It's a time when the behavior of the ovaries is erratic with regard to estrogen production. During peri-menopause, the ovaries produce estrogen in unpredictable amounts and at unpredictable times. Now, if FSH is the hormone which induces the ovaries to produce estrogen, wouldn't it make sense for FSH to vary greatly during this time also? Bingo!

FSH is all over the place during peri-menopause. It's an absolute rollercoaster! If you were to check the FSH level frequently and regularly during peri-menopause, you would notice an irregular, confusing pattern. Instead of having a predictable pattern consistent with normal menstrual cycles, it would rise and fall erratically. This chaotic behavior of FSH is linked to, and responsible for, the equally chaotic pattern of estrogen production by the ovaries. This relationship between estrogen and FSH (called feedback) is a form of communication between the brain and the ovaries. During peri-menopause, they're both confused.

I know that this all seems very scientific, but I want to ensure that you understand why the blood test for menopause doesn't give you an absolute answer. Use it as an additional measure to help you rule out medical problems which may have some of the same signs and symptoms of menopause. Use it to confirm arrival at the post-menopausal phase. But don't think of it as overriding your own intuition. I've always said: If my patient tells me one thing and the FSH tells me another, I believe my patient more than I believe the blood test. Remember, *you* know yourself better than anyone else does, and certainly better than a laboratory does.

There is one other phenomenon that I must bring to your attention. It is the effect of hormone therapy on the value of FSH. Because of the feedback relationship between estrogen and FSH, *any* estrogen in your body will cause a change in the value of FSH. So, if you're using birth control pills, hormones for menopause, or any other source of estrogen, the estrogen in these substances will affect the level of FSH, making it falsely lower than it really is. If you have reason to check your FSH level, you must discontinue all hormone products for approximately three weeks before checking it. Otherwise, it will be inaccurate.

Salivary Hormone Levels

Another method of evaluating hormone levels involves measuring the quantity of the hormones present in your saliva. The level in your saliva parallels the level in your body.[1] This method is more flexible, but also less accurate. It's not very familiar to doctors of allopathic medicine (M.D.s), and is quite familiar to doctors of osteopathic medicine (D.O.s) and doctors of naturopathic medicine (N.D.s). It's possible to test the levels of estrogen, progesterone, and testosterone in this manner. Be aware that salivary hormone levels will fluctuate more rapidly than blood levels of FSH.

Timing

Regardless of the testing method, it's likely that you'll need to repeat the test for purposes of comparison. Testing is best done in the early morning. It's also necessary to repeat the test at the same time in your cycle if you're having cycles. In counting days of your cycle, day one is the day that you notice the first sign of menstrual bleeding. The best time for testing is between days 20 to 23.[1]

Section II:

The Decision-Making Process and the Options

Chapter 5: The Balancing Act

Principles

Menopause is like a lot of other things in life that are just part of being human and female. We all go through it because it's a normal, natural process. However, no two women are alike. Not only are we different physically and physiologically, but we also differ in our psychological frameworks and our preferences. Even identical twins who share many things in common may differ as to their preferences in how to manage menopause. The key to success in progressing through and managing menopause is to use the following principles in analyzing the issues and making choices:

1. *You* know yourself better than anyone else does.
2. Biased information is of *no* use to you. Its goal is to **persuade** you to think in accordance with someone else's preference rather than to **inform** you so that you can think for yourself.
3. In making management choices for menopause, you must *balance* the benefits of each option with the risks of each option.
4. Once you have *complete and accurate* information, you will make the choice that is best for you at the time.
5. You may use *trial and error* to arrive at a decision.
6. Pursue each regimen for at least *three months* in order to allow your body enough time to adjust to that regimen. Changing your regimen more frequently than every three months will impair your ability to determine the best choice.

7. You have the right and the *freedom* to change your mind.
8. You don't have to continue management forever. You *may discontinue* at any time.

The Balancing Scale

In medicine, we analyze each alternative for management or treatment in terms of the benefits of that alternative weighed against the risks of that same alternative. We only recommend a management option if the benefits outweigh the risks. You'll probably find that you do the same thing as you consider your options.

Think of those scales with the plates hanging on either side of the fulcrum. They're designed to place things on the plates to see if they balance one another or if one is heavier than the other. That's what you need to do as you consider your options for menopause. Gather together all the factors that matter to you. On one side of the scale, place all the beneficial aspects of an option. On the other side, place all the detrimental or risky aspects of that same option. See how the scale tips. If the benefits outweigh the risks (the pros outweigh the cons), then it's an option worth considering. If not, you should see how another option balances out.

Sometimes, you'll place completely different things (rather than the benefits and risks of a single option) on the scale to see which one holds more weight for you. Let's say you're trying to decide whether to use traditional versus alternative and complementary medicine. You'd weigh them against one another to see which one you value the most.

You may place as much weight as you see fit on each factor. Face it: some things are more important to you than other things. You may value things differently than another person does. But be entirely honest with yourself. Don't belittle a factor out of denial about its importance. (For instance, if you're sedentary, admit it.) Remember that your personal attributes matter a lot. Include all of the following things in your balancing act, and add any others that you deem important:

1. Your health issues
2. Your family history

3. Your side effects of medications
4. Your quality of life factors
5. Your lifestyle
6. Your personal preferences
7. Your symptoms of menopause
8. Your ability to actually accomplish your goals with your chosen management style

Remember to take both *short-term* and *long-term* consequences into account in order to address both your present and your future benefits and risks. The goal for most women is to feel as good as possible both now and later. For instance, if your best choice from a medical standpoint would be estrogen, but you're so nervous about taking estrogen that you'd worry yourself silly, then it's probably not in your best interest to take it. You may be providing yourself with the best theoretical long-term benefit, but you'd be ignoring the short-term detriment of being so uneasy now. Honor your preferences.

It's amazing how much we differ in our value systems. The mere definition of "quality of life" is so variable from one woman to the next that we sometimes have difficulty appreciating or respecting one another's choices. You get to use your own definition of "quality of life" as you weigh the benefits and risks of the various options. For example, you may have had breast cancer, but still choose to use hormone therapy for a couple of years to get you through the early post-menopausal transition because your symptoms are devastating. For you, the possible risk of recurrent breast cancer may weigh less than the inability to function in your current life. Your friend who has also had breast cancer may feel as though she can deal with the daily onslaught of symptoms much better than she can with even a minute possibility of increasing her chances of recurrent breast cancer. You both have the right to do it your own way. Keep things in perspective, and trust your intuition.

Possible Options

In deciding how to manage menopause, you may consider the following options:

1. Do nothing
2. Manage your menopause with a primary focus on your **current symptoms** of menopause, and for purposes of improving your day to day quality of life (short-term focus)
3. Manage your menopause with a primary focus on **preventing future problems** (long-term focus)
4. Use a **combination** of measures to address both your short-term and your long-term goals

Questions to Ask Yourself

As you begin to consider your options for managing menopause, you may find it easiest to address your situation in a two-part process. First, ask yourself whether or not you wish to pursue any form of management or treatment at all. If your answer is, "Yes," then ask yourself what form of management you prefer. For example, do you prefer a pharmaceutical option such as hormones in the form of a pill, skin patch, cream, or vaginal ring? Alternatively, do you prefer an alternative or complementary type of treatment such as herbs or tofu? You might also ask yourself whether you prefer to find a single agent that suffices to alleviate all of your menopausal symptoms, or whether you have the patience and desire to find treatments for individual symptoms and health risks of menopause. To date, no single agent eliminates all menopausal symptoms and risks as effectively as estrogen. But that doesn't mean that estrogen is the answer for all women. The nice thing is that you have the opportunity to choose.

Categories of Management Options

The categories of the various management options generally fall into seven categories:

1. Doing nothing to manage menopause
2. Making diet and lifestyle choices that are beneficial for your menopause
3. Using the alternative or complementary medicine approach, including vitamins and minerals and/or botanicals and herbs
4. Using acupuncture or hypnosis

5. Using medical therapy with bioidentical, natural, or synthetic hormones
6. Using medical therapy with non-hormonal medications
7. Using some combination of the above

"Do I Want to Assume a Management Position?"

Remember my analogy of menopause and puberty? Menopause isn't a disease any more than puberty is. Of course, if someone had offered you the opportunity to manage puberty in order to make it more tolerable, you might have been a taker. And your parents might have insisted on it. Some women choose to let menopause progress along its natural course, without any manipulation. Some women adopt a hands-off approach since many of the symptoms of menopause are transitory. In some cultures, aging and all of its nuances are revered, and the attitude surrounding menopause is one of pride and acceptance rather than dread and inconvenience. In such cultures, few women voice any complaints about menopause. And they don't do anything to manage it, either.

Other women choose to do whatever they can to limit the discomfort, unpredictability, and inconvenience associated with menopause. They seek ways to smooth out the disruptions that menopause can create for their family, career, and sense of well-being.

There isn't a "right" way, and there isn't a "wrong" way. There are simply many ways. The most important thing is to know what's safe.

As you learn all that you need to know about menopause, you'll feel comfortable with making decisions about how you want to manage it. If you choose to let Mother Nature control it, you will have made that decision as an informed adult. If you choose to add to what Mother Nature has put in place, you'll have a variety of options to assist you in doing so.

In making choices, consider what you wish to achieve with the management of your menopause. Consider also the amount of effort you'll actually exert to accomplish your goals. Don't kid yourself here.

You know your limitations and your natural tendencies. Be realistic about what will fit your lifestyle and habits. Choose an option that will work for you. You're free to change your mind, and you can use trial and error to find the best management option. Think of *your* management of *your* menopause as a work in progress. *You* are your own manager. *You* have the power. Now use it.

If you choose to pursue some form of management for menopause that includes hormones, you may wish to start by having laboratory testing of all your hormone levels so that you can target replacement only for those which are deficient. Once you've established yourself on a regimen for three months, you may wish to retest your hormone levels to ensure that you have corrected the deficiencies without using more hormone replacement than necessary. Alternatively, you may wish to simply begin on a moderate hormone dosage which suffices for the majority of women and go from there. If you're treating symptoms with a substance other than a hormone, reanalyze how well you have resolved the undesirable symptoms. You may have to use a few products (one at a time) to discover one which works for you. Accept the fact that, over time, your needs may change. When they do, adjust your regimen accordingly.

One more thing, and this is important: **Your brain and your body may not agree with one another!** What I mean is that you may *think* you know what you prefer for management of your own menopause, but your *body* may not respond in the way you had hoped. This concept isn't easy for a lot of women to accept. It's most difficult if you're one of those people who wants to be in control.

Here's an analogy: Are you familiar with a birth plan? It's a document that a pregnant woman creates months before labor. A birth plan enables her to dictate what she *thinks* she'll want during labor in terms of pain medication (or lack thereof), personal care, baby care, etc. The problem is that, once she's actually *in* labor, she oftentimes wants something completely different than what she *thought* she'd want. Her brain is saying: "Remember the birth plan!" But her body is saying: "Are you nuts? Give me something for pain!"

That's understandable, because labor is unpredictable. Mother Nature controls labor. Months before labor, a perfectly comfortable pregnant woman can't predict what she's going to want when she's experiencing labor. That's especially true if she's never been in labor before. I often say (jokingly) that the only women who create birth plans are those who haven't ever been in labor before. There's a lot of truth in that statement, because women who've been in labor before know how unpredictable it is.

Whenever a pregnant patient says she's making a birth plan, I tell her to feel free to do so. But I also let her know that, during labor, if she wants something different from what her birth plan indicates, she should honor her wishes and ignore the birth plan.

So, the same applies to menopause. It's fine to have a management plan in mind. Just remember that your body may not respond to that plan. It doesn't mean you've failed or that you won't find a solution. It just means that you may have to be a little more open-minded. Listen to your body. It really does talk to you. It's a product of Mother Nature, and sometimes, your body knows what you need better than your brain does.

WORKSHEET TIMEOUT:

Pretend that you're preparing a "menopause plan" in the same way a pregnant woman would prepare a birth plan.

Skip to questions <u>#14 and #15</u> on your worksheet.

Since you're doing this <u>before</u> you know everything you'll know after reading the rest of this book, just put a <u>star</u> next to the options you think you want, realizing that you may very well change your mind once you've read the entire book. Don't circle anything yet.

You will come back to these questions later and answer them again once you have complete, unbiased, accurate information. So, don't worry about being locked in to your current choices.

Chapter 6:
Options: Medical, Non-medical, and Everything in Between

Diet and Lifestyle

While there are a wide variety of diet and lifestyle measures which have an impact on various aspects of menopause, some are more important than others. Those that are the most important appear again and again in the list of options for management. There are four that form the basis for managing almost every aspect of menopause. You'll see them over and over. So, let's just list them here. These four things have a positive impact on almost everything:

- Eating a healthy diet
- Engaging in regular exercise
- Maintaining appropriate body weight
- Refraining from smoking

If you did only these four things and nothing more, you'd be on the right path to a smoother menopause and a healthier life.

Foundation

In general, there are two broad categories of therapeutic options for managing menopause. The first is conventional medicine, which refers to the medical practices and teachings of medical doctors (M. D.s), who practice allopathic medicine, and doctors of osteopathy (D.O.s), who practice osteopathic medicine. Doctors of both allopathic and osteopathic medicine offer medical regimens that involve use of hormonal and/or non-hormonal medications. Pharmacists are also familiar with pharmaceutical products.

The second category is alternative and complementary medicine, which refers to practices, applications, and modalities that are not part of conventional medicine. The most familiar options involve the use of vitamins and minerals, botanicals and herbs, acupuncture, or hypnosis. The health professionals in the alternative and complementary fields include naturopathic doctors, herbalists, botanists, acupuncturists, and hypnotists.

Some professionals belong in both categories. These include D.O.s, dieticians, nutritionists, and fitness specialists.

All of these professionals in all of these categories of management options can offer assistance with diet and lifestyle changes. You may not even need professional assistance for that. You may just need self willingness.

As you can see, there are many professionals of varying backgrounds to assist you with your management of menopause. You don't have to do it alone, and you don't have to confine yourself to a single category of management options. You can shop around to find what you want and from whom you wish to gain assistance.

It's important to recognize the fact that these various categories exist. Not only does it provide you with a multitude of options from which to choose, but it honors the fact that women vary in their preferences. It also helps to direct you to the appropriate type of caregiver for guidance. As I mentioned earlier, this isn't a do-it-yourself manual for menopause, so it's highly likely that you'll need some assistance from someone in the health care industry.

You may prefer conventional medicine because of the strict regulations imposed by the Food and Drug Administration (FDA) upon pharmaceutical products. Such regulations ensure purity, consistency, stringent testing, and widespread familiarity among physicians about pharmaceutical products. You may like the fact that you can get a single prescription medication which will alleviate all your menopause issues.

Options: Medical, Non-medical, and Everything in Between

On the other hand, you may view pharmaceutical hormonal therapy as a means of treating menopause as if it were a medical disorder rather than a natural process of aging. Maybe you're dissatisfied with conventional medicine. Maybe you find alternative and complementary medicine more empowering because the products are available over the counter without a prescription. Maybe alternative and complementary medicine is more compatible with your personal, ethical, or religious values.

Users of alternative and complementary medicine have been identified as having a higher educational level, poorer health status, a holistic orientation to health, several chronic health conditions, and a transformational experience which changed their view of the world, such as a negative experience with traditional medicine.[1] Alternative and complementary medicine has actually become mainstream, representing the majority in terms of popularity and economic size.[2]

Proponents of botanical and herbal medicine argue that, because the cost of bringing a new drug to market is millions of dollars, manufacturers have little interest in plant by-products which they cannot patent.[2] They feel as though safe and effective plant regimens are set aside, while the public is subjected to more toxic and potent synthetic drugs.[2]

Only a minority of consumers reject conventional medicine completely. Most consumers of alternative and complementary medicine combine conventional medicine with botanicals, herbs, and other alternatives.[2] From the standpoint of hormones, the primary philosophical difference between conventional or traditional hormone replacement and alternative and complementary options is that the first concentrates on estrogen, while the second concentrates on progesterone.[3]

The good news is that you have options galore! Have an open mind and learn all you can. Then tailor the information to your circumstance, and make your menopause as great as you can make it.

Basic Principles for Utilizing Alternative and Complementary Medicine Options

If you choose alternative and complementary medicine as your method of managing menopause, there are some basic principles which you should keep in mind:

1. Remember that the word "natural" is not an assurance of safety or efficacy.[1]
2. Realize that dangerous drug-herb interactions do occur.[1]
3. Since there is no standardization of botanicals and herbs, the result is variability in content and efficacy from one batch to another. This is true for individual manufacturers as well as between manufacturers.[1]
4. Lack of quality control and regulation may result in contamination, adulteration, or misidentification of plant products.[1]
5. You should not take botanicals or herbs in doses that are higher than recommended or for durations longer than recommended.[1]
6. Always include all of your vitamin, mineral, botanical, and herbal products in your "list of medications."

Basic Principles for Utilizing Hormonal Options

If you choose hormonal therapy as your method of managing menopause, it is prudent to begin with low dose therapy initially for the following reasons:

1. To adjust the dose to the perfect level that provides the desirable results without excessive levels
2. To avoid or reduce side effects
3. To accommodate age-appropriate requirements

You are not eligible for hormones if you have any of the following:

1. You refuse to take hormones
2. You are pregnant
3. You have unexplained vaginal bleeding

Options: Medical, Non-medical, and Everything in Between

4. You have chronic liver disease
5. You have a history of blood clots
6. You have a cancer that is dependent on or worsened by hormones[4]

All right! Now you have the basic principles. Let's focus on some of the particulars. In order for you to make good choices for yourself, you'll need to have correct definitions for some things, and understand the differences between some things. Once again, this is an area that may cause you to raise your eyebrows a few times. Much of it falls into the category of things you thought you knew. You might discover that you had some misinformation.

Botanical and Herbal Therapy

Definitions

Botanical and herbal therapy refers to the use of plant products with special properties to manage physical symptoms. The distinction between herbal therapy and botanical therapy lies in the fact that **"herbal"** therapy refers to use of only the stems and leaves, excluding the seeds, flowers, fruit, buds, and roots. The term **"botanical"** includes foods and supplements derived from any part of a plant, including the seeds, flowers, fruit, buds, and roots, as well as the stems and leaves.[2]

Some plants contain unique substances which modify the physiology of the human body. Botanicals and herbs are distinct from drugs in that they are not subject to the strict standards for approval that the Food and Drug Administration (FDA) requires for pharmaceutical products. Plant products must only adhere to the production and marketing standards for *foods* rather than to those for drugs. As such, the purity, quality, and consistency of botanicals and herbs vary greatly.

Plants are available for therapeutic use in the form of herbs, oils, pills, teas, and tinctures. I will describe each of these for you.[1]

Bulk Herbs are raw or dried plants that are whole, pulverized, or powdered. Bulk herbs are also used to make teas and tinctures (liquid medicines). The powders can be put into capsules or formed into tablets. Think of bulk herbs as the original form from which you can make other botanical or herbal preparations.

<u>Oils</u> are concentrated, fat soluble chemicals which originate from herbs. They are usually designed for external use (on the skin), and may be very toxic if taken by mouth.

<u>Tablets</u> or <u>Capsules</u> are a compounded form of an herb to provide easy use and a fixed dose.

<u>Teas</u> are a means of extracting the part of an herb that is soluble (dissolvable) by adding hot water. The potency of a tea is dependent on the length of time that the tea steeps. And there's a difference between brewing and boiling an herb. <u>Brewing</u> involves bringing the substance to a boil and then removing it from the heat. <u>Boiling</u> involves bringing the substance to a boil and maintaining it for a period of time. Teas are available in the form of traditional teas, infusions, and decoctions.

1. <u>Teas</u> are brewed for 1 – 2 minutes. (You bring the water to a boil and then remove it from the heat, leaving the tea leaves in it for 1 – 2 minutes.)
2. <u>Infusions</u> are brewed for 20 – 30 minutes. (You bring the water to a boil and then remove it from the heat, leaving the tea leaves in it for 20 – 30 minutes.)
3. <u>Decoctions</u> are boiled in water for 20 – 30 minutes. (You bring the water to a boil and keep it boiling with the tea leaves in it for 20 – 30 minutes.)

<u>Tinctures</u> are alcohol-extracted concentrates that are added to water, and then placed directly in your mouth or under your tongue.

Other things that fall into the classification of botanical or herbal substances are highly concentrated extracts of plant chemicals, synthetic derivatives of plants, and some steroids.

Manufacture and Regulation of Botanicals and Herbs

The manufacture and regulation of botanical and herbal substances differs greatly from that of drugs. The differences are due to the fact that botanical and herbal products are classified as <u>foods</u> rather than as drugs. There are limits on the claims that may accompany these products on their labels and in their supporting literature, but the focus is on accurate advertising rather than on safety. <u>Dietary supplements</u> are neither foods nor drugs. As such, manufacturers don't have to provide *any* evidence to support the purported benefits before marketing the product. While the Food and Drug Administration (FDA) oversees the industry, the Federal Trade Commission is responsible for identifying inappropriate or unsubstantiated claims and enforcing the regulations.[1] What constitutes "science and research" in the medical arena is replaced by "advertising and marketing" in the botanical and herbal arena. This doesn't mean that botanical and herbal products are bad. It simply means that you need to be aware of the standards pertinent to their marketing and advertising.

Botanicals and herbs are subject to a high degree of variation in products. Because plants are grown in a field or a greenhouse, they may have different quantities of active constituents due to variations in growth conditions. As a result, products may differ greatly in the amount of active ingredient they contain.[1] If you're a gardener, you may have noticed some of these differences in your own plants. Some are big and robust and others are pitiful. The active ingredients in botanicals and herbs follow these same variations. You don't even have to be a gardener to appreciate this. Think about shopping for fruits and vegetables at the grocery store. Don't you usually pick up various heads of lettuce and examine them? I'll bet you do the same thing with fruit. Why? Because they *aren't* all created equal, that's why. Some are larger. Some are more robust in color. Some are more fragrant. Some are perfect in shape. Some are defective.

Your fruits and vegetables belong to the plant world. So do botanicals and herbs. The fact that an herbal company picked a bunch of herbs and put them in a bottle doesn't change the fact that the plants from which they originated differed from one another. That's why the botanical and herbal products you buy differ from one another.

Now, after buying your fruits and vegetables, don't you wash them before you eat them? Why? Because they're plants. They've been exposed to pollens, insecticides, dirt, hands, etc. In essence, they're contaminated, and you don't want to ingest the contaminants. The same is true for botanicals and herbs. While precautions exist to limit the contaminants that end up in the products you buy, there's no guarantee that there aren't traces left behind. You don't usually get sick from eating your fruits and vegetables, and you probably won't get sick taking botanicals or herbs. The point is that they aren't as pure, consistent, and contaminant-free as pharmaceuticals.

The botanical industry has *voluntary* guidelines, not mandatory ones. While some manufacturers have agreed to provide products that adhere to industry-defined standards, there is no mandatory oversight. Therefore, problems of adulteration, contamination, and dose standardization abound. This means buyer beware!

For the most part, the drug-like properties and effects of botanicals and herbs are directly related to the *quantity* of herb that you ingest. However, the strength of an herb may also depend on the *part* of the plant used. Pay attention to the nutrition information on botanical and herbal products. In general, the strongest, purest, and most effective botanical products consist of the whole plant.

Medical doctors are typically quite unfamiliar with botanicals and herbs and their effects. However, there are some botanicals and herbs which interact with drugs to enhance or negate the drug effect. Therefore, please be sure to inform all healthcare professionals about all the botanicals and herbs you use.

In assessing how well an alternative form of treatment works for the management of menopause, we first must determine how well the original, naturally-occurring biologic hormone worked. We then have to compare how well the botanical or herbal substance works compared to hormone replacement therapy.[5] When you read things comparing botanical and herbal products to pharmaceutical hormone therapy, that's essentially what they've done.

As for guidance with the use of botanicals and herbs for menopause, you'll likely find that an osteopathic doctor (D.O.) or a naturopathic doctor (N.D.) has more knowledge and a greater comfort level with botanical and herbal therapy than a medical doctor (M.D.) has. That's because botanical and herbal therapy is in the category of alternative and complementary medicine. This isn't a category addressed in the realm of allopathic medicine by conventional medical doctors (M.D.s). However, it is part of osteopathic training. Alternatively, you may find a certified botanist or herbalist very helpful in assisting you. You owe it to yourself to find a healthcare provider who has the knowledge and experience you need to assist you with the management of your menopause, regardless of your chosen regimen.

"Natural" Versus "Synthetic" Hormones

I include this section on "natural" versus "synthetic" hormones because it's an area that is fraught with confusion and misconceptions. The purpose of this book is to enable you to work with your physician, botanist, herbalist, or pharmacist as an informed patient. My goal is for you to have the correct terminology to request exactly what you want. In the area of natural versus synthetic hormones, it's quite common for women to use incorrect terms to describe their preferences. So, let's define each of these terms and elaborate a bit to make things crystal clear.

"Natural"

Natural refers to a substance found in nature which we utilize in its natural form. A plant possessing hormonal properties or effects, unaltered before packaging, is natural. An herb in its raw form is natural. An herb that is simply compressed into a tablet is still natural. So far, I'm sure you're with me. That's because so far I've only discussed plants and herbs. You think of them as natural. Naturally!

Here comes the confusing part. A *pharmaceutical product* may also be natural. That's right, you didn't misread that. It's possible for a prescription medication to be natural. An example is the pharmaceutical hormone "Cenestin." It's an estrogen tablet made from plant products. So, it's natural despite the fact that it's a pharmaceutical product.

Natural pharmaceutical products may be of either **plant or animal** origin. If that sounds odd, maybe you're forgetting that animals are found in nature. And animals form substances that are found in nature. So, natural pharmaceutical products may be of animal origin. While most natural products for menopause tend to be of plant origin, it's possible for a natural product to be of animal origin if it hasn't required significant alteration to be of use. As long as the substance of animal origin is close to its original form, it's still natural. An example is the estrogen pill called "Premarin." It's made from the urine of pregnant mares. Thus the name Premarin: Pre = pregnant, Mar = mare, In = urine. You see, pregnant mares are natural, and so is their urine. And it contains a lot of estrogen.

There's another twist to this, also. It's possible for the term "natural" to refer to something that is of *neither plant nor animal origin*. It may refer to something that is not even found in nature. How can that be? *Well, the term "natural" may refer to a substance which is **identical in structure to the molecules in the human body***. The scientific name for molecules which are identical to those in the human body is **"bioidentical."** When you're discussing something that you're going to put in your body, bioidentical substances may be the closest thing to natural that you can get. Think about it. Plants and animals are more different (and less natural) to your body than molecules similar to those in the body itself. Plants don't synthesize products that have the same structure as those in the human body. So, while plants are natural to Mother Earth, they aren't natural to the human body.[5] Likewise, animals and animal products are natural to the world, but not natural to your body.

All of these definitions of "natural" are valid. I'm simply pointing out the differences because, when it comes to menopause, there's a lot of miscommunication going on between women and their healthcare providers. Sometimes, it's difficult to explain exactly what you want. And sometimes it's even more difficult for your healthcare provider to understand, accept, and provide what you want.

One woman who desires "natural" hormones may want bioidentical hormones, while another woman wants something found in nature. There is a difference between the two. If you tend to want a natural product, read on. You'll be able to determine your preferences so that you can appropriately communicate your desires to your healthcare provider and receive exactly what you want.

"Synthetic"

"Synthetic" implies that the product is the result of a process which involves combining substances. The definition of "synthetic" focuses more on the process of *creating* a product than it does on where the components *originated*. The substances which are combined to create a synthetic product are either manufactured or artificially constructed.[5] The term "synthetic" may refer to **either natural or artificial** products. That makes sense, right? A natural product is synthesized when substances which are found in nature are combined in a manner to create a new product. An artificial substance is synthesized when chemicals interact to form a new product which contains non-natural components. The pharmaceutical industry has the ability to synthesize products from natural substances, chemically composed substances, or both. Some compounds are actually synthetic synthetics![5]

Sometimes, pharmaceutical companies convert natural substances into pharmaceutical products. In essence, they transform a natural substance into an unnatural substance. I don't intend for that to sound derogatory or judgmental in any way. It's just the best means of explaining how some useful pharmaceutical products originate. Most hormones that women take are made in a factory. In the case of estrogen, Cenestin, falls into this category. It's synthesized from plants. It's a synthetic combination of natural substances in the form of a pill. Premarin also falls into this category. It's extracted from the urine of pregnant mares (Pre = pregnant, Mar = mare, In = urine). This is an example of a natural substance of animal origin, converted (synthesized) into a pill. Both of these drugs are natural in the sense that they're derived from substances found in nature. Both are synthetic in the sense that the natural substance has been altered physically or chemically to a more useful form.

You're probably used to thinking about pharmaceutical products as "synthetic." Maybe you even think of them as "artificial." Well, although you now realize that such is not always the case, there are plenty of synthetic products which are "artificial," so to speak. An example is a product called Evista. It's a non-hormonal medication that prevents osteoporosis. It's synthesized entirely from chemicals in a lab. So, it's 100% synthetic, and has no natural components. The fact that it has no natural components doesn't make it inferior by any means. In fact, it's one of the most valuable drugs available for osteoporosis prevention and treatment.

Summary

If you prefer products derived from plants only, simply say so. Don't confuse yourself or your healthcare provider by misusing these terms. If it is easier to say "I don't want anything that's made from the urine of horses," say it in exactly those terms. If you prefer a product that's identical to the molecules in the human body, be sure to make that clear to your healthcare provider.

This distinction between natural and synthetic applies to every category of hormone in the realm of menopausal options. Hopefully, it will help you distinguish among the vast array of available options in managing your menopause. It's a very good thing that there are so many options. You may find that, while you tend to prefer one category or form of product over another from an intellectual or psychological standpoint, your body prefers a different one in terms of results. Don't think of natural and synthetic as being opposites. One isn't good and the other bad. Options are a good thing, and one doesn't have to be superior to another. All that matters is how they work ***for you***. It's good that you have both. You're free to try many options.

Bioidentical Hormones

One category of "synthetic" hormones is synthesized from substances which are identical to the molecules in the human body. We call these **<u>bioidentical hormones.</u>** These hormones tend to produce fewer side effects due to the fact that the human body recognizes them as less foreign, and metabolizes them more easily.

Options: Medical, Non-medical, and Everything in Between

In terms of natural versus synthetic, it sounds contradictory to say that bioidentical hormones are both synthetic and natural, but that is actually the case. They are synthetically-derived natural hormones. In other words, they are synthesized (therefore, "synthetic") from substances whose molecules are identical to those of the human body (therefore, "natural"), such that the body treats them as if it made them itself.

Most menopausal estrogen products which are not taken by mouth are bioidentical. They may be in the form of a skin patch or vaginal cream. Because they consist of the hormone estradiol, which is the same estrogen produced by the human body, they constitute bioidentical hormones even though they are also pharmaceutical products.[6]

Bioidentical hormones are actually natural in another sense. They may originate from plants, which are found in nature. I guess you could say that they're doubly natural. But the natural substances from plants are modified so that they are no longer in their natural form.

So, if you had to vote on whether the label "natural" or "synthetic" is more appropriate for describing bioidentical hormones, the label "synthetic" would win. But if you had to vote on whether a bioidentical substance or a substance occurring in nature is more compatible with the human body, the bioidentical substance would win.

I guess the decision as to which category you prefer rests on your focus. If your focus is on putting substances into your body which are the easiest for your body to handle, then go with bioidentical hormones. If your focus is on using natural products which have not been modified, go with botanical or herbal products. If you care most about strict standards for testing, go with pharmaceutical products.

Bioidentical hormones are produced by combining or adding substances together. That's why they fall into the category of synthetic substances. In the arena of pharmaceutical products, we refer to the process of combining substances as **compounding**. These "natural, compounded" hormones are synthesized from chemical substances that are the natural components of plants.[3] In a lab, they are converted to a form that the human body can use. After conversion, they are identical in molecular structure to the hormones that the human body manufactures itself. Thus, "bioidentical" means identical to the body.

There are special pharmacies, called <u>compounding pharmacies</u>, which will customize medications according to your doctor's specific prescription for your individual needs. We call these <u>custom-compounded medications</u>. They're available as creams, gels, capsules, implants, and suppositories.[7]

Custom-compounded formulations *aren't necessarily* bioidentical. They may be, but not always. Just separate the terms "bioidentical" and "custom." They don't mean the same thing, and they don't necessarily coincide.[7]

A commercial, prescription bioidentical medication isn't custom-made just for you. But it *is* tested and approved by the FDA. A custom-compounded formulation is designed just for you, but *isn't* tested and approved by the FDA.[7]

Finally, a custom-compounded medication *may* actually be synthesized from bioidentical substances, in which case, it's made just for you, from molecules identical to those in the human body, and it's FDA tested and approved.[7]

As I said with regard to communicating your wishes for natural versus synthetic products, just state specifically what you want. Don't even use the formal terms if you don't want to. If you want a formulation that's designed just for you, say so. If you want molecules identical to those in the human body, say so.

At this point, you might be wondering why molecules which are identical to those in the human body even make a difference. If you are, you're really thinking, and that's a great question. Here's the answer: All hormones exert their effect by "binding" with a receptor. Until the hormone binds with a receptor, it just floats around doing nothing. In other words, it's not active until it binds with a receptor. Think of the hormone and the receptor as puzzle pieces. The better they fit together with one another, the better they work and the fewer side effects they produce. Bioidentical hormones bind to receptor sites with a perfect fit, whereas other hormones have a less than perfect fit. Likewise, because they have the same molecular structure as the hormones that the body produces, they produce fewer side effects than synthetic hormones.[3]

Acupuncture

The term "acupuncture" describes a variety of practices which involve puncturing the body with thin needles in specific locations. The needles aren't just ordinary needles. They are much longer, and they've been augmented by low voltage current, sound waves, or laser beams. This is one of many forms of alternative medicine which deals with manipulating the flow of energy (qi) in the body.[8] While the exact mechanism by which acupuncture exerts its effect is unknown, many women experience significant benefits with regard to managing menopause. These benefits include relief of hot flashes, night sweats, insomnia, mood swings, and anxiety.

I know of no adverse effects of acupuncture. While there is no way to predetermine whether or not it will work for you, there's no reason to think of it as harmful. If you choose to give it a try and it makes you feel as though you've found nirvana, good for you. If not, you can choose another option.

Hypnosis

There isn't much scientific data on hypnosis for managing menopause, and it's not something that naturally comes to mind as an option for managing menopause. However, there's no harm associated with hypnosis, and if you want to try it, go ahead. If it doesn't work, you can move on to other options. There's a cliché that comes to mind: Don't knock it until you've tried it.

Chapter 7:
Categories of Hormones and Their Sources

The purpose of this chapter is to familiarize you with the various options that are available for each category of hormone. As you learned earlier, the hormones of interest are estrogen, progesterone, and testosterone. In addition to these individual hormones, some are important in combination. They include estrogen plus progesterone and estrogen plus testosterone. Each hormone has a variety of sources, including dietary, botanical, herbal, bioidentical, and pharmaceutical options. This chapter will provide you with an understanding of these sources, and present a variety of options for you to consider.

Despite the fact that I'll present the hormones one at a time, realize that they don't present themselves to your body that way. No hormone acts in a vacuum. Some of your symptoms result from combinations of hormones acting in harmony with one another. Other symptoms result from hormones that are counteracting one another. Still other symptoms may be the result of the predominant or the strongest hormone. Many times, the symptoms you notice will be the net effect of multiple fluctuating hormones.

At the beginning of the section on each of the hormones, I'll give you lists of the symptoms characteristic of both deficiencies of that hormone and excesses of that hormone. Don't expect your symptoms to match these lists perfectly. You aren't a robot. You're an evolving work in progress. Additionally, don't overanalyze these distinctions. While you may actually have symptoms from both categories (hormone excess and hormone deficiency), you may find that you exhibit one set of symptoms more strongly than the other.

Estrogen

Symptoms of Abnormal Estrogen Levels

In order to enable you to tailor the management of your menopause to your particular symptoms of menopause, you'll need to know the symptoms of estrogen excess versus the symptoms of estrogen deficiency. This may help you target the agents that'll serve you best at a specific time during peri- or post-menopause. Never forget, however, that menopause is a process. Rarely does one hormone function in isolation. Additionally, your symptoms may change over time.

Symptoms of Estrogen Deficiency

1. Less frequent or absent periods
2. Hot flashes
3. Night sweats
4. Insomnia
5. Fatigue
6. Forgetfulness
7. Mood swings
8. Irritability
9. Joint stiffness and joint pain
10. Dry skin
11. Hair loss
12. Vaginal dryness
13. Urinary problems (urinary tract infections, urinary incontinence)
14. Decreased sex drive

Symptoms of Estrogen Excess

1. Increased or excessive vaginal bleeding
2. Digestive issues such as nausea and vomiting
3. Food cravings
4. Breast pain and tenderness
5. Weight gain

6. Bloating
7. Depression
8. Persistent or recurrent vaginal yeast infections
9. Headache
10. Leg cramps (also a symptom of calcium deficiency)

Categories of Estrogen

There are three broad categories of estrogen. These include:

(1) <u>Plant</u> (botanical and herbal) sources of estrogen, which are natural, and not synthetic, when utilized in their original form;
(2) <u>Bioidentical</u> estrogen, which is both synthetic and natural (synthesized from naturally occurring substances into molecules which are identical to those in the human body); and
(3) <u>Synthetic</u> estrogen, derived either from natural substances (plant or animal) or from chemicals.

We'll discuss each of these in detail.

Introduction to Botanical and Herbal Sources of Estrogen

<u>Phytoestrogens</u>

Phytoestrogens are plants which have a hormonal effect similar or identical to that of estrogen. "Phyto" means plant, and "estrogen" means estrogen. So, these are plant sources of estrogen. There are three basic categories of plants which exert the hormonal effect of estrogen. They are: (1) Isoflavones; (2) Lignans; and (3) Coumestans. By far, the isoflavones are the most significant.

<u>Isoflavones</u> are soy or red clover derivatives in the form of herbs, tablets, or foods. The most familiar forms of isoflavones are soy supplements such as tofu, tempeh, meat substitutes made from soy, miso, soybeans, and garbanzo beans (chick peas).

Lignans are part of the cell wall of plants. They are absorbed into the body after breakdown by intestinal bacteria. Common sources of lignans include flaxseeds, pumpkin seeds, sunflower seeds, cranberries, black and green teas, garlic, broccoli, bran, and peanuts.[2] The greatest source of lignans is the husk seed that is used to produce oils, especially flaxseeds.

Coumestans aren't a significant source of phytoestrogens. They do have some hormone-like activity, however. High concentrations of coumestans are present in red clover, sunflower seeds, and bean sprouts.

A single plant may contain more than one category of phytoestrogens. For example, soybeans are rich in isoflavones, while soy sprouts are a potent source of coumestans.[2] Sunflower seeds are both lignans and coumestans.

Phytoestrogens are natural forms of estrogen, but are not identical to the estrogens in the human body. Phytoestrogens are *much weaker* than human estrogen, with potencies that are only 1/100 to 1/1000 as strong. Thus, phytoestrogens act like weak estrogens. Nonetheless, they have the same effects as human estrogen.

When we describe the way in which a substance produces an effect, we are describing how well it *fits* with another structure that allows it to exert that effect. When it comes to hormones and substances which exert an effect similar to that of a hormone, we often use the term "receptor." (You've already come across this term.) While this terminology may sound very scientific or medical, it's really very simple. Think about puzzle pieces. When you snap a puzzle piece together with another piece, you're doing the same thing that a hormone does with a receptor. Think of the hormone as the protruding portion of the puzzle piece, and think of the receptor as the opening into which you put the protruding part. When a hormone or hormone-like substance fills a receptor, it becomes activated. Activation enables the hormone to produce a response characteristic of that hormone.

"*Affinity*" is the word we use to designate how much of an attraction a hormone (or hormone-like substance) has for a receptor. Going back

Categories of Hormones and Their Sources

to the analogy of puzzle pieces, you may want to think of affinity in terms of how well two puzzle pieces fit together. There is really only one piece that fits perfectly. But you can try to snap another piece in place that fits, just not as well. Because it doesn't fit as well, it doesn't produce the exact result that the correct piece would have produced. In the end, the resulting puzzle picture will be different. You may still be able to recognize the overall picture, but parts of it will not be as clear.

In the case of hormones, the effect of joining the correct hormone to a receptor site will be different than that of joining the receptor with an incorrect hormone. The receptor has the highest affinity for the correct piece and a lower affinity for the incorrect pieces. If a substance has a strong affinity for a receptor, it is very attracted to it, and very likely to bind with it and produce an effect. If a substance has a weak affinity for a receptor, it is less attracted to it, and less likely to bind and produce an effect. The greater the affinity a receptor has for a certain type of hormone, the stronger the effect of that hormone once it occupies the receptor site. If a similar, but less perfect hormone occupies the receptor site, it produces a weaker version of the hormonal effect. The affinity of phytoestrogens for estrogen receptors is only 1/1500 to 1/11,000 as strong as that of the body's natural estrogen.[4]

Here's an analogy: All this talk of affinity and receptor binding may be thought of in terms of male-female relationships. The receptors are like promiscuous partners who attract a wide variety of mates. Despite the fact that they are most attracted to their perfect partner, they spend a lot of time attracting other prospects, also. Thus, they don't always bind with their intended specific partner. They bind with many other mates that are similar, but not "the one." Once bound with a less than perfect partner, they have a relationship, but it isn't as good as the relationship they would have had if they had attached to their ideal partner.

Phytoestrogens act by binding to estrogen receptors. Remember, though, that phytoestrogens are much weaker than the body's natural estrogen. So, it may seem as though it would take mass quantities of phytoestrogens to produce a noticeable effect. But such is not the case because of the unique manner in which phytoestrogens exert their effect. Rather than acting on estrogen receptors in exactly the same fashion as human estrogen does, phytoestrogens are more flexible in the way that they interact with receptor sites.

The result is that the effects of phytoestrogens are not always additive. Instead, they can have either enhancing or diminishing effects on the overall estrogen level. In other words, they work to balance the estrogen in the body. Another way of saying this is to say that they have both estrogenic (positive) and anti-estrogenic (negative) behavior. (I know this is confusing. Just keep reading. I promise I'll illustrate what I'm telling you.)

It all depends on how much human estrogen is circulating around. If the circulating level of estrogen is *low*, phytoestrogens have a positive estrogenic effect and *increase* the level of estrogen in the body. Alternatively, if the circulating level of estrogen is *high*, phytoestrogens have a negative estrogenic effect and *decrease* the level of estrogen in the body. The positive effect results because the phytoestrogen fills an estrogen receptor with estrogen, even though it is a weaker brand of estrogen. In this instance, *some* estrogen (even a weak one) is more than *no* estrogen. The negative estrogenic effect occurs because the weak phytoestrogen inhibits binding of the stronger human estrogen. As such, the weak phytoestrogen takes the binding site away from the stronger human estrogen, which lowers the overall amount of active estrogen.

The best way to visualize this is to give human estrogen and phytoestrogen molecules numerical values. Imagine that each of the human estrogen molecules has a value, let's say of 100, and that each phytoestrogen molecule has a value of only 1. You can see the positive or negative effect of a phytoestrogen by adding up the numerical values of the molecules that attach to a receptor site.

Let's illustrate this more clearly.

Here are some examples:

Example I: Let's say __*there's plenty of strong human estrogen in the body*__, and create a variety of scenarios to demonstrate various outcomes.

CATEGORIES OF HORMONES AND THEIR SOURCES

Scenario # 1:

If receptor A has 3 receptor sites for estrogen, and all 3 bind with human estrogen (100 each),
the total amount of estrogen is 300
(100 + 100 + 100 = 300).
This is the strongest possible result, giving the highest estrogen levels.

Scenario # 2:

If receptor B has 3 receptor sites for estrogen, and 2 bind with human estrogen (100 each),
while 1 binds with a phytoestrogen (1),
the total amount of estrogen is 201
(100 + 100 + 1 = 201).
This would constitute a negative estrogenic effect because the weaker phytoestrogen prevented a stronger human estrogen from binding. This resulted in an overall lower quantity of estrogen (represented by the lower numerical score of 201 versus 300).

Scenario # 3:

If receptor C has 3 receptor sites for estrogen, and 2 bind with phytoestrogens (1 each),
while the other 1 binds with human estrogen (100),
the total amount of estrogen is 102
(1 + 1 + 100 = 102).
This would also constitute a negative estrogenic effect because the 2 weaker phytoestrogens prevented stronger human estrogen from binding. This resulted in an overall lower quantity of estrogen (represented by the lower numerical score of 102 versus 300).

Scenario # 4:

If receptor D has 3 receptor sites for estrogen, and all 3 bind with phytoestrogens (1 each), the total amount of estrogen is 3 (1 + 1 + 1 = 3). In this case, the weak phytoestrogens prevented the strong human estrogen from binding. If your goal was to decrease the circulating level of estrogen (because you had symptoms of estrogen excess), phytoestrogens could help.

In summary, whenever there is plenty of circulating human estrogen, the binding of phytoestrogen will serve to lower estrogen levels.

Example II: Now let's change things a bit and say that *there is little or no human estrogen in the body*. Again, we'll create a variety of scenarios to demonstrate the results.

> Scenario # 1:
> If receptor E has 3 receptor sites for estrogen, and all 3 remain empty,
> the total amount of estrogen remains at 0.
>
> Scenario # 2:
> If receptor F has 3 receptor sites for estrogen, and 2 remain empty (0 + 0),
> while 1 binds with a phytoestrogen (1),
> the total amount of estrogen is 1
> (0 + 0 + 1 = 1).
> This would constitute a positive estrogenic effect because the 1 phytoestrogen is more than no estrogen. This resulted in an overall higher quantity of estrogen (represented by the higher numerical score of 1 versus 0).
>
> Scenario # 3:
> If receptor G has 3 receptor sites for estrogen, and 2 bind with phytoestrogens (1 each),
> while the other 1 remains empty (0),
> the total amount of estrogen is 2
> (1 + 1 + 0 = 2).
> This would also constitute a positive estrogenic effect because the 2 weak phytoestrogens

Categories of Hormones and Their Sources

constitute more than no estrogen at all. This resulted in an overall higher quantity of estrogen (represented by the higher numerical score of 2 versus 0).

Scenario # 4:

If receptor H has 3 receptor sites for estrogen, and all 3 bind with phytoestrogens (1 each), the total amount of estrogen is 3 (1 + 1 + 1 = 3).

In this case, the receptors have some estrogen rather than no estrogen. Since there's no human estrogen around, binding with a weak estrogen is better than binding with no estrogen. If your goal was to increase the circulating level of estrogen (because you had symptoms of estrogen deficiency), phytoestrogens could help.

In summary, whenever there is a deficiency of circulating human estrogen, the binding of phytoestrogens will serve to raise estrogen levels.

A beneficial side effect of phytoestrogens is that they don't increase your risk of breast cancer or uterine cancer. This may be due to their tendency to inhibit binding of the stronger human estrogen. Overall, it appears that isoflavones and lignans decrease the replication of cells, which is the process by which cancers occur.

Phytoestrogens contribute to lowering your risk of cancer in another way, also. Isoflavones and lignans increase the production of Sex Hormone Binding Globulin (SHBG).[3] SHBG attracts and binds free hormones which are floating around doing nothing productive. When SHBG binds these hormones, it harnesses the hormone in a way that keeps it from attaining harmfully high levels. This makes phytoestrogens a good choice if you have concerns about breast or uterine cancer.

The incidence of cancers and heart attacks decreases with increasing quantities of phytoestroens.[5] This is evident in the Asian diet, which contains an average of 40 – 80 mg of active isoflavones daily because of all the tofu and soybeans they eat. In contrast, the American and European diets tend to contain an average of less than 3 mg of isoflavones daily.[5] Cancer and heart attack aren't very common for Asians; but they're incredibly common occurrences for Americans and Europeans. There is no single synthetic or chemically-derived substance that matches the benefits of simply eating soy foods.

Phytoestrogens and other herbs exert their effects much more slowly than bioidentical hormones or synthetic hormones. It may take a full month to notice any difference in menopausal symptoms. As with all menopausal regimens, a three month trial is necessary to assess the full effect of phytoestrogens or herbs.

Foods as Hormonal Sources of Estrogen

The three most prominent estrogen-containing food sources that are useful in the management of menopause are: (1) Soy (tofu); (2) Flaxseeds; and (3) Foods that contain bioflavonoids.[6]

Soy

Soy may just be the magical menopausal wonder food. It offers all of the desirable benefits of hormones, but has none of the risks. You may use it in isolation or in combination with other agents in managing your menopause. Not only is it an excellent food source of protein and fiber, but it has so many positive effects on all parts of the body that it seems too good to be true.

Soy foods come in many forms. Soy beans (edamame), tofu, soy milk, soy based meat substitutes (soy burgers, etc.), soy based dairy substitutes (soy cheese, soy yogurt, soy ice cream, etc.), and soy protein powders are all becoming readily available on the shelves of most grocery stores world-wide. Generally, 1 gm of soy protein yields 1.2 – 1.7 mg of isoflavones, depending on the type of soybean that is the source of the protein.[4]

Different soy products have variable quantities of isoflavones. Processed soy products may have only 1/10 the isoflavone content as whole soy beans. Fermentation of soy (as in the case of tempeh) enhances the quantity of isoflavones.[3]

Categories of Hormones and Their Sources

Here's a list of the positive effects of soy with regard to menopause:

1. Helps regulate periods
2. Decreases hot flashes
3. Decreases night sweats
4. Decreases mood swings
5. Decreases irritability
6. Decreases PMS
7. Decreases dry skin
8. Decreases hair loss
9. Strengthens nails
10. Decreases weight gain by decreasing fat and increasing lean tissue mass
11. Decreases loss of calcium
12. Decreases the risk of breast cancer
13. Decreases the risk of uterine cancer
14. Increases healthy HDL and decreases lousy LDL, preventing heart attacks
15. Prevents bone loss and osteoporosis
16. Decreases the risk of colon cancer
17. Decreases migraine headaches

Hopefully, this list illustrates the reason I refer to soy as the wonder food. As you can see, soy covers all of the bases in managing menopause. With so many sources of soy foods available, it's easy to consume large quantities of soy while maintaining variety in your diet.

The benefits of soy are dose dependent. This means that the more soy you consume, the more beneficial effects you'll realize. Because foods contain different quantities of soy, and because some soy products contain more isoflavones than others, it's difficult to measure soy intake precisely. In general though, 100 – 160 mg of soy isoflavones daily provide the benefits enumerated above.

Flaxseed

Flaxseed is an example of a lignan. In general, lignans have many desirable effects, including the following:

1. They're anti-cancer agents.[6]
2. They're phytoestrogens, with the same ability to alter estrogen levels as soy isoflavones.[6]
3. They're antioxidants, which prevent tissue aging.[6]
4. They prevent heart attacks by decreasing lousy LDL and increasing healthy HDL.[6]
5. They're an excellent source of fiber.[6]
6. They're an excellent source of omega 3 fatty acids.[6]

Flaxseed products vary considerably, so you may wish to try different varieties or preparations. You can use flaxseeds as a garnish, eat them by the spoonful, or cook with them. The dose for purposes of menopause is 1 tsp - 1 tbsp daily. It's necessary to grind the flaxseeds in order to absorb all the nutrients they provide. Enjoy!

Bioflavonoids

Bioflavonoids are substances present in many fruits, such as orange and lemon peels, cherries, blueberries, grapes, and cranberries. In general, bright, colorful fruits and vegetables contain bioflavonoids. Additionally, some whole grains and herbs contain bioflavonoids.

Bioflavonoids are also available in the form of a nutritional supplement. The dose of supplement for relief of menopausal symptoms is 1000 mg daily.

Botanical and Herbal Estrogen

Dong Quai (Angelica sinensis)

Dong Quai is the best known of the herbs with phytoestrogenic activity. If you look at the ingredients in many of the herbal preparations for menopause, you'll notice that it's one of the ingredients in most of them. It has the effect of enhancing energy and inducing a sense of well-being.

There are many forms of Dong Quai that are available for management of menopause. These include: (1) The raw, dried herb; (2) The root; (3) Pills (tablets and capsules); and (4) Tinctures.

The starting dose of Dong Quai is 4.5 gm daily.[6] Most women require doses higher than this (up to 9 gm) to relieve the symptoms of menopause.[6] It doesn't work for everyone who uses it for menopause. Use caution with Dong Quai because it can thin the blood to an extent that is dangerous.

Chasteberry (Vitex agnus-castus)

The Chasteberry herb comes from the Chaste Tree. As the name implies, it's a fruit. It's widely available in health food stores and herbal shops. Chasteberry is popular for regulating irregular periods, suppressing PMS, treating insomnia, and alleviating depression. It acts on Follicle Stimulating Hormone (FSH) and Luteinizing Hormone (LH). The ultimate outcome of all this is that it increases the hormone balance in favor of progesterone.

Side effects of Chasteberry include suppression of appetite and skin rash. It is prohibited during pregnancy, nursing (lactation), and during treatment with certain psychiatric medicines, such as haloperidol (Haldol) and thioridazine (Mellaril). As always, inform all healthcare professionals if you're using Chasteberry.

The dose of Chasteberry in its natural fruit form is 1 tsp with 1 cup of water one to four times daily. The goal is to consume a daily dose equivalent to 20 mg of the crude fruit, or 30 – 40 mg of the fruit in decoction.[3] The dose in its liquid extract form is 20 – 75 drops one to four times daily. The liquid extract usually comes in a 1:3 ratio, but preparations differ. Always follow the instructions for the particular preparation you're using.

Black Cohosh (Cimicifuga racemosa)

Black Cohosh is a coarse perennial woodland herb with large compound leaves and a thick, knotted root system.[7] There are numerous common names for this plant. You may recognize it as Black Snakeroot, Black Root, Rattle Root, Rattle Top, Rattle Squawroot, Snake Root, Rattleweed, or Bugbane. With such a wide variety of names, you may just need to take a list of them with you if you go shopping for Black Cohosh.

Standardized extracts of commercial products of Black Cohosh, prepared from the dried root of the plant, are plentiful. Remifemin, which is a dried 40% isopropanol extract of the root, is the most popular of these. It is standardized to contain 1 mg of the active ingredient per 20 mg of extract. You've probably seen Remifemin on the shelf at a vitamin or nutrition store. It's a readily available commercial preparation of the herb.

Black Cohosh is also available in many other forms, including powdered root, tea, solid dry powdered extract, fluid extract, and tincture.

Women have been using Black Cohosh to manage the symptoms of menopause for many years. It's useful in decreasing hot flashes and night sweats. It reduces mood swings, PMS, depression, anxiety, insomnia, and vaginal dryness. It acts by binding to estrogen receptors and by suppressing the increase in Luteinizing Hormone (LH).

Black Cohosh is not effective in treating menopausal symptoms in women who are using tamoxifen.[7] So, if you're on tamoxifen for any reason, don't expect much from Black Cohosh. It is safe for women with estrogen-dependent cancers.

The most significant side effect of Black Cohosh is that it enhances the effects of medications used for high blood pressure, resulting in dangerously low blood pressure. It would be unwise to choose this option if you take medications for high blood pressure. Other, less severe side effects include nausea, vomiting, dizziness, headaches, breast pain, and weight gain.[6]

Four to twelve weeks of treatment with Black Cohosh may be necessary before recognition of any benefit. If you choose this agent, be sure to allow enough time to see how it works for you. Patience is the key.

The dosages of Black Cohosh are as follows:

Remifemin: 1 – 2 tablets (20 – 40 mg) twice daily
Powdered root: 1 - 2 gm three times daily

Black Cohosh tea: 1 – 2 gm three times daily

Solid dry powdered extract (in 4:1 concentration): 250 – 500 mg three times daily

Tincture (in 1:1 concentration): 4 mg or 1 tsp three times daily[6]

Licorice Root (Glycyrrhiza glabra)

Licorice Root is an herb that has many hormonal and non-hormonal uses. It contains both isoflavones and lignans as active ingredients, making it very versatile. In the case of menopause, it balances the estrogen to progesterone ratio. It also provides general protection against cancer and reduces fatigue.

Licorice Root has the significant side effect of increasing blood pressure. This imposes the requirement of careful blood pressure monitoring if you use Licorice Root.

The dose of Licorice Root is ¼ tsp solid extract one to two times daily.[6]

St. John's Wort (Hypericum perforatum)

St. John's Wort has antidepressant properties. The antidepressant effect of St. John's Wort depends on the quantity of hypericin in the formulation. If you compare labels on various brands of this herb, you'll see that the quantity of hypericin differs significantly from one to the next.

The dose of this herb is 2 – 4 gm (containing 0.2 – 1.0 mg hypericin) in capsule form, once or twice daily.[6]

Valerian (Valeriana officinalis)

Valerian is useful for insomnia. It decreases the time it takes to fall asleep and improves the quality of sleep.

You should not use Valerian if you have liver disease.

The recommended dose for Valerian is 1 – 2 capsules at night or 2 – 3 gm once or twice daily.[6]

Hops (Humulus lupulus)

Most people are familiar with Hops as an ingredient in beer. So, you might be wondering if you can just drink a lot of beer to manage menopause. Well, the answer is, "Yes, you can drink a lot of beer," and, "No, it won't help you manage menopause." It will help you gain weight, though.

Hops has estrogenic activity that results from the combined effect of its many constituents. Because of its hormonal properties, it's a common ingredient in skin softening creams. Hops is one of the six highest estrogen-binding substances in the category of botanicals and herbs. It has a moderate degree of estrogenic activity, and improves the symptoms of menopause (especially insomnia) as well as decreasing heart attacks and osteoporosis.[8]

You should not use Hops if you have an estrogen-dependent breast cancer or depression.[8]

Dosages are as follows:

Liquid extract: 1:1 45% ethanol
  (equal quantities of Hops and ethanol)
Tincture: 1:5 60% ethanol
  (five times more ethanol than Hops)
For most indications, a single daily dose of 0.5 gm is adequate.[6]

For insomnia:

1–2 gm of powder, or
0.5 ml liquid extract, or
1–2 ml tincture[6]

False Unicorn Root (Veratum luteum)

False Unicorn Root has little benefit for purposes of menopause. Its main effect is that it has diuretic properties and reduces fluid retention.

Categories of Hormones and Their Sources

The dosage is unknown.[7] I include it here to dispel any belief that it helps in managing menopause.

Motherwort (Leonurus cardiaca)

Use of Motherwort for menopausal symptoms is unfounded, but it has no known health hazards.

Dosages are as follows:

   4.5 gm of the herb daily
   2–4 gm infusion three times daily
   1:1 liquid extract of 2–4 ml three times daily
   2–6 ml tincture daily[6]

Joyful Change

Joyful Change is a Chinese tonic that contains numerous herbs, the combination of which is useful in menopause. It alleviates irregular periods, hot flashes, insomnia, and vaginal dryness.

Chai Hu Long Gu Muli Wang

Here's another Chinese remedy. This is a combination of herbs that improves insomnia and mood swings. One benefit of this substance is that it is safe enough to use indefinitely.

Bioidentical Estrogen

There are three forms of bioidentical estrogen, and they are the same as the three estrogens in the female body. These are: (1) **Estrone**; (2) 17 beta **Estradiol**; and (3) **Estriol**. In the human body, estradiol is the most important estrogen during your reproductive years. It's also the most potent of the three. Estriol is the main hormone of pregnancy, and it's produced by the placenta. After menopause, the main estrogen is estrone, and the primary source of it is fat cells.

The alternative and complementary medical community embraces estriol as the estrogen of choice. Estriol is the primary estrogen that the placenta produces. Theories abound claiming that high levels of estriol during pregnancy protect estrogen-sensitive tissues against cancer induced by estrone and estradiol.

Most compounding pharmacies prepare a "Tri-est" formulation. A Tri-est preparation achieves appropriate levels of all three components.[9] Most commonly, a prescription for bioidentical hormones contains a ratio of estrogens which mimics that in the human body before menopause. That ratio is 80% estriol, 10% estrone, and 10% estradiol.[10] An alternative to the Tri-est formulation is a "Bi-est" formulation which consists of 80% estriol and 20% estradiol.

Estriol, the largest component in both the Bi-est and the Tri-est formulations is the *weakest* of the three estrogens. Proponents of bioidentical hormones claim that it produces less risk and fewer side effects than the estrogens found in commercial pharmaceutical products.[11]

Bioidentical Estrogen

3 forms	Human	Tri-est	Bi-est
Estrone	10%	10%	0%
Estradiol	10%	10%	20%
Estriol (weakest)	80%	80%	80%

If you opt for bioidentical estrogen, your personal formulation could conform to the results of hormone testing and your symptoms of menopause. This allows maintenance of optimal levels of hormones and avoids higher dosages than necessary. Most of all, it acknowledges the fact that you're unique and require a formulation and dosage of hormones to mimic that in your own body.

Bioidentical hormones are available in the form of pills, skin patches, or vaginal preparations. With regard to efficacy, hormone delivery systems that involve absorption through the skin (creams, gels, or skin patches) are more direct than other forms. That's because they don't have to travel through the digestive tract and liver like pills that are taken by mouth. This shorter route also allows dosages to be as much as one 1/10 that of an oral dose.[10] Because of the higher dosages of estrogen in the form of pills, they are associated with higher rates of blood clots and diseases that result from blood clots (stroke and heart attack).

If you choose to utilize bioidentical hormones, you may wish to have your level of estradiol checked to ensure that your dose is appropriate. The acceptable level is 60 – 100 pg/ml. A level over 150 pg/ml is excessive.[9]

Compounding pharmacies are readily available. Simply request that your physician direct your prescription to a compounding pharmacy if you desire bioidentical hormones. These drug formulations may be more expensive and your insurance company may *not* be willing to pay for them. I know that economic issues may have an impact on your decisions. Therefore, I give you this information so that you can make choices that are suitable for both your preferences and your pocket book.

Not everyone agrees with the assertion that bioidentical hormones are better than other forms of hormone therapy. A review of the medical literature found no proven advantage of bioidentical hormones over other regimens.[11] There is no clear benefit to the heart, and there are no studies comparing the side effects of bioidentical to non-bioidentical hormones.

The world of compounded drugs is not subject to the same degree of oversight and regulation by the FDA (Food and Drug Administration) as the world of pharmaceutical drugs.[11] Rather than adhering to federal standards, it relies on state standards to ensure the quality and safety of these drugs.[11] They aren't routinely tested by any regulatory agency for purity and potency, and they don't have any labeling requirements.[11] They sort of float in a world between botanical/herbal agents and pharmaceutical drugs.

I don't like to label things as "better" or "worse." It's more accurate to accept the fact that they have differences. Because they're different, they provide you with more options, and that's good. So, use this information in the manner that suits you. Remember, no matter how much you like the idea of a particular option, it may or may not actually work for you. You have to listen to both your brain and your body. Believe me; they'll both talk to you.

Synthetic Estrogen

Synthetic estrogen is available in many forms, including pills, shots, skin patches, vaginal rings, vaginal creams, and vaginal tablets. The collective term for use of any type of pharmaceutical estrogen for menopause is **"Estrogen Replacement Therapy (ERT)."**

Estrogen Pills

Estrogen pills, taken by mouth, are the most readily available form of estrogen replacement therapy for menopause. Most of the studies on estrogen have analyzed the pill form of the hormone. The type of estrogen contained in pills is called "conjugated estrogen." The source of conjugated estrogen can vary from plant sources to animal sources. The most familiar form of conjugated estrogen comes from the urine of pregnant mares. It is called Premarin (Pre = pregnant, Mar = mare, In = urine).

Since women differ in their dosage needs, there are many dosages of conjugated estrogen available, ranging from 0.3 mg tablets to 2.5 mg tablets. While lower dosages may relieve some of the symptoms of menopause, a higher dose (usually 0.625 mg or its equivalent) may be necessary to confer the benefit of preventing osteoporosis.

Oral estrogen in pill form undergoes metabolism in the digestive system. Therefore, it passes through the liver. Since the liver is sensitive to estrogen, pills are not suitable for you if you have liver disease. The fact that oral estrogen passes through the liver forms the basis for a multitude of differences between oral and non-oral estrogen. Comparison between oral and non-oral forms of estrogen is the focus of many research studies. The non-oral forms of estrogen tend to demonstrate a safer overall profile in terms of their effect on the heart and the blood vessels. Thus, they present a lower risk for heart attacks and blood clots.

Oral estrogen has beneficial effects on healthy HDL but increases triglycerides and glucose. It also increases Sex Hormone Binding Globulin (SHBG), which results in an overall lower availability of estrogen in the body.[12] I know that sounds ironic, but it's precisely the reason that you have to take a higher dose of estrogen in pill form than you do in other forms.

Estrogen Shots

Estrogen shots aren't very popular due to the necessity of a monthly office visit and the discomfort of getting a shot. With so many other forms of estrogen available, shots are really unpopular. However, shots provide rapid absorption of estrogen into the blood stream and bypass the liver.

Estrogen Vaginal Rings

Vaginal rings are a newer form of estrogen administration. They offer convenience and ease of use. Most rings remain in the vagina for three months, after which you simply reach into your vagina, remove the ring, and replace it with another. Yes, you can do all of this yourself. It's easy and painless.

Vaginal rings are one of the most convenient ways to satisfy all of your needs in managing menopause. They provide estrogen to the entire body, and a little extra to the vagina. That's a perk because the vagina tends to need a bit more estrogen than other body parts. So, vaginal rings take care of the vaginal itching, dryness, painful intercourse, and urinary problems common to many menopausal women. Additionally, the blood stream absorbs estrogen through the vaginal skin and sends it throughout your body to take care of all the symptoms of menopause.

The disadvantages of rings are the possibilities of accidental expulsion, vaginal irritation, or discomfort. All of these are rare.

Estrogen Skin Patches

Skin patches deliver estrogen through the skin. Another name for them is "transdermal estrogen." You leave an estrogen patch on your skin for three days or a week, depending on the brand or the dose of estrogen it contains. Then you peel it off and replace it with a new one.

The amount of estrogen delivered into the skin by a patch depends on the size of the patch and its total dose of estrogen. The extent of absorption depends on where you place the patch. Some areas of your body absorb substances more efficiently than others. Usually this has to do with how much fat is present in the area. The more fat there is, the better the absorption. The best places for an estrogen patch are your abdomen, your buttocks, or your thighs.[12] Go figure! Aren't they the places you accumulate unwelcome fat? There are two standard dosages of estrogen in skin patches. They are 0.05 mg (comparable to 0.625 mg in a pill) and 0.1 mg (comparable to 1.25 mg in a pill).

Skin patches provide the same benefits of estrogen pills without the harmful effects on the liver. Additionally, unlike the oral pill form of estrogen, patches lower triglycerides and cause fewer blood clots.[13] The disadvantages of patches are that some women have difficulty making them adhere to their skin, and others have skin irritation from the adhesive on the patch. Reactions to the patch occur in 20% to 40% of women, usually in the form of a rash.[12]

Estrogen Vaginal Creams

Vaginal creams are especially beneficial for treating vaginal dryness and painful intercourse. They provide estrogen to the vaginal area in higher dosages than other forms of estrogen. That's a good thing, because the vagina is very selfish about estrogen. It tends to need more and to give you a really hard time if you don't supply it with what it needs.

Vaginal creams can penetrate the vaginal skin, allowing estrogen absorption into the blood stream. However, the degree to which they do so, and the amount of estrogen absorbed into the blood stream is difficult to control or determine.

The quantity of estrogen that is absorbed into the skin is less consistent with a cream than it is with a pill, so you many need additional estrogen to control your menopausal symptoms more predictably. Additionally, it's difficult to determine if the amount of estrogen absorbed from a vaginal cream is adequate in preventing osteoporosis.

But, vaginal creams can enter the blood stream and raise the level of estrogen in the blood.

Usually, you'll start by using the cream in your vagina daily for a short time. Then you can switch to using it only twice a week.

There is little data as to whether or not estrogen vaginal cream has any effect on the risk of uterine cancer, ovarian cancer, or colon cancer. We do know that estrogen vaginal creams do *not* increase the risk of breast cancer.[14]

Estrogen Gels

Estrogen gels rely on absorption of estrogen through the skin. The actual amount of hormone absorbed, and thus the actual dose of estrogen, depends on how large an area of skin the gel covers. The actual site of application doesn't seem to matter.[12] They're different from creams in that they have the consistency of a gel, and you don't put them in your vagina.

Some gels come in a pump that you depress for a specific dose of estrogen. You just rub it on your arm, abdomen, thigh, or shoulder, where it dries in a couple of minutes. It enters the blood stream quickly. Of course, you don't want to go in the shower, bathtub, sauna, steam room, or hot tub immediately afterwards and wash it all off.

It's best to apply the gel at the same time every day to a large area of skin to ensure consistency in the dose you get.[15] You should not put these estrogen gels in your vagina or on your breast.[15]

Advantages of estrogen gels are that they don't harm the liver like oral pills, and there are no problems with adherence to the skin or rashes like patches.[15] They increase healthy HDL, but also increase triglycerides and glucose.[15] They cause less blood clotting than oral estrogen.

You may use estrogen gel with or without progesterone, and the progesterone can be in any form. Like oral estrogen, estrogen gel prevents osteoporosis.

Estrogen Vaginal Tablets

A dose of 25 mcg per day of vaginal estrogen in tablet form does not raise the blood level of estrogen significantly.[14] These aren't as likely to give you as high a dose of estrogen as pills, patches, rings, creams, or gels. Other than that, they're most similar to the vaginal creams in the way they work.

Estrogen Pellets

Estrogen pellets for implantation below the skin surface are another option. They release a constant stream of estrogen. They are for purposes of long-term rather than short-term use.

Do you see how many options there are? Notice that the benefits and risks of various forms of estrogen vary. It's your job to pay attention to these differences, not only for estrogen, but for all the hormones. Focus on the factors that matter the most to *you*. It really is possible for you to tailor your management to your needs and desires.

Selective Estrogen Receptor Modulators (SERMs)

Selective Estrogen Receptor Modulators are **_non-hormonal_** medications which have some effects that are similar to estrogen and others that are not similar to estrogen. SERMs (Selective Estrogen Receptor Modulators) are just what their name implies.

These substances are synthetic products which bind with estrogen receptors. There are different kinds of estrogen receptors, in different parts of the body. SERMs are "selective" because they *bind with some estrogen receptors in some parts of the body and not in others*. Therefore, the location of the receptor(s) to which a SERM binds determines the overall effect of the drug on the body.

They're "modulators" because they *modulate or manipulate the effects of estrogen*. Some of their effects are the beneficial effects of estrogen, while others are the detrimental effects of estrogen. They're an excellent option if you want some of the benefits of estrogen, but don't want to use estrogen in particular or hormones in general. So, here come the SERMs.

I know this sounds confusing thus far. Not to worry. I'll clear things up for you shortly.

With regard to SERMs, there are four body parts bearing estrogen receptors. They are (1) the breast, (2) the heart, (3) the bones, and (4) the uterus. A SERM can be friendly or unfriendly to each of these four body parts.

A SERM is friendly to the breast if it decreases the risk of breast cancer. It's unfriendly to the breast if it increases the risk of breast cancer.

A SERM is friendly to the heart if it decreases the risk of a heart attack. It's unfriendly to the heart if it increases the risk of a heart attack.

A SERM is friendly to the bones if it decreases the risk of osteoporosis. It's unfriendly to the bones if it increases the risk of osteoporosis.

A SERM is friendly to the uterus if it decreases the risk of uterine cancer. It's unfriendly to the uterus if it increases the risk of uterine cancer.

A SERM can also have a neutral effect on any of these body parts, and neither increase nor decrease the risk for disease.

Now, let me introduce you to the SERMs.

Tamoxifen (Nolvadex)

Most people are familiar with tamoxifen as a chemotherapy drug for breast cancer. That's its most common use. The most beneficial aspect of tamoxifen is the fact that it decreases the risk of breast cancer occurrence and recurrence. Thus, women can use it both for prevention and treatment of breast cancer. Tamoxifen is most beneficial in the first five years of use, after which the beneficial effects may plateau. (So, tamoxifen is friendly to the breast.)

Some of the secondary effects of tamoxifen are useful in managing symptoms of menopause. These include its ability to prevent bone loss, decrease lousy LDL, and decrease heart attacks. (That means tamoxifen is friendly to the bones and the heart.)

Tamoxifen is an attractive choice for you if you are concerned about or are at high risk for breast cancer, osteoporosis, and/or heart attack.

The most significant disadvantage of tamoxifen is that it has an adverse effect on the uterus, increasing the risk of uterine cancer. It does so by thickening the lining of the uterus. (This is pretty unfriendly, wouldn't you say?) As such, you'd have to have evaluation of your uterine lining via ultrasound and/or uterine biopsy on a regular basis if you were to use tamoxifen. While this may be a nuisance, it provides peace of mind if you use tamoxifen. Of course, if you've had a hysterectomy (removal of your uterus), you don't have to worry about this significant side effect and the inconvenient surveillance it requires.

Other undesirable side effects of tamoxifen include blood clots, visual disturbances, and an increase in hot flashes. These events aren't as common or as predictable as thickening of the lining of the uterus is. But they're significant when they occur.

Raloxifene (Evista)

Raloxifene is most appealing if you have significant concerns about osteoporosis. It increases bone density to a degree equal to that of estrogen. Interestingly, it is more effective in preventing osteoporosis in the hip than in the spine. (So, raloxifene is friendly to the bones.)

Because it decreases lousy LDL and increases healthy HDL, it decreases the risk of heart attack. (So, it's friendly to the heart.) Another advantage of raloxifene is its lack of effect on breast tissue so that it does *not* increase the risk of breast cancer. Finally, it has no effect on the uterus. (It's neutral with regard to the breast and the uterus.) All of these perks are fairly significant, don't you think?

The disadvantage of raloxifene is that it has the same tendency to create blood clots as estrogen. So, you can't use both raloxifene and estrogen at the same time. That would be incredibly risky, and you'd be overshadowing the benefits with the risks.

Raloxifene is a good choice for you if you have concerns about osteoporosis of the hip, breast cancer, uterine cancer, and/or heart attack. The usual dose is 60 mg daily.

You may recall that I used this drug (Evista) as an example when I was explaining synthetic substances.

Bisphosphonates

There are a variety of bisphosphonates. You may recognize some of the names listed below:

1. Alendronate (Fosamax)
2. Risedronate (Actonel)
3. Ibandronate Sodium (Boniva)

The bisphosphonates are much more specific than raloxifene for the purpose of preventing osteoporosis. They attach to estrogen receptors in bone only. They prevent both hip and spine fractures, while having no effect on the breast, the uterus, or the heart. (They're friendly to the bones, and neutral to the breast, uterus, and heart.)

Unfortunately, the bisphosphonates do *not* alleviate any of the symptoms of menopause. The good news is that it's reasonable to use an estrogen product *with* a bisphosphonate.

There are specific requirements as to how you have to take a bisphosphonate. First, you must take it first thing in the morning with a large glass of water. Second, you have to refrain from eating for at least 30 minutes. Third, you must sit or stand upright for at least 30 minutes after taking it because it has a tendency to creep back up into the esophagus and irritate it. If you take the daily dose, you may get tired of these rules, so luckily, these drugs have a once a week dosage option. Boniva is a brand of bisphosphonate that you take only once a month. For the monthly medications, you have to lengthen the time you sit or stand upright and refrain from eating to 60 minutes.

Bisphosphonates are a good option for you if you have primary concerns about osteoporosis, regardless of other issues. You may use a bisphosphonate alone or combine it with other agents in the management of menopause.

Tibolone

Tibolone is a synthetic hormone. While it's theoretically a "hormone" rather than a "non-hormone," it behaves very much like a SERM. So, I'm introducing it to you along with the SERMs. That way, you can compare and contrast it with the SERMs.

Like the SERMS, the actions of tibolone depend on its metabolism and activation in various tissues of the body. It does not increase the risk of uterine cancer, breast cancer, or blood clots.

It does prevent osteoporosis (making it friendly to the bones).

It alleviates hot flashes, night sweats, vaginal dryness, forgetfulness, and mood swings. It sounds great, but despite all these attributes, Tibolone doesn't produce adequate relief for many women.[16]

Tibolone is suitable only once you've become *post*-menopausal.[17] You can't use it in those unpredictable peri-menopausal years. Side effects include vaginal bleeding and breast pain.[17] It might not be your idea of fun to have vaginal bleeding as a side effect of a medication you take for menopause after your periods cease.

So, let's say you're opposed to taking hormones or you can't take hormones for some reason. Yet, you really want some of the advantages of hormones. You could consider taking a SERM, and you could tailor your choice to the one that's best for your needs and desires. Pretty friendly, isn't it?

Progesterone

Symptoms of Abnormal Progesterone Levels

Just as in the section on estrogen, this section begins with lists of the symptoms of progesterone deficiency and progesterone excess. The purpose of these lists is to enable you to target the predominant hormonal environment of your body at various times during the process of menopause. You may be able to look at all of these lists together and determine which hormones are causing you to feel a certain way. Then you can choose the options which adjust that particular hormone accordingly. Remember, some of your symptoms may be due to interactions between hormones rather than to the presence or absence of a single hormone in isolation.

This section on progesterone is particularly important for you if you are just entering the peri-menopausal phase, because a decline in progesterone levels initiates peri-menopause. The decline in progesterone then results in a relative excess of estrogen. While there's not an absolute excess of estrogen, the imbalance between estrogen and progesterone has the *effect* of estrogen excess.

Symptoms of Progesterone Deficiency

Irregular or heavy periods
Premenstrual syndrome (PMS)
Anxiety
Migraine headaches

Symptoms of Progesterone Excess

Fatigue or drowsiness
Depression

Categories of Progesterone

As with estrogen, there are three categories of progesterone. These include: (1) Botanical and herbal sources of progesterone; (2) Bioidentical progesterone; and (3) Synthetic progesterone.

Progesterone has some unique properties because of which I call it the "chameleon hormone." A chameleon is that lizard-like animal that can change colors to blend with the surrounding environment. It's able to change appearance to look like a number of other things. I use the term "chameleon" to describe progesterone because progesterone has the ability to convert itself into other hormones. It's able to transform into testosterone or estrogen under certain circumstances. You could think of progesterone as the hormone with an identity problem.

This ability of progesterone to convert itself into other hormones is the reason why some advocates for progesterone promote it as the solution for all menopausal symptoms for all women. Now, you already know that I'm not so bold as to suggest *any* regimen for *all* women. I have no biases or preferences with regard to menopausal management options. Each woman is unique, and each woman has changing needs during the process of menopause. So, while progesterone may alleviate some or all of the symptoms of early peri-menopause, it may cease to do so as menopause progresses. It may work great for some women and not for others. Just remember that if something doesn't work for you, it's not because you're abnormal. You're just unique, and that's good. That's why there are so many choices.

Progesterone is also unusual in the sense that the bioidentical and synthetic forms may produce very different results in the same woman. Some women notice more unpleasant side effects with synthetic progesterone than they do with bioidentical progesterone. Bioidentical (micronized) progesterone may cause sedation, while synthetic pharmaceutical progesterone may cause moodiness. Other women tolerate both types of progesterone equally well. You may find that you prefer one over the other. When you get to the section on diseases, you'll find that one form of progesterone may be better than another for managing your risk for certain diseases. Like I said, progesterone is quite malleable.

Of course, one of the most important aspects of progesterone is how well it protects your uterine lining. Progesterone via the vaginal route results in adequate levels to prevent uterine cancer. Other routes vary, with oral and transdermal progesterone (skin patches, creams, and gels) being more variable. In any case, if you use both estrogen and progesterone, the balance between the two hormones is critical. We'll discuss this in detail later.

Botanical and Herbal Progesterone

Chasteberry (Vitex agnus-castus)

Chasteberry has the effect of increasing the production of progesterone in the body. Instead of just adding progesterone from an outside source, it results in an increase in your body's natural progesterone. The whole herb and the powdered drug are available as capsules, drops, film tablets, and compound preparations.

Dosages are as follows:

> Capsules: 40 – 100 mg
> Liquid extract: 1:1 aqueous – alcoholic extract, 30 – 40 mg
> Dried extract: 100 gm containing 0.2 gm dried extract in a ratio of 1: 5 in either ethanol or water[6]

Wild Yam (Dioscorea villosa)

Wild yams in the form of food have a significant biologic effect, but are *not* a reasonable source of hormonal supplementation in their natural form. That's because it requires huge quantities of raw yams to provide even a small progesterone effect.[9] The root of the Wild Yam plant is a precursor for manufacturing progesterone and estrogen.

Wild Yam progesterone creams and gels abound. You can rub them on your abdomen, buttocks, or thighs. They're available in health food stores, vitamin shops, and grocery stores. Usually, you can find a variety of brands in a single location.

Wild Yam may have an additive estrogenic effect when combined with estrogen. In other words, the progesterone in the Wild Yam could decide to transform itself into estrogen rather than maintaining its identity as progesterone. This is an example of the chameleon properties of progesterone. What this means is that you could get more estrogen than you intend if you use progesterone cream made from wild yams. You may think you're balancing your estrogen with progesterone, while, in fact, you're getting a double dose of estrogen! That's why you've got to tell your healthcare provider if you're using this stuff.

Despite its identity problem, Wild Yam progesterone creams and gels are quite popular.

Dosages are as follows:

    Capsules: 200 mg, 400 mg, 505 mg, 535 mg
    Liquid: 1:1 or 1:2 of 250 mg/ml

Bioidentical Progesterone

Bioidentical progesterone comes from hormones in plant compounds which are chemically identical to the progesterone that your ovaries produced.[18] The first attempts at creating an oral preparation of bioidentical progesterone were unsuccessful because it was poorly absorbed from the stomach or rapidly metabolized and inactivated in the liver.[18] It required excessively high doses to achieve adequate levels in the blood stream.[15]

In order to improve the delivery of progesterone in an oral formulation, researchers developed a new form of the hormone, called "micronized progesterone."[18] Micronized progesterone is simply a form of the hormone that increases the available surface area of the hormone. In so doing, it improves its absorption. Suspending micronized progesterone in oil improves its absorption even further.[18] Because of these two varieties of micronized progesterone, we now have bioidentical progesterone in capsules for oral use.

U.S.P. (United States Pharmacopeia) Progesterone (ProGest, Prometrium, Crinone)

The term for bioidentical progesterone is "U.S.P. Progesterone." This is progesterone that is sold in bulk to compounding pharmacies. It's available in various forms, including a cream (ProGest), a gel (Crinone), and an oral pill form (Prometrium). The oral form is the most convenient.

Progesterone Cream

Progesterone cream is made from wild Mexican yams. The yams actually contain a precursor of progesterone which gets converted into the bioidentical form of the hormone in a laboratory.

Progesterone cream is available without a prescription in the form of a 2% cream that you can apply anywhere on your body. You really have to read the labels on progesterone creams because they vary greatly in potency. Some contain less than 2 mg of progesterone per oz of cream. Others contain between 2 and 15 mg per oz.[18] Some actually contain as much as 400 mg per oz.[18] These creams often claim to have actions that are typical of estrogen and testosterone as well as progesterone.

Synthetic Progesterone

Progesterone Gel

Progesterone gels that are currently available in synthetic form (as opposed to botanical or herbal forms) contain dosages of progesterone that are excessive for menopause. They are appropriate for infertility patients who are using drugs to assist them in achieving pregnancy. Others are designed for inducing labor in pregnant women. So, I don't think you'd find them very useful for menopause! I've included them for purposes of clarification only.

Progesterone Pills

Progesterone pills for use during menopause are available in a variety of dosages. Since progesterone is merely a companion drug to estrogen for women who have a uterus, the dosages of progesterone are designed to balance the dosages of estrogen. Think of progesterone as just a piggy-back to estrogen, and it's only necessary if you have your uterus. If you've had a hysterectomy (removal of your uterus), you don't need any progesterone.

It's uncommon to use *synthetic* progesterone all by itself for menopause. Contrast this to the common use of botanical or herbal forms of progesterone all by themselves. If you recall, I mentioned earlier that the alternative and complementary approach to menopause focuses on progesterone rather than on estrogen. That focus explains this discrepancy. In general, use of progesterone alone for menopause results in unpredictable degrees of conversion of the progesterone to estrogen and testosterone, so the medical community just focuses on estrogen and testosterone directly.

Synthetic, pharmaceutical progesterone is more resistant to metabolism in the liver than bioidentical progesterone. So, the pharmaceutical brands allow lower doses, better absorption, and better prevention of uterine cancer. There is a ten-fold variation in the levels of pharmaceutical progesterone and bioidentical progesterone following oral intake. That's a big difference.

Progesterone Shots

Progesterone shots produce predictable levels of the hormone in the blood stream, but are painful and inconvenient.[16] There aren't many women using progesterone shots, given all the other options out there.

Progesterone-Only Birth Control Pills

Birth control pills that contain only progesterone, rather than estrogen and progesterone, are great for controlling the erratic periods that characterize early peri-menopause. The fact that they also provide birth control is a special bonus because that's the time when it's most difficult to know when you're fertile. If you get pregnant then, you have what we call a "change of life baby." And it *will* change your life all right!

The other benefit of progesterone-only birth control pills is that they decrease the risk of uterine cancer. They may or may not improve your symptoms of menopause. They may even make them worse or cause symptoms of progesterone excess.

Progesterone-Containing Intrauterine Device (IUD)

IUDs containing progesterone are designed for the purpose of contraception rather than for menopause. Who knows, though. With time and research, these could prove beneficial for preventing uterine cancer in peri-and post-menopausal women by preventing build-up of the uterine lining.

Synthetic Estrogen Plus Progesterone

The collective term for estrogen *and* progesterone therapy together in the management of menopause is "**Hormone Replacement Therapy (HRT)**." Compare that to the term for estrogen therapy without progesterone, which is "Estrogen Replacement Therapy (ERT)." You will have less confusion if you make this distinction and use these terms correctly rather than using them interchangeably.

Until 2002, these estrogen plus progesterone regimens represented the gold standard of management for menopause. Some of the medications in this category were the most commonly prescribed drugs in the United States. Since then, there has been a flurry of excitement surrounding these regimens and a decrease in their use. At present, they're coming back into vogue. I'll elaborate on all of that later in a discussion of hormone studies and their implications.

Variables

There are a variety of different types of combined estrogen and progesterone products. They differ in two major ways. First, they vary in terms of the ***dosage*** of the hormones they contain. That's because the younger you are, the higher the dose your body requires to meet its needs. Second, they vary in the type of hormone *regimen* they entail. By "regimen," I mean that some of them involve taking the hormones in a manner that mimics your cycles, and allows you to have a period. Others are designed so that you don't have a period.

Now I know that you wish you could just take whichever one you wanted, but it's not quite that easy. Why? Because Mother Nature gets in the way. Simply put, you can't just turn off your periods with hormones when you want to. You've got to work with Mother Nature. Not only is she bigger than you, but if you mess with her, she'll make you regret it.

So, what we have for combined estrogen and progesterone are three categories of hormone regimens. You should probably think of them, and maybe even use them, in order. So that's the way I'll list them and discuss them. Here they are, in order:

1. Low dose birth control pills or skin patches
2. Cyclic estrogen plus progesterone HRT
3. Continuous estrogen plus progesterone HRT

Low Dose Birth Control Pills

As you know, birth control pills come in a monthly package designed to mimic a 28 day menstrual cycle. You take a pill each day and have a period towards the end of the package. They contain both estrogen and progesterone, and the doses of those hormones either mimic your cycle or produce something similar enough for you to have cycle control and pregnancy prevention. Some of the newer birth control pills entail taking active pills for 84 rather than just 21 days. They make it possible for you to have a period once every three months rather than once every month.

Low dose birth control pills are regular birth control pills with the lowest possible doses of hormones to prevent pregnancy. But, they still have much *higher dosages* of estrogen and progesterone in them than the estrogen and progesterone pills designed for menopause. Think of it this way: The younger you are, the more estrogen you need. It takes

Categories of Hormones and Their Sources

more estrogen and progesterone to prevent pregnancy than it does to manage menopause. So, low dose birth control pills represent the first phase of combined estrogen plus progesterone.

I know it sounds like an oxymoron to call the "high dose" alternative "low dose birth control pills," but that's just the way it is. Don't let the "low dose" part of the name confuse you. They're high dose relative to the hormones designed specifically for menopause (called "HRT").

You may find low dose birth control pills an ideal choice if you're in the very early phases of peri-menopause. Remember, that's a time when you still have to use birth control if you don't want to get pregnant, and this is an easy way to accomplish two things at once. You would take your low dose birth control pills, have very predictable, light periods, prevent pregnancy, and miss out on any of the symptoms of menopause. I'm sure you'll be jealous of all your friends who get to experience the full effects of those signs and symptoms of menopause.

There is one huge stipulation for using birth control pills after the age of 35. *You can't smoke.* I mean not at all. If you do, it's a deal breaker. You're simply not a candidate for birth control pills after age 35 if you're a smoker. "Smoker" means smoking tobacco in any form (cigarettes, cigars, pipes). It also includes marijuana or any other non-tobacco products you may smoke from time to time. The risks are just too great for blood clots, stroke, and heart attack.

If you're not a smoker, and have no health risks that are birth control pill unfriendly, you can use low dose birth control pills for many years. You can even use them until age 55, and then switch to hormone replacement therapy (HRT) in the lower doses appropriate for menopause. You might have the choice of trying the continuous regimen and hoping that Mother Nature doesn't have a different plan for you. If she does, you'll have bleeding on that regimen and will need to switch to the cyclic regimen for a couple of years. You can try the continuous regimen again later. Either way, the transition from peri-menopause to post-menopause will be very smooth for you, and you may miss out on the whole thing. (Oh darn!)

As with all birth control pills, the low dose pills regulate periods, make your flow lighter, mask all the symptoms of menopause, and prevent osteoporosis. They are metabolized in the digestive system, so they can affect the liver. Don't take low dose birth control pills if you have liver disease.

Low dose birth control pills have an added advantage of treating a variety of problems in addition to those associated with menopause. Of course they prevent pregnancy at a time when your cycles are erratic, but they do even more than that.[19] Let me enumerate some of these extra benefits for you. The list may surprise (and delight) you. Low dose birth control pills improve or eliminate all of the following:

1. Irregular menstrual periods
2. Heavy bleeding with periods
3. Anemia due to heavy periods
4. Growth of fibroids (benign tumors) in the uterus
5. Premenstrual syndrome (PMS)
6. Mood swings
7. Ovarian cysts
8. Ectopic pregnancy (pregnancy outside of the uterus, most commonly in the fallopian tube)
9. Pelvic inflammatory disease (PID)
10. Non-cancerous breast diseases
11. Acne [19]

Low dose birth control pills also have some long-term effects that are beneficial.[19] First, they are associated with a 50% decrease in your risk of ovarian cancer.[19] This statistic pertains to you individually rather than to the population at large, so this counts for a lot. Use of low dose birth control pills for more than ten years reduces the risk of ovarian cancer in the general population by as much as 80%.[19] This protection gradually increases in the first year, and persists for more than 20 years after discontinuing the pills.[18]

Another long-term perk of low dose birth control pills is an overall reduction in the risk of uterine cancer by as much as 70% with 12 or more years of use.[19] They also produce a long-term reduction in the

Categories of Hormones and Their Sources

risk of hip fracture, and have the desirable effect of increasing healthy HDL and decreasing lousy LDL.[19]

You are *not* a candidate for use of low dose birth control pills under certain conditions.[19] If you personally have any of the following, your risks will outweigh any benefits from low dose birth control pills, and you'll need to take advantage of a different option:

- Personal history of blood clots
- Heart attack in the past
- Previous stroke
- Breast cancer
- A nasty smoking habit over age 35[19]

For a non-smoker with none of these risk factors, low dose birth control pills are truly an example of "one-stop shopping" with regard to management of peri-menopause.

Low Dose Birth Control Skin Patches

There are skin patches that do the same things that pills do. They serve the same purpose and the same population of women as the low dose birth control pills. If you prefer a patch over a pill, and you meet all the other criteria that I just described for low dose birth control pills, then be my guest and use a patch.

In some ways, the skin patch has advantages over pills. Oral pills containing estrogen plus progesterone significantly increase the risk of blood clots, but skin patches containing estrogen plus progesterone don't.[20] This is due to the fact that pills taken via the oral route pass through the liver as they are broken down into a form the body can use, while skin patches deliver hormones in a form that bypasses the liver.[20] The higher the dose of hormones, the more significant this is. So, it's more significant with low dose birth control preparations than it is with even lower dose hormone replacement therapy (HRT) regimens for menopause.

The disadvantage of low dose birth control skin patches is that the patch can come off when you least expect it. Sometimes, you don't even notice that it's no longer attached to your skin. If so, you may go for days without hormones. And if you're using it for both birth control and hormone replacement during peri-menopause, you could have a great big surprise, called pregnancy. So, check to ensure that your patch is where you put it.

Cyclic Estrogen Plus Progesterone

The cyclic regimen is the one you'll need if you haven't reached post-menopause by going for 12 full months without a period. It's a regimen that mimics your cycle, but prevents all the yucky symptoms of menopause.

The idea behind cyclic estrogen and progesterone is to give you estrogen replacement alone during the first half of your cycle, and then to give you estrogen plus progesterone during the second half of your cycle. That allows you to benefit from the estrogen in getting rid of your symptoms of menopause, and benefit from the progesterone in shedding your uterine lining. So, it protects you against uterine cancer.

The pharmaceutical companies have designed some nifty products that make hormone replacement easy. These products usually come in a cycle pack that is very similar to a birth control pill pack. Each pack covers a single cycle of one month, and they're easy to take. You just punch out a pill exactly as you do with birth control pills.

Of course, you can do the same thing by getting two separate prescriptions of estrogen and progesterone, and just remembering what to take each day. But that can be tricky. You have to remember which days you're supposed to take just the estrogen and which days you're supposed to take both estrogen and progesterone. That's the way it was for years and years, though, so take your pick. There is one advantage to having two separate prescriptions for estrogen and progesterone. You can vary the dosage combination of the two. Not only that, you can also vary how many days you take the progesterone. It's possible that you'll only need a few days of progesterone to induce shedding of your uterine lining rather than the larger number of progesterone days in the cycle packs.

Cyclic estrogen plus progesterone is a way of giving you the hormones you need before you reach post-menopause. The dosage of hormones in these pills is not enough to prevent pregnancy. It's just enough to get rid of the symptoms of menopause and prevent osteoporosis.

These products do come in various dosages and brands. Some are made from animal products; others are made from plant products. It seems that when one pharmaceutical company produces something, they all follow. Therefore, you can usually find more than one brand of each product. Sometimes they differ only slightly. At other times, they harbor significant differences.

You may wish to use cyclic estrogen plus progesterone when you're just transitioning into post-menopause. You may find that there's a lot of guesswork as to exactly when you become post-menopausal, especially if you've been on any kind of hormones around that time. If so, these cyclic forms of estrogen plus progesterone may be just the answer for you. You can take them for a couple of years and then change to the continuous regimen. That is, if Mother Nature agrees.

Continuous Estrogen Plus Progesterone

Once you've definitely reached post-menopause, and Mother Nature doesn't intend for you to have any more periods, you're ready to consider continuous estrogen plus progesterone. This regimen doesn't allow for *any* vaginal bleeding. If you bleed at all while on them, you need an evaluation to ensure that nothing's wrong. That's why you don't want to start them too soon. An evaluation for unexpected vaginal bleeding includes an ultrasound to check out your uterus and ovaries, and a biopsy to examine the lining of your uterus. It really isn't very fun.

Continuous estrogen plus progesterone regimens are also available in those nifty little cycle packs. The difference is that every pill in the pack is identical, and contains both estrogen and progesterone. The dosages are standard, and the ratio of estrogen to progesterone is fixed. You just punch out a pill every day.

Alternatively, you can get a prescription of each hormone separately and just take one of each every day. If you do it this way, you have more flexibility with the dosages of each. So, if you've discovered that you need more or less of one hormone than the standard dosage, you can more easily make an adjustment that suits your individual needs. It's not that difficult to remember to just pop two tablets in your mouth every day if they're the same all the time.

You may find that you can decrease the dosage of this regimen over time. Or, you may need to keep it the same. You may try to discontinue it after a few years if you wish. Then again, you may want to stay on it forever. It's really an individual thing. You have to weigh all your own benefits and risks in the short term *and* the long term in making these decisions.

HRT Skin Patches Containing Estrogen and Progesterone

Skin patches containing estrogen and progesterone serve the same purpose as pills containing estrogen and progesterone. The difference is that they're in the form of a patch that you place on your skin. They contain standard dosages of each hormone, and you change the patch according to the prescribed schedule.

In some ways, there are advantages to the skin patch. Oral pills containing estrogen plus progesterone significantly increase the risk of blood clots, but skin patches containing estrogen plus progesterone don't.[20] That's because pills taken via the oral route pass through the liver as they are broken down into a form that the body can use, while skin patches deliver hormones in a form that bypasses the liver.[20] Unless you have other risk factors for blood clots, the incidence of blood clots due to hormone therapy for menopause is relatively low.[20]

The disadvantages of skin patches are that they cause skin irritation or a rash for some women, and they don't adhere well to the skin in others. You've probably seen a patch that fell off some unsuspecting woman's skin somewhere. I've seen these by poolsides on occasion. Maybe you didn't recognize what it was at the time. The menopausal woman who was wearing it probably didn't recognize that she lost it, either. But, eventually she got the feeling that "something" was missing.

Testosterone

Symptoms of Abnormal Testosterone Levels

Although there are obvious symptoms of testosterone imbalance, it's still wise to perform laboratory testing for free testosterone before you take testosterone supplements. Blood tests and saliva tests are available for this purpose.

Symptoms of Testosterone Deficiency

1. Lack of energy
2. Decreased sex drive
3. Difficulty having an orgasm
4. Thinning of the pubic hair
5. Decreased muscle mass
6. Bone loss (osteoporosis)
7. Decreased feelings of well-being

Symptoms of Testosterone Excess

1. Mood swings
2. Acne
3. Facial hair (whiskers)
4. Deepening of the voice
5. Weight gain
6. Increased sex drive

Categories of Testosterone

Botanical and Herbal Testosterone

Cayenne (Capsicum species)

This herb is available in the form of a cream for purposes of increasing circulation and for use as a female orgasm stimulant. The active ingredient is called capsaicin.[7]

MENOPAUSE

Possible side effects are burning, stinging, and redness of the skin. These are normal reactions to capsaicin, and they resolve over a few days, even with continued use. There are no known health hazards associated with the use of Cayenne.

There is a limit on the frequency of usage of Cayenne. Use it only for two consecutive days, and refrain from using it again for two weeks after that. If you use it in excess of these parameters, it can cause blistering and ulceration.

The appropriate concentration of the cream is 0.25% - 0.75% capsaicin.

Cubeb (Piper cubeba)

Some people believe that Cubeb is the answer for a decrease in your sex drive. The assertion that Cubeb increases sex drive is unproven, but there aren't any known health risks in the designated dosages, which are as follows:

Powder: 2 – 4 gm daily
Extract (1:1): 2 – 4 ml daily
Tincture (1:5): 2 – 4 ml daily

Damiana (Turnera diffusa)

Damiana is a common ingredient in products for menopause. It alleviates menopausal symptoms and increases sexual function.[8]

It binds weakly with estrogen receptors and more strongly with progesterone receptors. This means that it acts more like progesterone than estrogen. It is used as an aphrodisiac.

There are no health hazards in proper dosages.

Dosages are as follows:

Capsules: 380 mg, 384 mg, 395 mg, 450 mg
Fluid extract 1:1

CATEGORIES OF HORMONES AND THEIR SOURCES

Bioidentical Testosterone

Dehydroepiandrosterone (DHEA)

DHEA is a precursor of testosterone that is produced by the adrenal glands. As with most androgens, the level of DHEA is low before puberty. It peaks at age 25, and begins to decline at age 30. By the age of 70, it's almost undetectable. It has the effect of improving lean body mass, glucose tolerance, and the immune response.[9]

DHEA is available with or without a prescription. The bioidentical form provided by compounding pharmacies is a cream for use on the skin or in the vagina. Some women use it on the clitoris to enhance its sensitivity. Adherence to prescribed dosages is important to avoid the masculine side effects of testosterone excess. DHEA that is available over the counter is variable in purity and quality, so be very careful if you use it. Adherence to recommended dosages with the over the counter preparations is much more tricky.

Bioidentical testosterone is also available in the form of a patch for application to the skin.

Negative side effects of DHEA include liver damage, undesirable hair growth, and acne. Very high doses can increase the lousy LDL and decrease the healthy HDL.[9]

You shouldn't use DHEA if you've had breast cancer.

Testosterone Cream

The only place to get testosterone cream is from a compounding pharmacy. You can rub a little into your vagina or on your clitoris for increased sensitivity during sexual stimulation. It's not immediate, and may take one or two weeks before you notice a difference. Don't use too much or you'll have increased sensitivity all the time.

Synthetic Testosterone

Synthetic testosterone is available in various forms. The most common product combines testosterone with estrogen for use in women. The trade name for that medication is Estratest. It's available in half strength and full strength tablets.

Testosterone is available in isolation, but isn't approved for use by females. Now that doesn't mean that isolated testosterone is unavailable. Many doctors will still prescribe it for women, even though it isn't approved for women. Some of the available forms include oral pills, shots, skin implants, and skin patches.

Side effects of testosterone include hair growth on the face and chest, acne, and deepening of the voice. It can also harm the liver, raise lousy LDL, lower healthy HDL, and raise triglycerides.

Chapter 8: Dosage Dictionary

One of the confusing things about hormones, pharmaceutical medications, herbs, and botanicals is the *units of measure* for how much of something you should take. Dosages of medications are usually given in the metric (International) system, while botanical and herbal remedies use both the metric and the imperial (U.S.) system. While you really don't have to understand the exact meaning behind an obscure dosing unit, it's nice to have some idea about how much of something you're taking.

Remember that you can't compare things unit for unit because the strength of the substance makes a huge difference in determining the necessary dose. Since we're discussing quantities here, think of the differences in the dosages of one substance to another just as you do the differences in quantities of ingredients needed for a recipe. It's like the difference in the quantities of flour versus vanilla extract needed to bake a cake. The flour isn't as concentrated, so you need more. The vanilla extract is concentrated, so you only need a little bit. I guess the message here is that you really can't compare dosages. The nature of the active ingredient is what determines how much of a drug, botanical, or herb you'll need to get the desired effect.

In an attempt to give you just enough to get an idea of the quantities for dosing, I'll explain the basics about both the metric (International) and the imperial (U.S.) systems. I'll limit my explanation to the units pertinent for mass and capacity, which pertain to measurements for solids and liquids, respectively. That should suffice for the kinds of substances you'll encounter with medicines, botanicals, and herbs.

The Metric System (Systeme International or SI)

The metric system involves a base unit that equals one. All quantities above or below that base unit are in multiples of ten. That's it. It's really that simple. It's the most universal system throughout the world, so it also goes by the name "Systeme International," and has the abbreviation SI.[1]

For mass, which is the unit for solids, like tablets, the scale looks like this:

10^{-12}	picogram	(pg) =	1/1,000,000,000,000 gram*
10^{-9}	nanogram	(ng) =	1/1,000,000,000 gram
10^{-6}	microgram	(mcg) =	1/1,000,000 gram*
10^{-3}	milligram	(mg) =	1/1,000 gram*
10^{-2}	centigram	(cg) =	1/100 gram
10^{-1}	decigram	(dg) =	1/10 gram
10^{0}	gram	(gm) =	1 gram*
10^{1}	decagram	(dag) =	10 grams
10^{2}	hectogram	(hg) =	100 grams
10^{3}	kilogram	(kg) =	1,000 grams
10^{6}	megagram	(Mg) =	1,000,000 grams

The * indicates the units you'll see frequently as dosage units for medications.

For capacity, which is the unit for liquids, the scale looks like this:

10^{-12}	picoliter	(pl) =	1/1,000,000,000,000 liter
10^{-9}	nanoliter	(nl) =	1/1,000,000,000 liter
10^{-6}	microliter	(mcl) =	1/1,000,000 liter
10^{-3}	milliliter	(ml) =	1/1,000 liter*
10^{0}	liter	(l) =	1 liter*
10^{1}	decaliter	(dal) =	10 liters
10^{2}	hectoliter	(hl) =	100 liters
10^{3}	kiloliter	(kl) =	1,000 liters

Another unit of the metric system that is common for medical quantities is the mole (mol). It refers to the amount of a "substance."

In this case, the substance is a molecule, atom, or other microscopic particle. Because the mole is so small in the first place, only the negative exponents apply to it. So, the scale looks like this:

10^{-12}	picomole	(pmol)	=	1/1,000,000,000,000 mole
10^{-9}	nanomole	(nmol)	=	1/ 1,000,000,000 mole
10^{-6}	micromole	(mcmol)	=	1/1,000,000 mole
10^{-3}	millimole	(mmol)	=	1/1,000 mole
10^{-2}	centimole	(cmol)	=	1/100 mole
10^{-1}	decimole	(dmol)	=	1/10 mole
10^{0}	mole	(mol)	=	1 mole

Sometimes, you'll see a combination of these terms in the form of a ratio. Usually, it will be a solid/liquid. Some examples are ng/ml, ng/dl, pg/ml, and pmol/l. All this refers to is a certain amount of a solid substance dissolved in a certain amount of a liquid. If it pertains to the value of a lab test that involved drawing your blood, then blood will be the liquid. It will designate how many molecules of a substance are dissolved in a certain quantity of blood. In essence, it determines how concentrated the product is. It seems complicated, I know. The nice thing is that you don't really have to pay a lot of attention to these details.

The U.S. System (Imperial System)

The U.S system doesn't follow the philosophy of multiples. You just have to know the quantities and the conversions from one to the other. It's easy if you're used to it. But if you're not, it probably doesn't make a lot of sense, and there's no easy mathematical way to figure it out.[1]

Here are the dosage units you'll see for mass as they pertain to solids and liquids. The U.S/Imperial system doesn't use a different base name for solids and liquids as does the metric system.

Ounce (oz)	=	480 grains (gr)
Grain (gr)	=	1/480 ounces (oz)
Tablespoon (tbs)	=	3 teaspoons (tsp)
Teaspoon (tsp)	=	1/3 tablespoons (tbs)

Now, if you want an idea of how the metric measurements compare to the imperial measurements, here are some equivalents.[2]

For mass and weight of solids:

1 kilogram (kg)   = 1000 grams (g)   = 2.2046 pounds (lb)
1 gram (g)   = 0.035 ounce (oz)
1 milligram (mg)   = 0.001 gram (g)   = 0.015 grain (gr)
1 microgram (mcg) = 0.000001 gram (g) = 0.000015 grain (gr)

For capacity of liquids:

1 liter (l)   = 1.057 quarts (qt)
1 deciliter (dl)   = 0.10 liter   = 0.21 pint (pt)
1 centiliter (cl)   = 0.01 liter   = 0.338 fluid ounce (fl oz)
1 milliliter (ml)   = 0.001 liter   = 0.27 fluid dram
5 milliliters (ml)   = 1 teaspoon (tsp)
15 milliliters (ml) = 1 tablespoon (tbs)
100 milliliters (ml) = 4 ounces (oz)   = 0.5 cup (c)

There are also special units for apothecaries in the Imperial System. (As if we needed to make things more complicated!) Of course, most of these will be unfamiliar to you, but my goal is to tell you too much rather than too little. If you happen to see or hear one of these measures, you'll have an idea what it means.

For weights and mass of solids, the Apothecaries' units are as follows:

1 scruple = 20 grains
1 drachm = 3 scruples
1 ounce   = 8 drachms   = 480 grains
1 pound   = 12 ounces   = 5760 grains[2]

For capacity of liquids, the Apothecaries' units go like this:

1 fluid drachm = 60 minims
1 fluid ounce = 8 fluid drachms
1 pint   = 16 fluid ounces[2]

Dosage Dictionary

Okay, that's it. I've had enough, and hopefully you have, too. Don't let this section perplex you. Just know that it's here. It may help you in understanding how much or how little of something is in the product you choose to use for management of menopause. Some people care about these details; others don't. My goal is to prevent you from feeling like you have no idea what the dosage measurements mean.

Section III:

Signs, Symptoms, and Diseases of Menopause and Aging Along With All the Management Options

Introduction

Now let's address a variety of management options for each aspect of menopause individually. In order to make this information more useful and make this book more user-friendly, it's not only laid out in paragraph format, but also charted to summarize all the information in a comparative manner. The chart is at the beginning of the book.

This symptom-based section will allow you to target specific symptoms and manage them individually. It will address each medical or non-medical option, and discuss each individually. Each sign or symptom of menopause will include options in a variety of categories, including dietary choices, lifestyle changes, vitamins and minerals, botanical and herbal products, hormonal medications, and non-hormonal medications. For each option, I'll give you the benefits, the risks, and any considerations that are noteworthy. This will empower you with the knowledge necessary to make wise choices.

Some of the information may seem redundant. That's intentional. I want you to be able to use any section of this book in isolation if you wish. I'd rather repeat myself or tell you too much than to leave something out.

The chart at the beginning of the book summarizes the information and allows you to compare one option to another. It's a great way to narrow down your choices to arrive at a final decision as to your best fit.

Chapter 9: Periods With a Personality Change

With regard to your menstrual cycle, the typical sign that you're beginning the peri-menopausal phase is periods that become farther and farther apart. This means that the time frame between the beginning of one period and the beginning of the next period lengthens. Usually, this entails skipping some periods altogether. You may begin to have a period every two months (every 60 days) rather than every month (every 28 – 30 days). Usually, the length of time between periods increases to longer and longer intervals (every three, four, or five months) until they finally cease completely. Usually, the time from the initial decrease in frequency to complete cessation of periods is nearly two years.

The frequency of menstrual cycles is precisely what allows us to distinguish peri-menopause from post-menopause. By definition, post-menopause requires the absence of all menstrual activity for 12 ***consecutive*** months. Until this occurs, you haven't yet completed the menopausal transition process.

Of course, if you've had your uterus removed (Total Hysterectomy or Subtotal/Partial Hysterectomy), you aren't going to rely on this as a sign of peri-menopause. Nor are you going to know precisely when you've reached post-menopause. That's okay. As you'll see, there will be plenty of other indicators of peri-menopause. Most likely, there will be more than you'll find welcome. You'll just monitor the other signs and symptoms of menopause to determine when you're transitioning into your post-menopausal phase of life.

It would really be nice if your periods just followed a simple pattern of becoming less frequent. However, you know that Mother Nature isn't that simple or that direct. So, instead of a smooth transition, there's a lot more to this change in your periods. I like to refer to this aspect of the transition as "periods with a personality change."

Just as puberty and adolescence ultimately accomplished the goal of turning you into an adult, your inconsistent cycles will ultimately disappear altogether. However, they may be quite erratic along the way. In reality, 90% of women have four to eight years of cycle changes before reaching post-menopause. During that time, there are a variety of changes you may notice in your periods. You may experience any of the following:

- Lighter periods
- Heavier periods
- Longer periods
- Shorter periods
- Skipped periods

A common misconception is that *any* irregularity in your periods indicates peri-menopause. That's one of those misconceptions that can get you into trouble. Some changes are **not** consistent with peri-menopause. Instead, they constitute **_abnormal bleeding_**. They include the following:

- Heavy bleeding with *clots*
- Bleeding which lasts *more than 7 days*
- Bleeding which is *more than 2 days longer* than your normal periods
- Periods which are *less than 21 days apart* (counting from the first day of one period to the first day of the next period)
- Spotting or bleeding *between periods*
- Bleeding *after intercourse*

If you have any of these instances of abnormal bleeding, you need an evaluation to omit the possibility of other medical problems. The lesson here is that you should *never* automatically assume that anything goes when it comes to periods with a personality change.

No doubt, peri-menopause may entail totally erratic periods. For some women, there's no predictability at all with their periods as they enter the transition into menopause. I'm not saying that every pattern other than periods that get farther and farther apart is inconsistent with peri-menopause. I'm simply saying that *you can't assume* it's peri-menopause. You need to have your doctor evaluate you to make sure it's nothing else.

Management Options

There really isn't any "management" for periods that occur less frequently. It's what you should expect, and maybe even celebrate. The most important thing for you to do is to record when your periods occur. That way, you can adequately track how many you've skipped. It's important to know when you've gone 12 consecutive months without a period, and you need to be accurate about it if you still have your uterus. If you don't it's not as important, as you'll see in the chapter on uterine cancer.

Hormonal Medication Options

Of course, there are ways for you to mask this symptom altogether. Such would be the case if you choose to take birth control pills or a birth control patch. If you do, your periods will remain regular, light, and predictable. That's especially convenient if you need contraception. As long as you're a non-smoker, you can take hormonal birth control until age 55 and then transition to something else. By that time, you can be pretty sure that you're not fertile and that you're post-menopausal.

Chapter 10: Hot Flashes

Incidence

Hot flashes represent the most common manifestation of menopause. Over 80% of peri-menopausal women experience hot flashes. Hot flashes differ depending on whether menopause is natural or surgical. Surgical menopause makes hot flashes more common. As many as 95% to 100% of women who are menopausal as a result of surgery (Bilateral Oophorectomy), chemotherapy, or radiation therapy have hot flashes, as compared to only 80% of women undergoing natural menopause.[1] For many women, the hot flashes of menopause will disappear over time without any intervention. However, while present, hot flashes may be debilitating. They tend to be not only most common, but also most severe in women who become menopausal as a result of surgery, chemotherapy, or radiation therapy.[2] While there is much talk about hot flashes, a true understanding of what actually constitutes a menopausal hot flash is rare. Hot flashes tend to follow a consistent pattern that is unique for each woman. If you need therapy to control hot flashes, you'll have the opportunity to choose from a multitude of options to manage them.[3]

Descriptive Aspects

A typical hot flash is a *sudden*, temporary sensation of heat or burning that passes over the surface of your body, leaving a film of sweat. Actually, sometimes it's more like a stream, or a river, or a waterfall of sweat. It usually begins at your head, passes down your neck, and progresses in wave-like fashion over your entire body. It's usually accompanied by redness and flushing of your face. The skin on your neck, shoulders, chest, and upper arms may redden, also. You may actually perspire during the episode, and immediately thereafter experience a sensation of chill or cold.[2] It's possible that you'll notice an increase in your heart rate during a hot flash. We call this rapid heart rate "heart palpitations." You may also experience a decrease in your ability to concentrate during the time frame surrounding a hot flash.[1] The frequency and severity of hot flashes may vary over time.[2] They persist for more than one year in 95% of women, and for one to five years in 65% of women.[1]

Triggers

Hot flashes occur at the oddest times. Just when you need to be calm, cool, and well composed, a hot flash will zap you. You may actually find that stress or embarrassing moments are just the perfect triggers for your hot flashes. Other triggers include hot environments, hot foods, spicy foods, heavy clothing, smoking cigarettes, caffeine, and alcohol.

Hot flashes are like the voice changes in an adolescent boy. As his voice starts to become deeper due to testosterone production, he sometimes makes a croaking sound when he speaks. His voice cracks at just the wrong time. It's quite funny sounding, and almost everybody laughs. It would be wonderful if we could all just laugh about hot flashes the way we laugh about the croaking voices of adolescent boys. But, unfortunately, we haven't yet become comfortable with menopausal blunders to the same extent we have with adolescent blunders. With time and familiarity, we will.

Variables Affecting Hot Flashes

The frequency and intensity of hot flashes vary widely across populations. Culture, diet, body weight, ethnicity, environmental stressors, and even socioeconomic status affect the incidence and severity of hot flashes.[1] *Cultural differences* exist because some cultures consider hot flashes fairly normal, so they aren't as unexpected. *Diet* makes a difference because hot, spicy foods have a tendency to induce hot flashes. So, watch out when you eat that hot Thai food. *Body weight* is a big factor because extra weight leads to poor heat tolerance. It's no surprise that hot flashes are much more miserable for obese women. *Ethnicity* matters because some ethnic groups just don't have as much hair or as many sweat glands on their bodies. Asians are a perfect example of this. Only 19% of post-menopausal Japanese women complain of hot flashes, compared with 60% of post-menopausal American women. *A stressful environment* is one of the best triggers for hot flashes. Just think about how most people, menopausal or not, sweat when they're nervous. Finally, *socioeconomic status* plays a role because of the ability to control environmental temperature and comfort at higher socioeconomic levels, and not at lower ones. Taken together, all this would indicate that you're least likely to have a problem with hot flashes if you're a rich, thin, Asian woman who loves to eat bland food, and you have no stress in your life.

Persistent heat intolerance or feeling hot most of the time is *not* the same thing as a hot flash. The word "flash" implies that the hot flash of menopause is a fleeting event. The duration of a hot flash ranges from just seconds to several minutes. No doubt, it'll seem as if your hot flashes last longer than that, especially if you don't recognize what's happening. Just knowing what to expect with a hot flash will help you stay calm and get through it more smoothly.

This distinction between a hot "flash" versus just being hot most of the time is critical. It's one of those distinctions that can prevent you from confusing a symptom of menopause with an actual disease. For example, being hot much of the time is consistent with thyroid disease. Don't make the mistake of assuming that a hot flash is the same as being hot most of the time. If you do, you'll ignore your thyroid problem, and that could be severely detrimental.

Causes of Hot Flashes

In medical terminology, hot flashes are called "vasomotor symptoms." While the exact cause of hot flashes is uncertain, there are two theories as to why hot flashes occur. One theory proposes that there is a resetting of the temperature control center in the brain to a lower comfort zone. The other theory proposes that there is a small temperature elevation preceding each hot flash along with a lower resting temperature.

Hot flashes are a result of *changing* levels of estrogen rather than low levels of estrogen. The absolute level of estrogen doesn't predict or correlate with hot flashes.[1] Peri-menopause is the time when the levels of estrogen are changing. Therefore, hot flashes may be more severe during peri-menopause than they are during post-menopause. This is one of the symptoms of menopause that may be temporary or permanent. If it's permanent, it may improve over time.

Management Options

Diet and Lifestyle Options

Certain lifestyle changes may provide relief from your hot flashes. These measures may succeed in alleviating hot flashes some of the time, but not all of the time.[3] Here are some suggestions:

Reduce Hot Flash Triggers

Identify and minimize your personal hot flash triggers. Some common triggers include heat (warm rooms, hair dryers), strong emotions, hot beverages, hot or spicy foods, alcohol, caffeine, and cigarette smoking.[3] I'm not suggesting that you become emotionally withdrawn and go sit in a cool room drinking cold drinks and bland foods. But for some women, these little changes make a huge difference. Of course, you don't have to do all these things all the time. Do what seems sensible at the time. If you're attending an important business meeting in which you are the center of attention, maybe you should forego the coffee.

Keep Cool

Keep your body cool by dressing in lightweight clothing, wearing layers that you can shed, fanning yourself, and lowering the ambient temperature of your home.[3]

Regular Exercise

The key word is "regular." Hot flashes occur much less frequently in women who exercise regularly. Exercise reduces stress and promotes better sleep. However, it's important to be aware of the possibility of triggering hot flashes through exercise if you aren't physically conditioned for it.[3] Now, it may sound contradictory to advise activity that makes you sweat to keep you from sweating, but it really does work. This is similar to recommending exercises that you think will kill you in order to make you live longer. Go figure!

Stress Reduction

Practice stress reduction. Some of the best ways to do this include meditation, yoga, massage, biofeedback, positive visualization, and a relaxing lukewarm bath.[3] Relaxation exercises can reduce the number of hot flashes you have. Even simple deep breathing periodically throughout the day for one minute sessions can reduce hot flashes.[4]

Paced Respiration

Pace your respiration at the start of a hot flash. This means breathing slowly and deeply, from the abdomen.[3] It helps to think relaxing thoughts while you are doing this. Yoga teaches this kind of breath control, and you may find it helpful to investigate the yogic form of breathing, called pranayama.

Vitamin and Mineral Options

Vitamin E

Vitamin E, in a dose of 800 IU/day or less, is safe. However, the effect on hot flashes is equal to that of placebo.[3] There are more benefits from vitamin E as a result of its immune-enhancing effects than from its ability to quell hot flashes.

Botanical and Herbal Options

In general, it's important to know that purity of herbs varies significantly between brands and between different batches of the same brand. Therefore, proper dosages may be difficult to achieve.[2] You may have to try various brands of herbs or vary the quantity that you take. Be patient with this. It's worth the effort. If you find a brand that works for you, stick with it. Don't continue experimenting with other options just for fun after that. It probably won't be fun.

Phytoestrogens

Phytoestrogens are naturally occurring plant-based compounds that produce the same effect as estrogen.[2] There are three types of phytoestrogens:

1. Isoflavones (soy, chickpeas, lentils, and red clover)
2. Lignans
3. Coumestans[2]

For purposes of hot flashes, the isoflavones are by far the most useful. Isoflavones are soy or red clover derivatives in the form of herbs, tablets, or food. <u>Soy supplements</u> are available by many names. Soy supplements are tablets or herbs with phytoestrogens in them. <u>Soy foods</u> include tofu, tempeh, meat substitutes made from tofu, dairy products made with soy, and soy beans. Generally, soy foods are less effective in reducing hot flashes than soy supplements.[2]

Studies have shown that isoflavones generally reduce hot flashes only slightly.[3] Nevertheless, the incidence of hot flashes varies in frequency in a manner that is inversely proportional to the amount of soy in your diet. So, the more soy you consume, the fewer hot flashes you'll have. In Europe, hot flashes occur in 70% to 80% of women. I don't think they've become familiar with soy there. The incidence is 57% in Maylasia, 18% in China, and 14% in Singapore.[5] In Japan, where the consumption of phytoestrogens is approximately 200 mg per day, the women have the lowest incidence of hot flashes.[1]

Some of the common red clover product names are Promensil and Rimostil.[1]

Hot Flashes

Black Cohosh (Cimicifuga racemosa)

Black Cohosh is a perennial plant related to the buttercup.[2] This is one of the more common herbs for managing hot flashes. You may notice that it's an ingredient in many of the herbal products available for menopause in general, or hot flashes in particular. The most popular product containing Black Cohosh is Remifemin.[3]

The dosages vary, especially in products containing a combination of herbs. In some studies, women reported mild improvement in hot flashes after taking 40 mg of Black Cohosh alone.[3] In addition to hot flashes, Black Cohosh may also relieve vaginal dryness, insomnia, depression, and anxiety.[6]

Side effects are rare, and include nausea, vomiting, occasional gastric discomfort, headache, dizziness, breast pain, and weight gain.[2] Safety beyond six months of use is unknown,[3] but there are many women who have used it for much longer than that.

Evening Primrose (Oenothera biennis)

The Evening Primrose plant (also called Evening Star) produces seeds that are rich in Gamma Linolenic Acid, which is an essential fatty acid. It also has some anticoagulant properties which serve to thin the blood. It's available in health food stores as a dietary supplement.[2] It is no better than placebo in the treatment of hot flashes,[2] but some women find it beneficial for breast pain, bladder symptoms, and PMS-like symptoms.[7]

Dong Quai (Angelica sinensis)

Dong Quai is a type of angelica common in Chinese herbal medicine.[2] It seems as though there is more talk about using Dong Quai for hot flashes than actual use for hot flashes. That's because it hasn't been shown to have an effect on hot flashes.[2] Use caution with Dong Quai because it can thin the blood to an extent that is dangerous.[2]

Hormonal Medication Options

Estrogen

Estrogen provides the most effective relief for hot flashes.[3] The dose necessary to relieve hot flashes varies from person to person, and you may need a higher dose to prevent your other symptoms of menopause than you do for hot flashes. If you're looking for the most straightforward, guaranteed, simple way to prevent hot flashes and any other symptoms of menopause, estrogen would be the treatment of choice. Estrogen is available in the form of shots, pills, vaginal rings, skin patches, and skin gels.

Progesterone

Progesterone is available in oral (pill), intramuscular (shot), and topical (cream) forms. In general, the pill and the shot forms of progesterone are effective in treating hot flashes.[3] Progesterone creams are less predictable in their ability to relieve hot flashes.[3] Ironically though, the alternative and complementary medicine community seems to promote progesterone cream more than any other form of progesterone for the treatment of hot flashes.

The most significant side effect of progesterone is increased breast discomfort. This effect is directly proportional to dose: the higher the dose, the greater the breast tenderness.[2] Other side effects include irregular vaginal bleeding and premenstrual syndrome (PMS) in women who are still having periods. PMS includes breast discomfort, mood swings, bloating, and temporary weight gain of just a few pounds.[2]

Tibolone

Tibolone is a steroid that hasn't been approved by the Food and Drug Administration (FDA).[2] In addition to minimizing hot flashes, it prevents osteoporosis and dryness of the vagina.[2] The main side effect is vaginal bleeding because it causes the uterine lining (endometrium) to shed.[2] Long term effects of this drug are unknown.[2]

Non-hormonal Medication Options

SSRI Antidepressants

A variety of antidepressants appear to be effective in relieving hot flashes. While they are not specifically approved or indicated for hot flashes, they're in such widespread use for depression that many women enjoy this added benefit. They belong to the class of antidepressants called Selective Serotonin Reuptake Inhibitors. Some of the medications that have proven beneficial are fluoxetine (Prozac), paroxetine hydrochloride (Paxil), and venlafaxine (Effexor).[3] They typically decrease the number of hot flashes, but not the intensity. Overall, they don't tend to work as well as estrogen for hot flashes.[8]

Common side effects include abnormal sexual function (like difficulty achieving orgasm), dry mouth, constipation, nausea, and reduced appetite.[2] Because of the reduced appetite, some of these medications also have the effect of making weight loss easier.

Neurontin (Gabapentin)

Neurontin is actually a drug for convulsions or seizures. Nevertheless, it effectively reduces hot flashes. There are very few studies demonstrating this effect.[3] The most significant side effect is dizziness.[2] There aren't many women using this drug solely for the purpose of reducing hot flashes.

Bellergal

Historically, this was one of the first preparations used for hot flashes. Over time, there have been so many other options available for hot flashes, that it isn't used much any more. That's a good thing due to its severe side effects and its addictive potential.[2] In essence, it's history.

Antihypertensive Agents

Three drugs used for the treatment of high blood pressure have some effect on hot flashes.[2] However, the effect is one of a reduction in intensity rather than complete elimination of hot flashes.[9] These medications are clonidine, lefoxidine, and methyldopa.[2]

All three agents are difficult to tolerate because of side effects such as nausea, depression, headache, dizziness, dry mouth, and fatigue.[2] Here again, there aren't many women taking these drugs for the sole purpose of reducing hot flashes. More commonly, women with high blood pressure use these drugs for their blood pressure control, and get to enjoy the added benefit of reducing hot flashes as a perk.

Veralipride

This drug inhibits hot flashes, but hasn't been approved by the FDA.[2] It causes major side effects, including breast pain, leakage of breast milk, and tremor.[2] You shouldn't even consider this one.

CHAPTER 11: NIGHT SWEATS

Description

Night sweats simply represent hot flashes which occur during sleep. Now, you would think that you'd get a break from all this hormonal chaos during sleep, but not so. Night sweats may occur occasionally, nightly, or multiple times in a single night. They tend to occur during peri-menopause, and in times of hormone adjustment or stress, While they don't always awaken you from sleep, they are likely to leave your "pajamas" and/or sheets plenty damp. You may awaken from the uncomfortable sensation of lying on wet fabric.

Alternatively, you may awaken with feelings of anxiety and a sudden need to just throw all the covers off of you. These episodes aren't just pure sweating. There's a clammy feel to the skin, and you may have racing of your heart (palpitations). Like hot flashes, you may go from burning hot to freezing cold in a matter of seconds. So, night sweats may be a significant source of interrupted sleep. Night sweats result from the same physiologic process that causes hot flashes.

Management Options

Diet and Lifestyle Options

Control Your Sleep Environment

The best thing to do for night sweats is to sleep naked. That way, when you have an episode of sudden awakening and you're drenched, you can just throw off the covers and you'll cool down more quickly. Of course lowering the temperature of the bedroom or turning on a fan will also help. Don't drink anything hot just before bed, and try to go to sleep in a calm, stress-free mood.

There are companies which have taken advantage of niche marketing, and created special products for menopausal women with night sweats. I know of one that makes nightwear out of special fabric. It's called "Cool Sets" (www.coolsets.com). Another one makes special sheets and pillow cases that channel moisture away from the skin. It's called "Derma Therapy Bedding" (www.menopausebedding.com).

All of the botanical, herbal, and medical therapies that help with hot flashes may also help prevent night sweats. This may be more successful if you take them close to bedtime rather than in the morning. If you have already read the management options for hot flashes, you'll find this section essentially a carbon copy of that one, with just a few differences.

Vitamin and Mineral Options

Vitamin E

As with hot flashes, vitamin E may be no more beneficial than a placebo.[1] However, it is not harmful, and it does offer other benefits. The dose is 800 IU/day or less.

Botanical and Herbal Options

Remember that purity of herbs varies significantly between brands and between different batches of the same brand. Therefore, proper dosages may be difficult to achieve.[2] You may have to use trial and error with brands and dosages. Be patient with this. It's worth the effort. If you find a brand that works for you, stick with it. Don't continue experimenting with other options just for fun after that. In other words, don't dissect a rose. If you're doing well, don't change anything!

Phytoestrogens

Phytoestrogens are naturally occurring plant-based compounds that produce the same effect as estrogen.[2] There are three types of phytoestrogens:

1. Isoflavones (soy, chickpeas, lentils, and red clover)
2. Lignans
3. Coumestans[2]

The isoflavones are by far the most useful for night sweats just as they are for hot flashes. Isoflavones are soy or red clover derivatives in the form of herbs, tablets, or food. If they are in tablet or herb form, we refer to them as a soy supplement, and they are available by many names. Soy foods include tofu, tempeh, meat substitutes made from tofu, dairy products made with soy, and soy beans. Generally, soy foods are less effective in reducing night sweats than soy supplements.[2]

Even though studies have shown that isoflavones generally reduce night sweats only slightly,[1] the frequency of night sweats is inversely proportional to the amount of soy in your diet. So, the more soy you consume, the fewer night sweats you'll have. The incidence of night sweats in women of various countries mirrors the incidence of hot flashes. The percentage of women with night sweats is 70% to 80% in Europe, 57% in Maylasia, 18% in China, 14% in Singapore,[3] and rare in Japan.[4] The low incidence in Japanese women is due to the consumption of large quantities of phytoestrogens, averaging 200 mg per day.[4]

Some of the common red clover product names are Promensil and Rimostil.[4]

Black Cohosh (Cimicifuga racemosa)

Black Cohosh is a popular ingredient in herbal products for menopause. It is one of the most common herbs in use for both hot flashes and night sweats. Remifemin is the most familiar product containing Black Cohosh.[1]

There is a range of dosages of Black Cohosh in products containing a combination of herbs. Some women report mild improvement in night sweats after taking 40 mg of Black Cohosh alone.[3] In addition to hot flashes and night sweats, Black Cohosh may also relieve vaginal dryness, insomnia, depression, and anxiety.[5]

While rare, there are numerous side effects with Black Cohosh, including nausea, vomiting, occasional gastric discomfort, headache, dizziness, breast pain, and weight gain.[2] Safety beyond six months of use is unknown,[3] but there are many women who have used it for much longer than that.

Evening Primrose (Oenothera biennis)

While there is no proof that Evening Primrose is better than placebo in the treatment of hot flashes and night sweats,[2] some women find it beneficial for breast pain, bladder symptoms, and PMS-like symptoms.[6] Beware of the fact that Evening Primrose has some anticoagulant properties, which thin the blood.

Dong Quai (Angelica sinensis)

Dong Quai has not been shown to have an effect on night sweats,[2] but it's a common ingredient in Chinese herbal medicine.[4] Use caution with Dong Quai because it can thin the blood to an extent that is dangerous.[2]

Hormonal Medication Options

Estrogen

Estrogen is extremely reliable and effective in relieving night sweats.[3] The response is almost immediate. The dose necessary to quell night sweats may be minimal, too low to prevent your other symptoms of menopause. If you have neither the time nor the patience to determine if other options will work for you, start with estrogen. Any form will do the trick, including shots, pills, vaginal rings, skin patches, and skin gels.

Progesterone

All progesterone is *not* created equal for management of night sweats. Pills and shots are effective,[1] while creams are less predictable.[3] That may be due to the variability in the quantity of progesterone in progesterone creams. Nonetheless, the alternative and complementary medicine community promotes progesterone cream over all other forms of progesterone for night sweats.

The most significant side effect of progesterone is breast tenderness. This effect is directly proportional to dose: the higher the dose, the greater the breast tenderness.[2] Other side effects include irregular vaginal bleeding and premenstrual syndrome (PMS) in women who are still having periods. PMS includes breast discomfort, mood swings, bloating, and temporary weight gain of just a few pounds.[2]

Tibolone

Tibolone is not in common use for night sweats. That's primarily because it hasn't been approved by the Food and Drug Administration (FDA).[2] However, it does minimize night sweats, as well as prevent osteoporosis and dryness of the vagina.[2] The main side effect is vaginal bleeding because it causes the uterine lining (endometrium) to shed.[2] Long term effects of this drug are unknown.[2]

Non-hormonal Medication Options

SSRI Antidepressants

The Selective Serotonin Reuptake Inhibitors appear to be effective in relieving night sweats. There are so many women taking them for depression that we've discovered secondarily that they help reduce night sweats. Some of the medications that have proven beneficial are fluoxetine (Prozac), paroxetine hydrochloride (Paxil), and venlafaxine (Effexor).[1] They typically decrease the number of night sweats, but not the intensity. Overall, they don't tend to work as well as estrogen for night sweats.[7]

Common side effects include abnormal sexual function (like difficulty achieving orgasm), dry mouth, constipation, nausea, and reduced appetite.[2] Because of the reduced appetite, some of these medications also have the effect of making weight loss easier.

Neurontin (Gabapentin)

Neurontin is an anticonvulsant drug for seizures that just so happens to effectively reduce night sweats. There are only a few studies demonstrating this effect.[3] The most significant side effect is dizziness.[4] It's not in common use for night sweats, and you wouldn't take it specifically for that purpose.

Bellergal

Bellergal is only of historical interest. Long ago, it was one of the first preparations used for hot flashes and night sweats. Over time, there have been so many other options available for night sweats that it isn't used much any more. Because of its severe side effects and its addictive potential, it has been replaced with a host of other agents.[4]

Antihypertensive Agents

Certain antihypertensive agents reduce the intensity of night sweats.[2] However, they do not completely eliminate them.[8] These medications are clonidine, lefoxidine, and methyldopa.[2]

If you have high blood pressure and happen to be using one of these medications, you'll probably notice a reduction in the intensity of your night sweats as an ancillary benefit. All three agents are difficult to tolerate because of side effects such as nausea, depression, headache, dizziness, dry mouth, and fatigue.[2]

Veralipride

While you may hear about Veralipride, don't even consider it for night sweats. It does inhibit hot flashes and night sweats. But it hasn't been approved by the FDA,[2] and it causes significant side effects like breast pain, leakage of breast milk, and tremor.[2]

Chapter 12: Insomnia

Description

In the context of menopause, insomnia refers most commonly to difficulty in *falling* asleep. Other features may include waking up in the middle of the night and being unable to go back to sleep, and/or waking up with the chickens and being unable to go back to sleep. It's as if your body's clock is confused. It's a time of sleep cycle confusion. In part, your body's clock is off, such that day and night are not distinct. You have difficulty getting sleep at the designated time. But you still *need* more sleep during the peri-menopausal transition than you did before it began. Your body is hard at work to change from one stage of life to another.

Hormones, Aging, and Sleep

No matter how old you are, hormones and sleep just seem to be related to one another. Let's see now; how is sleep affected during adolescence and pregnancy? Have you ever noticed how adolescents can sleep for hours and hours and hours? It's common for them to log 12 to 20 hours in one sleep session. On weekends, they may sleep until noon or well into the afternoon hours. They just can't seem to get enough sleep. They outgrow it after adolescence. So, when the sex hormones are on the *rise* during adolescence, sleep comes easy, and it's continuous, with hardly an interruption. At the opposite end of that spectrum, when sex hormones are waning during peri-menopause, sleeping is difficult and full of interruptions. Hmmmm. Could it be that sex hormones are sleep inducers?

What about pregnancy? You know it involves huge *increases* in the quantities of sex hormones circulating in the body. One of the tell tale signs of early pregnancy is extreme sleepiness. Progesterone also has a direct effect on sleep. In fact, you can actually think of progesterone as the drowsy hormone, because it induces drowsiness. The drowsiness characteristic of the first trimester of pregnancy is due to increased levels of progesterone. Pregnant women will tell you that it's all they can do to stay awake even when they're sitting or standing. The sleepiness of pregnancy is most prominent when all those hormones are flooding into the blood stream during the first trimester. Once the hormones are fairly stable and the second trimester begins, the extreme sleepiness lessens. No doubt, there's still an increased need for sleep throughout pregnancy, but it's when those hormones are rapidly changing that it's most noticeable.

Of course, once that baby is born, mom has to get by on very little sleep. How convenient! Those high levels of hormones are on the *decline* then, and a new mom manages to survive on short stretches of sleep of an hour here and an hour there. Go figure! I guess Mother Nature allows for a hibernation of sorts during pregnancy in order to prepare you for months of sleep deprivation after delivery.

Age seems to have an effect on sleep, also. Babies need lots of sleep. Could it be that they have some of those hormones from pregnancy hanging around for a while which cause them to sleep so much? Maybe hormones in breast milk increase the need for sleep. There's a hormone called Growth Hormone that is particularly important during infancy. It's also present in high quantities during adolescence. You have very little of it in old age. While it's not a sex hormone, it still has a strong relationship to our need for sleep. There's no doubt that you need more sleep any time Growth Hormone is at work.

Ever noticed how elderly people seem to wake up earlier than everyone else? They rise with the chickens! That's because their sex hormones (estrogen in females and testosterone in males) are on the *decline*. Granted, most of us go to bed earlier as we age, but we certainly don't sleep as much as babies, adolescents, or pregnant women do.

Simply put, aging is associated with an increase in sleep difficulties.[1] The prevalence of insomnia increases with age, and it's twice as common in women as in men.[2]

So, there must be something to this correlation between hormones, aging, and sleep. Peri-menopause, it seems, is another natural hormonal transition that creates an adjustment in our sleep patterns.

Well, it shouldn't surprise you that estrogen is a major determinant of sleep.[2] Its effects on sleep are numerous and complicated. At the most basic level, it decreases the time it takes to fall asleep (sleep latency), decreases the number of times you awaken from sleep, and increases the total amount of time you sleep.[2] On the contrary, as estrogen *decreases* during the transition into menopause, you experience lengthening of the time it takes to fall asleep, an increase in the number of times you awaken from sleep, and a decrease in the total amount of time you sleep.

There's one more substance to mention here. The body chemical that is most important in sleep is Gamma Aminobutyric Acid (GABA). It's not a hormone, but it interacts with hormones. So, it deserves some attention. GABA is involved with the initiation and maintenance of sleep. But it doesn't act alone. The female hormones have an effect on GABA, and estrogen increases the amount of GABA in the body.[3] Once again, estrogen has a huge role. The lower levels and the fluctuating levels of estrogen mess up our GABA levels. With inadequate GABA, you have difficulty initiating and maintaining sleep.

Consequences

Insomnia initiates and augments many of the other symptoms of menopause. Inadequate sleep contributes to irritability, fatigue, inability to concentrate, lack of energy, and mood swings. It's a vicious cycle. Anxiety and depression may result from a shift in body image, and that has a negative impact on sleep patterns, also.[2]

Some women suffer from insomnia as a result of disordered breathing during sleep.[2] Another term for this is "*sleep apnea.*" You may have heard that term. It means that there are short episodes in which active breathing stops, requiring a momentary awakening to jump-start the breathing process again. Excess weight can be the primary cause of sleep apnea. And, of course, hormones are involved. Progesterone is the culprit when it comes to breathing. Progesterone stimulates respiration, and decreased progesterone levels may result in sleep apnea.[2]

Management Options

Diet and Lifestyle Options

Dietary Measures

Avoiding caffeine (which is a stimulant and bladder irritant) and alcohol (which disrupts normal sleep) can serve to improve sleep markedly. Some people actually use alcohol as a means of inducing sleep, but the result is greater daytime sleepiness.[2] Alcohol is detrimental to sleep because it actually worsens insomnia, and causes breathing disturbances during sleep. I guess you're beginning to see that the same lifestyle recommendations repeat themselves for various aspects of menopause. Funny; they're the same lifestyle changes that you'll see for healthy living in general.

Sleep Hygiene

Sleep hygiene refers to the habits that surround sleep patterns. It doesn't mean that you should bathe in your sleep. There are a variety of categories included in sleep hygiene. They include: (1) Stimulus Control Measures; (2) Sleep Routines; and (3) Sleep Restriction.

Stimulus Control Measures

Stimulus control measures are practices that encourage associating the bed and bedroom with sleep, and avoiding use of the bed or bedroom for other activities (other than sex, of course). It's unwise to read, eat, watch television, and talk on the phone in the bed. This is really a form of operant conditioning in which the simple sight of the bed or bedroom makes your body go into sleep mode.

Sleep Routines

Temporal control measures are practices which establish a routine sleep pattern. Adhering to the same bed time and waking time every day places your body on a cycle that regulates the sleep center in your brain. Your body will desire sleep habitually at the designated time each night, significantly decreasing the risk of insomnia.

Sleep Restriction

Sleep restriction limits the amount of time devoted to sleep so that your body is ready to engage in a full night of continuous sleep. Daytime napping isn't allowed, and a full night's sleep is limited to only about six hours at first. With time, the length of a full night's sleep increases.

Regular Exercise

Regular exercise works wonders to enhance sleep. Note, however, that you shouldn't exercise near bedtime, because it might just make it difficult for you to wind down. Exercise tires the body and relaxes the mind in a beneficial way, even if insomnia isn't severe. In fact, regular exercise has the combined effect of giving you more energy during the day and increasing your quality of sleep at night.

Relaxation

Ahhh! Relaxation therapy works wonders for sleep. It's only natural that when you're relaxed, you feel ready to drift off to sleep. There are many varieties of relaxation therapy, including yoga, meditation, and auditory (sound) therapy. You may have a personal thought or practice that serves to relax you. If you visualize your own relaxing stimulus, it may put you in a state of calm that allows you to drift off to sleep.

Vitamin and Mineral Options

Melatonin and 5-HTP

Melatonin and 5 - HTP (5-Hydroxytryptophan) are natural substances produced by the human brain. 5 - HTP is actually a precursor of melatonin. Both substances function by causing your body to respond to darkness, and to feel sleepy at night and alert during the day. However, the levels decrease with age, and people with insomnia tend to have very low levels.[2] Some menopausal women actually have a shift in the timing of melatonin secretion, which disrupts the normal sleep / wake cycle.[2] The dose of melatonin is 0.5 - 3.0 mg one to two hours before bedtime. The dose of 5 - HTP is 100 mg three times daily, increasing to 200 mg three times daily.

Botanical and Herbal Options

Kava Kava (Piper methysticum)

Kava Kava is a sleep-inducing herb that is immediately effective. You don't have to wait for weeks or months to notice the effect it has on helping you get to sleep. You'll recognize a difference in days, if not sooner. It improves the quality of sleep and lessens the time to fall asleep. It's a common ingredient in many herbal products for menopause. While it's available in health food stores, it's dangerous if you have liver problems.

Valerian (Valeriana officinalis)

Valerian is effective in inducing sleep and preventing interrupted sleep. It is safe and non-addictive. The effects of Valerian are increased with alcohol, so don't combine the two.[4] You may add Valerian to Kava Kava if necessary, or use it in isolation. The dose is 150 - 300 mg at bedtime. The Valerian needs to be a standardized 8% valerenic acid. Side effects of Valerian include headache, excitability, and heart rate changes.[4]

INSOMNIA

Hops (Humulus lupulus)

Hops is especially effective for insomnia due to its calming effect, but there are no recommendations for its use in menopause.[4] Hops improves the quality of sleep, decreases sleepiness the next day, decreases the recall of bad dreams, and decreases the frequency of waking up during the night. In essence, Hops really works in the sleep department. The dose is 1 – 2 gm of powder, or 0.5 ml of liquid extract, or 1 – 2 ml tincture.

Passion Flower (Passiflora incarnata)

Passion Flower is the proud recipient of lay press claims to be one of "nature's safe, natural tranquilizers." Advertising claims tout it as having the ability to relieve anxiety, muscle tension, insomnia, restlessness, and headache. It's marketed as the herb of choice for temporary insomnia, and it doesn't produce a hangover effect. From a scientific standpoint, however, the Food and Drug Administration (FDA) doesn't recognize this herb as safe or effective because there is no supporting scientific evidence.[4]

Don't confuse Passion Flower with Passion Fruit. They are both parts of the same plant, but it's the flower that helps in managing insomnia. Passion Fruit is a tasty tropical fruit. There are also many food items, like ice cream, that are the flavor of Passion Fruit.

Others

Other botanical and herbal products for insomnia include **Black Cohosh**, **Chasteberry**, **Joyful Change**, and **Chai Hu Long Gu Muli Wang**.

Hormonal Medication Options

Progesterone

Progesterone has a calming, sedative effect. It's the high progesterone levels in pregnancy that create an overwhelming desire and need for increased sleep during the first trimester. Thus, it is effective in treating insomnia. Progesterone cream produces the most rapid effect, making application at bedtime your best bet. The dose is ¼ - ½ tsp of 2% skin cream.

Non-hormonal Medication Options

There are two classes of medications that are most commonly prescribed for the treatment of insomnia.[1] They are sedative hypnotics and antidepressants. Some of these drugs have names that are quite a mouthful to say. Don't worry about your pronunciation. You shouldn't request a specific drug, anyway. Instead, discuss your symptoms and let your healthcare provider suggest the best options.

All medications for insomnia should be utilized on a short-term basis. You should also utilize them within the context of an overall treatment plan that includes behavioral measures, such as the sleep hygiene practices I described earlier. The guiding principles for sleep medications include the following: (1) Use safe, effective drugs; (2) Take the lowest dose for the shortest period of time (less than two weeks); and (3) Gradually discontinue the medication if the time frame or the dose have been excessive.[1] If you take a medication for insomnia for more than two weeks, consult your healthcare provider.

Sedative Hypnotic Medications

Benzodiazepines

The benzodiazepines increase total sleep time, decrease the time it takes to fall asleep, and decrease the frequency and duration of awakenings.[2] These medications may be addictive. As such, they require higher dosages over time and create withdrawal when discontinued.[2] Thus, they carry the potential for abuse.

The benzodiazepines require cautious use in elderly people because the side effects mimic some of the common concerns of aging. These side effects include memory impairment, excessive sleepiness, falls, and accidents. There's also an association between the use of benzodiazepines and bone fractures due to falls.[1]

Here's a list of the generic names and the brand names for the most popular benzodiazepines:

1. Estazolam (ProSom)
2. Flurazepam (Dalmane)
3. Quazepam (Doral)
4. Temazepam (Restoril)
5. Triazolam (Halcion)
6. Ramelteon (Rozarem)

These drugs vary greatly in the time that they remain in the blood stream, ranging from several hours to several days. The ones that remain in the blood stream longer are more commonly associated with daytime drowsiness, difficulty concentrating, and accidents like falls.[2] The benzodiazepines with the shortest duration in the blood stream are the safest. Some of these drugs may have lingering effects in making you sleepy beyond eight hours. That means they have a long duration in your blood stream and are less safe. If you can switch to one that lingers for less than eight hours, do so. People vary as to how long these drugs remain in their blood streams.

Imidazopyridines

Also included in the sedative hypnotic class of drugs are the non-benzodiazepines. Another name for this class of drugs is imidazopyridines. These medications are not associated with becoming dependent on the drug, requiring higher doses over time, or withdrawal upon discontinuing them.[2] The generic and brand names for these are as follows:

1. Zaleplon (Sonata)
2. Zolpidem tartrate (Ambien)
3. Eszopiclone (Lunesta)

These medications remain in the blood stream for a very short time, resulting in a low risk of daytime drowsiness or difficulty concentrating,[2]

Ambien and Lunesta last longer than Sonata, making them better for sleeping through the entire night.[2] Sonata lasts a short enough time that a second dose in the middle of the night may be necessary. All of these medications act quickly, so it's important to take them just before going to bed.[2]

Side effects may include headache, dizziness, drowsiness, and nausea.[2]

These agents are safe for short term use. There's no tendency for addiction with these drugs, no need to increase the dosage over time, and no withdrawal upon discontinuing them.[2]

Antidepressant Medications

Tricyclic Antidepressants

The tricyclic antidepressants are an older category of antidepressant medications that have been used for insomnia. The most popular of these is amitriptyline (Elavil). It has sedative properties, but also has significant side effects.[2] It remains in the blood stream for a prolonged time, which results in daytime drowsiness.[2]

SSRI Antidepressants

The SSRIs (Selective Serotonin Reuptake Inhibitors) are a newer class of antidepressants that are safer than tricyclics. However, there is no evidence that they're effective in treating insomnia when there's no accompanying depression.[2]

Among the SSRI antidepressant medications, trazodone and mirtazapine are the two that are used most commonly for insomnia.[1]

Trazodone increases the ease of sleep, decreases waking episodes, and improves your subjective perception of the quality of sleep.[1] It has mild to moderate sedative properties. While most women will fall asleep more easily with it, they don't necessarily wake up feeling more refreshed.[2] It may also make it difficult to concentrate the following day.[2] The most significant side effect of trazodone is low blood pressure on standing up, and it can cause an irregular heart rate.[2] It's unsafe to take trazodone with other antidepressant medications.[2]

Mirtazapine improves sleep latency, which is just another way of saying that it helps you fall asleep faster.[1]

Over the Counter Medications

Antihistamines

Most over the counter sleep medications are antihistamines. The most common active ingredient is diphenhydramine. They provide mild to moderate sedation, including a hangover effect the following day.[2] These drugs aren't recommended for elderly individuals due to their side effects, which include low blood pressure on standing up, constipation, blurred vision, confusion, and urinary retention.[2]

Chapter 13: Fatigue

Description

With the aforementioned insomnia causing inability to fall asleep, and night sweats awakening you during sleep, it's logical, although unfortunate, that fatigue would naturally result. This includes a sense of feeling tired as well as lacking energy for your normal activities. Small things may seem like a big chore. You may not even have energy for the fun things, although you have the desire to participate. It's as if your brain says: "Let's go!" And your body says: "I'm too wiped out."

The fatigue that is typical of menopause is mostly a result of sleep difficulties during the night. You may not even be aware of the fact that you're having difficulty sleeping. You may only be aware of the resulting fatigue. So, many of the goals for reducing fatigue are about getting more sleep.

Another aspect of fatigue pertains to your energy level. Many hormonal events in the female life cycle have an impact on energy level.

Many pre-pubertal girls experience fatigue just before they have their first period (menarche). It's not uncommon for them to say they feel tired in the days or weeks beforehand.

Most women notice significant limitations in their energy level during pregnancy. This is apparent very early in pregnancy, long before weight gain, altered center of gravity, or a large uterus come into play. Fatigue begins very early in pregnancy, at the time when hormone fluctuations take place.

With both menarche and early pregnancy, there is a steadily increasing influx of new hormones. The body is hard at work to prepare for a new phase of life. Well, menopause is no different. The waning hormones during peri-menopause require the body to adjust to a new situation, and once again, you experience fatigue. For many women, this is temporary, and stabilizes once the transition is complete.

Your job is to find the best means of getting plenty of sleep at night and boosting your energy during the day.

Management Options

Many of the management options for fatigue mirror those for insomnia. Given the fact that fatigue results from inadequate sleep, some of the management solutions for fatigue are all about getting more sleep. Others are about boosting your energy. There are some critical differences in the usefulness of some of the management options listed for insomnia, especially the non-hormonal medication options.

Diet and Lifestyle Options

Exercise

Here we go again! It sounds like an oxymoron to say that exercise will decrease your fatigue, but that's the way it is. Regular exercise will actually give you more energy. Have you ever noticed how energetic athletic people are? You may have thought that they're athletic because they're energetic, but that's not true. In fact, the opposite is true. They're energetic *because* they exercise. The exercise *gives* them energy! So get out there and get in exercise mode. It works wonders to decrease your fatigue.

Now, the level and the type of exercise in which you engage are important. You want to maximize the energy-producing effect of exercise and minimize exacerbation of your fatigue. If you're already quite an athlete, you'll probably need to simplify and shorten your workouts to avoid excessive fatigue. Alternatively, if you're not used to exercising, start with gentle, less intense activities. You want to feel energized after your workouts, not exhausted and worn out. You might want to consider yoga or Pilates.

Vitamin and Mineral Options

Melatonin and 5-HTP

Melatonin is a natural substance produced in your brain. It causes your body to respond to daylight and darkness, so that you feel sleepy at night and alert during the day. Thus, it is useful for both insomnia and fatigue. However, the levels decrease with age, and people with insomnia tend to have very low levels.[1] Some menopausal women actually have a shift in the timing of melatonin secretion, which disrupts the normal sleep / wake cycle.[1] The dose of melatonin is 0.5 - 3.0 mg one to two hours before bedtime.

5 - HTP (5-Hydroxytryptophan) is a precursor of melatonin. The dose of 5 - HTP is 100 mg three times daily, increasing to 200 mg three times daily.

Botanical and Herbal Options

Kava Kava (Piper methysticum)

Kava Kava will help prevent insomnia. It's a sleep-inducing herb, and it's immediately effective. It's beneficial for managing fatigue simply because so much of the fatigue of menopause is due to interrupted and deficient sleep. The good thing about Kava Kava is that you don't have to wait for weeks or months to notice the effect it has on helping you to get more sleep. You'll recognize a difference in just days, if not sooner. You'll notice an improvement in the quality of your sleep and a shortening of the time it takes you to fall asleep. It's a common ingredient in many herbal products for menopause, and it's available in health food stores. Remember, it's dangerous if you have liver problems, so make sure you don't have liver disease before taking it.

Valerian (Valeriana officinalis)

Valerian is the most popular herb for inducing sleep. It also prevents interrupted sleep. The secondary benefit is that you'll experience less fatigue when you get a higher quantity and quality of sleep. It's safe and non-addictive. Combining Valerian with alcohol is dangerous because alcohol magnifies its effect.[2] Combining it with Kava Kava is fine. The dose is 150 - 300 mg at bedtime. The Valerian needs to be a standardized 8% valerenic acid. Side effects of Valerian include headache, excitability, and heart rate changes.[2]

Hops (Humulus lupulus)

While not specifically recommended for use in menopause,[2] Hops can be of great use because of the link between insomnia and fatigue. Hops improves the quality of sleep, decreases sleepiness the next day, decreases the recall of bad dreams, and decreases the frequency of waking up during the night. Because Hops works so well in inducing a good night's sleep, it prevents fatigue the following day.

Passion Flower (Passiflora incarnata)

Once again, the usefulness of this product for fatigue stems from the fact that it enhances sleep. It's marketed as the herb of choice for temporary insomnia, and it doesn't produce a hangover effect. Advertising claims tout it as having the ability to relieve anxiety, muscle tension, insomnia, restlessness, and headache. From a scientific standpoint, however, the Food and Drug Administration (FDA) doesn't recognize this herb as safe or effective because there is no supporting scientific evidence.[2]

You're probably familiar with Passion Fruit. This is the flower of the same plant.

Others

Other botanical and herbal products for fatigue include **Dong Quai** and **Licorice Root**.

FATIGUE

Hormonal Medication Options

Progesterone

Progesterone has a calming, sedative effect. That's great at night, but not so great during the day. It's the high progesterone levels in pregnancy that create an overwhelming desire and need for increased sleep during the first trimester. So, it's great in helping you get sleep, but timing is important. Progesterone cream produces the most rapid effect, making application at bedtime your best bet. The dose is ¼ - ½ tsp of 2% skin cream. For fatigue, be sure to use progesterone only at night. If you use it during the day, you might augment your fatigue.

Non-hormonal Medication Options

There are two classes of medications that are most commonly prescribed for the treatment of insomnia.[3] By using them to enhance sleep, you'll avoid fatigue during the day. They are sedative hypnotics and antidepressants. Keep in mind that your goal is to sleep soundly throughout the night and awaken refreshed and full of energy. If you're using drugs to help you sleep, you have to be sure they wear off before you're ready to start your day. You also have to be sure they don't leave you feeling physically groggy or mentally foggy.

All medications for insomnia should be utilized on a short-term basis. You should also utilize them within the context of an overall treatment plan that includes behavioral measures, such as the sleep hygiene practices I described earlier. The guiding principles for sleep medications include the following: (1) Use safe, effective drugs; (2) Take the lowest dose for the shortest period of time (less than two weeks); and (3) Gradually discontinue the medication if the time frame or the dose have been excessive.[1] If you take a medication for insomnia for more than two weeks, consult your healthcare provider.

Sedative Hypnotic Medications

Benzodiazepines

While the benzodizepines are quite useful for insomnia, they can actually *augment* fatigue. They *will* help you get more sleep. The problem is that they may leave you so drowsy that you're too fatigued to function at the level you desire.

The benzodiazepines increase total sleep time, decrease the time it takes to fall asleep, and decrease the frequency and duration of awakenings.[1] The problem is that these medications may be addictive. As such, they require higher dosages over time and create withdrawal when discontinued.[1] Thus, they carry the potential for abuse. That's not going to help you overcome fatigue.

The benzodiazepines require cautious use in elderly people because the side effects mimic some of the common concerns of aging. These side effects include memory impairment, excessive sleepiness, falls, and accidents. There's also an association between the use of benzodiazepines and bone fractures due to falls.[3]

Here's a list of the generic names and the brand names for the most popular benzodiazepines:

1. Estazolam (ProSom)
2. Flurazepam (Dalmane)
3. Quazepam (Doral)
4. Temazepam (Restoril)
5. Triazolam (Halcion)
6. Ramelteon (Rozarem)

These drugs vary greatly in the time that they remain in the blood stream, ranging from several hours to several days. The ones that remain in the blood stream longer are associated with daytime drowsiness, difficulty concentrating, and accidents like falls.[2] The benzodiazepines with the shortest duration in the blood stream are the safest. Some of these drugs may have lingering effects in making you sleepy beyond eight hours. That means they have a long duration in your blood stream and are less safe. All in all, the benzodiazepines aren't very efficient for fatigue. And if you use them for fatigue, you won't be very efficient, either.

Imidazopyridines

The best sedative hypnotic drugs for fatigue are the non-benzodiazepines. Another name for this class of drugs is imidazopyridines. These medications are not associated with becoming dependent on the drug, requiring higher doses over time, or withdrawal upon discontinuing them.[1] The generic and brand names for these are as follows:

1. Zaleplon (Sonata)
2. Zolpidem tartrate (Ambien)
3. Eszopiclone (Lunesta)

These medications remain in the blood stream for a very short time, resulting in a low risk of daytime drowsiness or difficulty concentrating.[1] That's ideal for getting enough sleep *and* preventing fatigue the next day. Ambien lasts longer than Sonata, making it the better of the two for sleeping through the entire night.[1] Sonata lasts a short enough time that a second dose in the middle of the night may be necessary. All of these medications act quickly, so it's important to take them just before going to bed.[1]

Side effects may include headache, dizziness, drowsiness, and nausea.[1] Of course, if you experience drowsiness the day after using any of these, you've defeated the purpose of using them for fatigue!

These agents are safe for short-term use. There's no tendency for addiction with these drugs, no need to increase the dosage over time, and no withdrawal upon discontinuing them.[1]

Antidepressant Medications

Tricyclic Antidepressants

The tricyclic antidepressants are an older category of antidepressant medications that have been used for insomnia. The most popular of these is amitriptyline (Elavil). Although it has sedative properties, it also has significant side effects.[1] It remains in the blood stream for a prolonged time, which results in daytime drowsiness.[1] So, while you might find amitriptyline useful for insomnia, it will probably worsen your fatigue.

SSRI Antidepressants

The SSRIs are also more of a problem than a solution for fatigue. They're safer than tricyclics, and they're effective in treating insomnia when there's accompanying depression.[1] Naturally, we wonder how they treat fatigue. Well, they don't have much to offer in that realm.

Trazodone increases the ease of sleep, decreases waking episodes, and improves your subjective perception of the quality of sleep.[3] It has mild to moderate sedative properties. While most women will fall asleep more easily with it, they don't necessarily wake up feeling more refreshed.[1] It may also make it difficult to concentrate the following day.[1] The most significant side effect of trazodone is low blood pressure on standing up, and it can cause an irregular heart rate.[1] It's unsafe to take trazodone with other antidepressant medications.[1]

Mirtazapine improves sleep latency, which is just another way of saying that it helps you fall asleep faster.[3]

Over the Counter Medications

Antihistamines

You definitely don't want to take antihistamines for fatigue because they produce mild to moderate sedation, including a hangover effect the following day.[1]

Chapter 14: Forgetfulness

Description

Well, with all that transpires in the course of menopause, you may think it would actually be kind of Mother Nature to impair our ability to remember any of it. Some people have said that such is the case for childbirth, but most of us don't believe that. While you won't forget everything about your menopausal experience, you'll certainly forget a lot of other things. I've often considered that the "pause" in the word "menopause" could refer to all the pauses you'll make when you can't recall what it is that you were going to say or do. Possibly, this mid-life change called "menopause" is a misnomer. Maybe we should call it "mental pause."

When it comes to menopause, the most common type of forgetfulness is a *fleeting* type of forgetfulness. Most women describe instances when they have something on their mind, such as a task or an errand they need to accomplish, and a second later, they can't remember what they were thinking about. You may find that you walk to the refrigerator, but upon opening the refrigerator door, you can't remember what you needed in the first place! If you're like I am, you'll go upstairs for something and be unable to recall what it was you needed once you're there. You may be in mid-sentence and forget what you were trying to say. It's these fleeting moments of forgetfulness that are typical of menopause.

If and when you first experience this phenomenon, you'll feel as though you're going crazy. Once you're aware that it's only a normal symptom of menopause, you'll become familiar with it, and, although annoying, realize that you're normal. I suggest that you get in the habit of writing things down as they pop into your head. That will constitute your "To Do List." Refer to your list often. In some cases, you'll refer to your list nearly every hour of the day to stay on track. Don't trust your memory; it isn't as reliable as it once was. If you're like I am, you'll remember things just as you're drifting off to sleep. You won't want to wake up enough to write them down, but you know you'll never remember them in the morning. Let me warn you, it's worth the effort to go ahead and jot them down before you go to sleep. Keep a notepad and pen at your bedside. You'll be amazed at how often you use them.

This type of clouded thinking is not exclusive to menopause. It also occurs before periods (premenstrual) and after pregnancy (postpartum). This type of forgetfulness is *not* the same thing as Alzheimer's disease, so please don't misconstrue it as such. The typical forgetfulness of menopause is laughable and easily managed with a number of agents available for the management of menopause in general or for the sharpening of memory in particular.

Management Options

Diet and Lifestyle Options

Diet

Your diet has a strong effect on your brain. For your brain to function adequately and efficiently, you've got to feed it. Certain foods are especially beneficial for enhancing brain function. The most basic principle is to start each day by feeding your brain its breakfast. Your brain takes a break from its active tasks during sleep, so it requires breakfast to get started. The perfect breakfast should consist of lean protein, whole grains, and vitamin C. After breakfast, it's better to eat small meals frequently than it is to eat large meals infrequently. The overall diet that is most beneficial for your brain is one that is low in fat and high in protein, fruits, vegetables, and whole grains. With regard to fats, unsaturated fats are actually very good for your brain. These include olive and sesame oils, salmon, and sardines.

Soy in any form is great brain food. Not only does it contain estrogen, but it's high in protein, low in fat, and high in fiber. Thus, it meets all the qualifications for foods and hormones that your brain likes. Additionally, it's safe and has no side effects.

Alcohol Restriction

Alcohol in excessive amounts dulls your brain in both the short term and the long term. Limiting alcohol to moderate amounts (two drinks maximum in a single day) is a reasonable behavior modification to enhance memory.

Smoking Cessation

Smoking cessation is a huge must in an effort to improve brain function. Just as smoking clogs the arteries to your lungs and heart, it also clogs the arteries to your brain. The end result is that there's less blood flow to your brain. Since the blood carries oxygen to your brain, smoking results in less oxygen available to your brain. An oxygen-deprived brain functions about as well as oxygen-deprived lungs.

Just think; this is a great time and a perfect incentive to quit smoking. If you've smoked for years, use this time in your life to reinvent yourself, invest in your future, and decide that it's time to abandon old bad habits and adopt new good ones.

Vitamin and Mineral Options

Vitamins B1 (Thiamine), C, and E are critical to sharp brain function. **Zinc, selenium, and folate** are also extremely important for your brain. If you're unlikely to consume daily recommended dosages of these in your diet, take supplements. There are a variety of multivitamin preparations designed especially for women, some of which are specific for menopause. We're all different, and we have different needs. Your individual needs change from time to time, too. The differences in various brands of multivitamins simplify the process of ensuring that you obtain the correct balance of vitamins. Take advantage of these products. If you need additional quantities of certain vitamins, add them to the regimen.

Botanical and Herbal Options

Ginkgo (Ginkgo biloba)

Ginkgo (*Ginkgo biloba*) is probably the most widely known herb that enhances brain function. It acts by increasing blood flow to your brain. It does this by thinning your blood, so be sure to mention this as one of the "medications" you take when a healthcare professional asks you about your medications. You wouldn't want to have surgery without alerting the surgeon to the fact that you were on a blood thinner, so treat this as you would any other blood thinner.

The majority of the studies on Ginkgo have demonstrated a benefit in thinking and memory. Usually, though, it takes about 12 weeks for you to notice an obvious improvement in memory. It's worth the wait if you're having severe or devastating problems with forgetfulness. Ginkgo also slows the rate of progressive deterioration in dementia.[1]

The dose is 40 - 80 mg three times daily.

Gotu Kola (Centella asiatica)

Gotu Kola also increases blood flow to the brain. Studies have shown that general mental ability, academic activities, and test scores improve with the use of Gotu Kola.[1] The dose is 90 mg daily, taken in the morning, because it has the side effect of inhibiting sleep.

Hormonal Medication Options

Estrogen

Estrogen, in any form, enhances brain function significantly. The absence of estrogen is the reason for the forgetfulness of menopause, so it makes sense that replenishing estrogen also replenishes memory.

If you're looking for the most obvious, certain, and simple solution to your memory problem, estrogen is the answer.

Estrogen protects against the memory loss that is typical of the normal aging process.[2] It's normal for elderly women to remember distant memories from the past, but it's difficult for them to learn new things and recall new information.[2] Haven't you noticed how elderly women can tell you all about their childhood, their college days, and their families, but they can't seem to recall what you told them yesterday? New verbal information presents the greatest impediment, and estrogen protects verbal memory ability.[2]

Progesterone

Progesterone enhances brain function in much the same way that estrogen does. It's an excellent option if you cannot or choose not to take estrogen.

Progesterone is available in the form of tablets, creams, and gels. Tablets provide a more predictable and controlled quantity than creams or gels. Tablets usually require a prescription, whereas creams and gels are readily available without a prescription. The dose for progesterone is 25 - 50 mg daily, increasing to 100 - 200 mg daily if needed.

Testosterone

Dehydroepiandrosterone (DHEA) is a form of testosterone that enhances brain function in much the same way that estrogen does. It is metabolized into progesterone in the body.

DHEA is commonly available without a prescription. It's a weak androgen, but it has the potential of causing acne, deepening of the voice, male pattern hair growth (on the chin, chest, face), and male pattern baldness in some women. These aren't very common, and they're noticeable early enough to discontinue the drug before any long-term effects occur, but I'm sure you would want to know this possibility beforehand. The dose of DHEA is 5 - 25 mg daily. Side effects are significant for women with epilepsy. Thus, if you're epileptic, consider other alternatives.

At this point, are you beginning to see how you can pick and choose the options that are most suitable for your situation? Keep your preferences in mind as you continue to read about the other signs and symptoms of menopause.

Chapter 15: Mood Swings, Irritability, and Depression

Description

Mood Swings

Once again, I ask you to recall that wondrous process called puberty. Remember the mood swings? All female hormonal events, including puberty, premenstrual syndrome, and definitely pregnancy, involve mood swings. So, it is the process of hormonal *change* that brings about mood swings. Maybe you warned the people around you about your tendency to be moody when you were premenstrual or pregnant. Maybe you should warn them again.

As female hormones fluctuate, either in a cyclical fashion (as during menstrual cycles) or erratically (as in peri-menopause), mood swings result. Our mood remains stable when our hormones stabilize. So, give it some time. Most likely this is one of those symptoms that will go away eventually. Understanding this phenomenon will help you tolerate or manage your mood swings.

Irritability

Irritability is very closely related to mood swings. It's a reflection of the threshold for emotional upset. In other words, events that you previously tolerated without upset now seem irritating to you. It's almost as if your personality changes. You're less flexible with and tolerant of others.

Have you heard stories about middle-aged women telling people off, making rude comments, or going berserk in public? There are some really funny scenes of such things in movies. These women aren't crazy. And many times, they're absolutely correct in their assessment of the situation. What they lack is self control. Instead of being able to just let something go, they let someone have it. It's funny in the movies. It's not funny when you're the one losing control.

Depression

It seems that depression, while not universal, is more familiar than we'd like during menopause. Sometimes it stems from stressful life events rather than from hormonal changes. It's a time when there may be adolescents in the house, kids leaving for college, elderly parents with health problems, emergence of personal health issues, and the need for retirement planning. There's a lot to juggle as you enter your early 50s.

Incidence

Depression is common during the process of menopause. Studies reveal that 52% of women who experience depression during menopause have never had depression previously.[1] The incidence of depression tends to increase in the year before and the year after achieving post-menopausal status. If you have a history of depression, you're four to nine times as likely to have depression during menopause as women who don't.[1] Additionally, if you experience hot flashes, you are 4.6 times as likely to experience depression during menopause.[1] Depression is most likely when peri-menopause lasts longer than 27 months and when hot flashes are moderate to severe.[1]

Mechanisms

There are two mechanisms for depression.

The first seems obvious and logical, given the combination of symptoms typical of menopause. From a psychological standpoint, you may not welcome menopause simply because it represents a time in your life when you may not feel as sexy or desirable as you did before. Maybe you don't embrace this as a positive transition, and thus feel depressed about the inevitability of menopause and aging.

Such a negative perception of menopause is very culture-specific. Some cultures, such as the Japanese, view menopause and aging as events that deserve great reverence. Menopause receives respect as a right of passage no differently than puberty, marriage, and childbearing. As a result of this positive, healthy attitude, Japanese women have few complaints about menopause. They welcome the changes of menopause just as they do any other life event. In essence, there are many benefits in simply having a positive attitude.

The second mechanism by which you may designate depression as a symptom of menopause is simply to acknowledge the fact that many of the symptoms that are diagnostic for menopause are also diagnostic for clinical depression. For instance, common symptoms of depression include insomnia or excessive sleeping, fatigue, irritability, moodiness, weight gain or weight loss, inability to enjoy activities that you used to enjoy, changes in appetite, and lack of sex drive. Thus, it may just be that the typical "depression" of menopause mimics some aspects of true psychological depression.

Depression and insomnia tend to be linked. Episodes of depression and insomnia coincide with periods of the most rapid decline in estrogen. Thus, it's not the absolute level of estrogen that causes these two symptoms of menopause, but rather the rapidity of change in a downward direction.[2] Anything that causes depression increases the risk of insomnia, and vice versa.[2]

The chemical substance in the human body that is most closely identified with depression is serotonin. Female hormones have an effect on serotonin. Both natural and surgical menopause decrease serotonin levels.[2] Just think of serotonin as a happy substance. Without it comes sadness.

So far, the symptoms we've discussed create a vicious cycle. You can't get to sleep easily, so you lie awake for hours. Once you fall asleep, you have night sweats which wake you up again. By the time morning arrives, you're fatigued. When you're fatigued, you can't think. So, you can't seem to remember anything, and your forgetfulness leads to mistakes and oversights. That makes you cranky. The crankiness and sleep deprivation make you moody. Needless to say, your moodiness does nothing positive for your social life or family relationships. All of this leaves you depressed, and that makes it difficult for you to sleep…

Insomnia ⟶ Night Sweats ⟶ Interrupted Sleep ⟶ Fatigue
↑ ↓
Depression ⟵ Irritability ⟵ Mood Swings ⟵ Forgetfulness

Just try explaining all this to someone (your husband, boyfriend, or child) who has no idea what menopause is. They're probably going to tell you that if it were all that bad, people would talk about it more and they would know to expect major changes in your personality. With their current lack of information, they may wonder if you've been replaced by an irritable twin. Make it easy on yourself. Hand them this book. (By the way, the last chapter of this book is "For the Guys." You'll be doing yourself, and your guy, a big favor if you give the book to him so that he can read the last chapter. But, finish reading it yourself, first.)

Management Options

I've grouped mood swings, irritability, and depression because they represent a different degree, frequency, and severity of the same process. In general, they reflect an inability to deal effectively with stress, monitor your response to stress, or manage your emotions. The management options are the same for all of these symptoms of menopause. In general, mood alterations, and especially depression, don't respond to treatment or management immediately. It may take as long as two months for a change in mood to be evident or for permanent improvement to be noticeable.[3]

Diet and Lifestyle Options

Diet

You can improve the stability of your moods simply by **avoiding foods and beverages that have a stimulatory effect**. Included in this category are caffeinated drinks, like coffee, tea, and soft drinks. Of course, you need to balance this by also **avoiding drinks that have a sedative effect**, like alcohol. Alcohol has the effect of prolonging episodes of depression.

Adhering to a **low sugar diet** avoids the sugar surges that sometimes change behavior in the short term, and then create a craving for another sugar boost a couple of hours later. That means avoiding chocolate, sweets, and simple carbohydrates, like bread and pasta. So, we're back to the same recommendation that you encountered earlier. It consists of a high protein, high fiber, low fat diet. I know you've heard this before. All health recommendations just seem to come back to the same thing.

Regular Exercise

Regular exercise has the effect of reducing stress. Maybe it's because you have the opportunity to focus and work through your stresses while you exercise, and you're able to deal with them more efficiently afterwards. Maybe it's because exercise raises the level of endorphins, which have the effect of making you feel good. Maybe it's because you feel good about doing something healthy for yourself. Whatever the mechanism, regular exercise definitely helps normalize mood and decrease irritability.

Vitamin and Mineral Options

Vitamin Deficiencies

A number of vitamin deficiencies can contribute to mood problems, ranging from irritability to mood swings to depression. The vitamin levels to evaluate include **vitamin B6, vitamin B12, folate, biotin, and vitamin C**. Also important are the minerals **calcium, magnesium, copper,**

and the omega 6 fatty acids. If you discover that you're deficient in any of these, take supplements to correct the deficiency. All supplements should have the recommended amount on the label. Use it to guide you as to how much you should take.

5 - Hydroxytryptophan (5-HTP)

5 - HTP is a derivative of the amino acid tryptophan. It's produced by the human body and converted into serotonin, which affects brain function and mood. Nausea is a possible side effect of 5 - HTP. The dose is 100 – 200 mg three times daily.

Inositol

Inositol has a role in altering serotonin levels in the brain. It's not one of the major management tools for mood problems in menopause because there are other options that have proven more effective. Nevertheless, it deserves mention. The dose is 12 gm daily, increasing to 18 gm daily if necessary.

S-adenosyl-L-methionine (SAMe)

SAMe is a natural substance that is present in the cells of your body. It's a metabolite of the amino acid L-methionine. It's useful for promotion and support of both mood and emotional well-being.[3]

There are numerous studies demonstrating an association between psychiatric disorders and deficient SAMe metabolism, particularly depression. Some of these studies compare SAMe to antidepressant medications. The results reveal that SAMe is as effective as antidepressants in controlling depression.[3]

SAMe is unlike antidepressant medications in that it has a more rapid onset of action. This means that you don't have to wait weeks or months to notice an improvement in your mood. Improvement is evident in only one or two weeks with SAMe, versus four to eight weeks with antidepressant drugs.[3]

Another benefit of SAMe is that it doesn't produce the common bothersome side effects typical of some antidepressant drugs, like insomnia, nervousness, nausea, and sexual dysfunction.[3]

SAMe is most available in 200 mg tablets. The usual dose for management of depression ranges from 400 – 1600 mg daily, with 800 – 1600 mg necessary for most women. It's best to take this in divided doses of half the total amount twice daily.[3]

Botanical and Herbal Options

St. John's Wort (Hypericum perforatum)

St. John's Wort is a very popular and effective herb for depression. It has the effect of reducing both anxiety and depression. Its antidepressant activity is dependent on and due to the hypericin component. Pay attention to the purity and quantity of this ingredient in any St. John's Wort products that you investigate. This herb is useful in mild depression, but it has no place in the treatment of moderate or severe clinical depression. Studies using St. John's Wort specifically for menopause have shown marked improvement in subjective and physical symptoms using formulations containing 300 mcg of hypericin per tablet.[4]

The side effects of St. John's Wort are similar to, but less severe than, those of some antidepressant medications. These include dry mouth, dizziness, and constipation.

An important thing to be aware of with the use of St. John's Wort is that anesthesiologists have noticed that it can inhibit or exacerbate anesthesia and sedatives. So, they recommend discontinuation of St. John's Wort three weeks before any surgery that requires anesthesia.[5] Even without surgery, be sure to inform your healthcare provider if you take St. John's Wort (or any other botanical or herbal substance).

There are many forms of St. John's Wort. Here are the various dosages of each for purposes of mood swings, irritability, and depression associated with menopause.[4]

Capsules or tablets: 300 mg of standardized extract three times daily
Dried herb: 2 – 4 gm taken three times daily
Tea: 2 – 3 gm of dried herb in boiling water
Liquid extract: 1:1 in 25% ethanol: 2 – 4 ml taken three times daily
Tincture: 1:10 in 45% ethanol: 2 – 4 ml three times daily

California Poppy (Eschscholtzia californica)

California Poppy has a sedative effect. It reduces anxiety, and thus smoothes out mood swings, reduces irritability, and helps prevent depression. It is not in widespread use, and there are very few studies on it.[4]

California Poppy is available as a tea, which is prepared using 2 gm of the herb in 150 ml of water. Alternatively, there's a liquid extract, which is taken as a single dose of 1 – 2 ml.[4]

Valerian Root (Valeriana officinalis)

Valerian Root is a common valerian or garden heliotrope. The active ingredient in it is Gamma Aminobutyric Acid (GABA). It eliminates anxiety, which is a common aspect of depression. You may take Valerian Root in addition to St. John's Wort.

Although there are no reports of toxicity with Valerian Root, there have been some instances of abnormal muscle tone and visual disturbances with it.[6]

The dose for mood disturbances is 100 – 300 mg of standardized extract containing 0.8% valerinic acid.

Others

Other botanical and herbal products for alleviating mood swings, irritability, and depression include **Black Cohosh, Chasteberry,** and **Chai Hu Long Gu Muli Wang.**

Hormonal Medication Options

Estrogen

Have you ever noticed how intimately related your moods are to your estrogen levels? Everything that affects the amount of estrogen circulating in your body also affects your overall mood and your changes in mood. That's why adolescence and pregnancy are notorious for moodiness, and it's also why menopause has the same characteristic. Adolescent and postpartum depression are well known entities because depression is common with the changing levels of estrogen at those times.

Since declining amounts of estrogen are pertinent to menopause, replenishing estrogen has the effect of erasing mood swings, irritability, and depression. Once again, if you're looking for a single solution, estrogen should do the trick.

You can treat any of your mood problems with any form of estrogen that gets absorbed into the blood stream, including shots, pills, patches, gels, or vaginal rings.

Testosterone

What about testosterone? Well, there isn't much data on using testosterone for mood alterations in women, but when testosterone is combined with estrogen, it enhances your sense of well-being and energy.[7] On the other hand, some women become much more moody, and even angry or mean, when they take testosterone alone or with estrogen.

Non-hormonal Medication Options

Two classes of antidepressant medications are available. They are both in common and widespread use today.

SSRI Antidepressants

The Selective Serotonin Reuptake Inhibitors (SSRIs) are the most popular antidepressants in use currently. You may recognize the names of some of these medications. They include fluoxetine (Prozac), fluoxetine hydrochloride (Serafem), paroxetine (Paxil), and sertraline (Zoloft). They're used for irritability, mood disturbances, hormonally induced depression, and clinical depression.

While they serve to improve all of these conditions, they also have significant side effects. Some of the common ones are headache, nausea, appetite suppression, weight loss, decreased sex drive, and difficulty achieving orgasm.

Despite their side effects, these medications have better safety and tolerability than the older antidepressants.[8] They represent the most popular pharmaceutical option for mood problems in menopause. Elderly women tend to show a less significant response to SSRIs than younger women.[8]

Tricyclic Antidepressants

The tricyclics are an older class of antidepressants. They include imipramine (Tofranil) and amitryptyline (Elavil). These drugs also improve depression, but with a different set of bothersome side effects, such as dry mouth, constipation, dizziness, blurred vision, heart palpitations, and memory loss. With the forgetfulness that is typical of menopause, you probably don't need anything that further increases your memory loss right now.

CHAPTER 16:
CRAVINGS FOR SWEETS, CARBOHYDRATES, ALCOHOL

Cravings and Hormones

It seems that all of life's hormonal changes come with dietary cravings. Have you ever noticed how adolescents seem to eat a diet composed of almost nothing but carbohydrates? They consume pizza, pasta, bread, potatoes (mostly French fries), desserts, macaroni and cheese, cereal, and rice to the extent that most of their meals consist of nothing but these types of foods. They do this for years at a time.

Give some thought to pregnancy. Almost everyone knows that pregnant women crave strange foods. The cravings of pregnancy aren't nearly as predictable as the cravings of puberty and adolescence, and they vary widely from one woman to another. If you've been pregnant yourself, maybe you remember your own cravings. They may have been different from one pregnancy to the next. What's happening in pregnancy is that your body needs some ingredient or chemical substance that the object of your cravings supplies. It may not make sense to you, but it's Mother Nature at work. The food that was the object of your cravings tasted so delicious! It stimulated your taste buds excessively, and the great taste made you want even more.

Even your monthly cycles involve cravings at certain times. Typically, it's the hormonal changes that occur just before your period starts that make it prime time for cravings. The timing of those cravings is one of the reasons that we have a name for the time preceding periods. No doubt, you've had or heard of PMS (premenstrual syndrome). Most women crave chocolate, caffeine, carbohydrates, and sweets during that time. Some crave salty foods. Along with the irritability, moodiness, bloating, and breast tenderness that are typical of the premenstrual phase, I'm sure you can see why this is a challenging time each month.

Well, here comes menopause, and guess what? Cravings are common with this hormonal change, also. Once again, sweets and carbohydrates are common cravings, just as they are with puberty and PMS. However, there's another item on the menu of cravings during menopause. It's alcohol! That one can be dangerous. Maybe the craving for alcohol stems from the long list of symptoms that you have to contend with to progress through the process of menopausal change. Maybe it's a coping mechanism for dealing with stress.

The problem with craving these things during peri-menopause and post-menopause is that the cravings aren't necessarily temporary. If you give in to these cravings permanently, you'll end up consuming an awful lot of calories that are a chore to work off. So, you may need to temper these cravings. It's not like adolescence when your metabolism was so fast that you could eat anything and maintain your figure. It's not like pregnancy when you were growing a baby to account for your weight increase. And to top it off, menopause *slows* your metabolism, which results in weight gain. I know, I know. Ugh!

Management Options

Management options for the cravings associated with peri- and post-menopause require a lot of **self control**. Of course, there are **behavior modification techniques** and **hypnosis**, too. Most women don't have to resort to such extremes. You can probably control this by limiting your food intake and exercising more. There's no magic herb or pill for this. It's just important to be aware that cravings are common, and the things you crave aren't beneficial to your overall well-being.

Chapter 17: Breast Pain

Description

Once again, I have to ask: Remember PMS? Oh yes, that full, achy feeling in the breasts with the added attraction of nipples that are so sensitive that even your clothing bothers them. And remember the first trimester of pregnancy, when you wouldn't allow your partner to even touch your breasts because they were so tender? Well, here it is again. Hormones are the culprit once more. During peri-menopause, it's an irregular, milder occurrence than it is in pregnancy. With all the other things going on during peri-menopause, you probably will find that breast pain is one of the more minor symptoms. The good news is that this is one of the symptoms that will probably be only temporary.

Management Options

The breast pain associated with menopausal hormone changes isn't severe. It's really more of a nuisance. It doesn't compare with the breast tenderness of pregnancy, and it's no worse than the breast tenderness that you had just before your periods. It really doesn't require management or treatment. You might want to wear a bra to support your breasts, but you don't have to do anything special. It certainly doesn't call for medications. Evening Primrose oil *may* decrease breast tenderness, but there isn't much of a consensus on it.

If you're inclined to choose a single option that suffices for all symptoms of menopause, it should take care of your breast tenderness along with everything else. In most cases, that would be some form of estrogen plus progesterone. However, there are women who notice *more* breast tenderness when they take estrogen than they do without it. It's the imbalance between estrogen and progesterone (with more estrogen and less progesterone) that causes breast tenderness just before your period begins. Don't assume that you'll have breast tenderness with hormone replacement therapy just because you had breast tenderness with birth control pills. Because the dosages of estrogen and progesterone for menopause are so much lower than they are in birth control pills, you can't predict the response your breasts will have to them without trying them.

Chapter 18: Joint Stiffness and Joint Pain

Description

This sounds like arthritis, doesn't it? The fact is that arthritis, stiffness, and joint pain are common aspects of aging. The only type of arthritis that applies to aging or menopause is **osteoarthritis**. So, while there are various other types of arthritis, please confine your thoughts and this information to osteoarthritis only. Both males and females experience stiffness and pain in the joints as they age. It's a phenomenon of *aging* much more than it is a phenomenon of peri-menopause or post-menopause.

I've included joint pain and joint stiffness in the list of signs and symptoms of peri-menopause because it's common to notice them for the first time as you enter peri-menopause. It's also possible for them to be rather sudden. This has to do with…you guessed it…the declining levels of estrogen. Estrogen acts like a joint lubricant. Without it, your joints don't move as smoothly. You aren't undergoing rapid aging. It just seems that way because you're noticing so many new things in a relatively short period of time.

Men are different. They age more gradually. They don't have a male menopause that is as condensed or as recognizable as ours. They notice joint discomfort more slowly. It may even start earlier for them, especially if they were extremely athletic. Their testosterone levels wane over time, from age 18 onward. So, the guys do catch up with the gals in the creaky joint department.

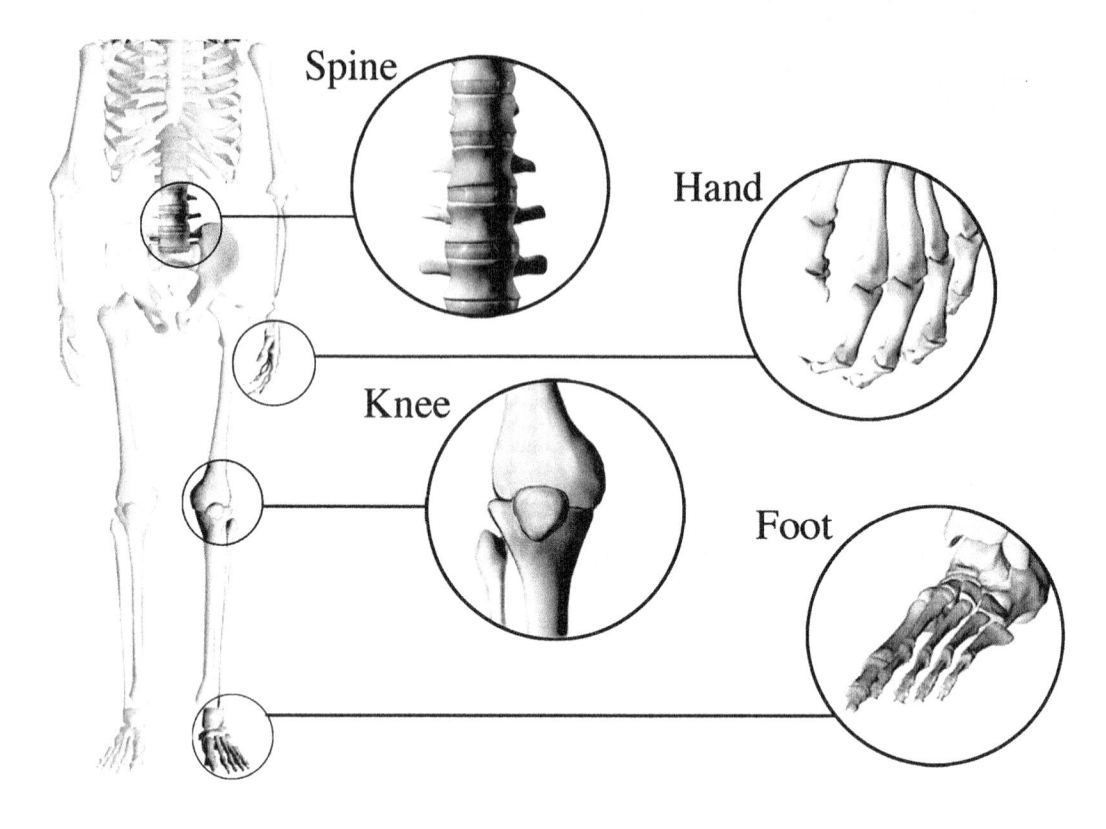

Medical Illustration Copyright © 2007 Nucleus Medical Art,
All rights reserved Figure 7: Joints affected by osteoarthritis

The best way to envision the pain and stiffness of arthritis is to think of a door and its hinges. If you were to stop opening and closing the door, its hinges would rust over time. The rusty hinges would make attempted movement of the door difficult. There would be resistance to movement. If, on the other hand, you were to continue moving the door, it wouldn't have the opportunity to rust. It would stay freely mobile, and the rust wouldn't build up.

Our joints are like the hinges of a door. A substance called *"cartilage"* covers the ends of the bones that form the hinge. Over time, some of this cartilage begins to flake off and collect in the joint space. Once there, it acts like rust to clog the joint space and make movement of the joint difficult. The joints provide us with the ability to move freely as long as we don't let them become immobile. However, because arthritis involves joint stiffness accompanied by pain, many people will resist the urge to move their painful joints. By remaining immobile, the joints have more opportunity to "rust."

We tend to become less active with age. Have you ever noticed how elderly people limit their movements? They rearrange things so that they don't have to walk as far, reach as high, bend over as much, or twist as often. All those limitations just serve to make their joints *more* stiff and "rusty." Be sure you don't limit your range of motion. Keep moving.

Management Options

Diet and Lifestyle Options

Exercise

Earlier, I likened the pain and stiffness of joints to a door with rusty hinges that prevent the door from opening and closing smoothly. The most important aspect of my analogy is that if you continue moving the door, the hinges won't rust. They'll remain mobile and there won't be as much resistance to movement.

Exercise is movement for your joints. Now, I'm not suggesting that you move your joints quickly, suddenly, or in any manner that causes increased pain. High impact activities are probably not a good idea. What I am suggesting is that you exercise in a manner that keeps your joints mobile and prevents further immobility.

There are a variety of exercise options that are gentle, slow, and beneficial for your joints. They increase the range of motion of your joints and give you more flexibility in the process. These include thorough stretching, yoga, Pilates, T'ai chi, and swimming. To top it off, they're all very relaxing, also.

There's no reason to restrict yourself to just these exercises if you're able to do more. With time, you'll notice that you're able to engage in a wider variety of exercises because your increased flexibility and mobility allow you to do so. If possible, add walking, cycling, and light weight-lifting to your regimen. Modify as necessary for your ability level and for the specific joints that are stiff. You'll be amazed with the results.

Heat

Heat works wonders for joint flexibility and comfort. You can sit in a hot tub, apply hot cloths to your joints, sit in a steam room or sauna, or attend a hot yoga class (Bikram yoga). If you live in a warm climate, you're fortunate, and if you live in a cold one, find some heat.

There are a variety of products for applying heat to various parts of your body. They're designed to fit around your knee, your back, your neck, your shoulders, etc. Most are activated by air exposure when you open the package, and they remain hot for about eight hours. There are even some small ones for hands and feet. Sometimes, they can make the difference in your ability to participate in activities which would be off limits otherwise.

Diet

Diet plays an important role in the way your joints feel and function. There are joint-friendly foods and joint-enemy foods. Knowing this will allow you to make food choices that suit your needs.

Here's a list of foods which are beneficial to joint health:

1. Fish containing omega 3 fatty acids
   (Omega 3s have the effect of reducing inflammation [swelling] of the joints. The best types of fish are fresh tuna, salmon, and halibut. Eat fish at least twice, and preferably, three times per week.)
2. Fruits and vegetables containing polyphenols, like grapes and olives
3. Vegetables which contain calcium, such as broccoli and cabbage
4. Celery and sweet potatoes for their anti-inflammatory properties
5. Spirulina, wheat grass, and barley grass
6. Kelp, for its rich iodine content

Joint Stiffness and Joint Pain

Now, for the foods which aggravate joint stiffness:

1. Acidic foods or foods which cause an acidic reaction in the body
   (There are lots of these, including tomatoes, tomato sauces, pasta sauces, red peppers, vinegar, foods made with vinegar, pickles, and pickled foods.)
2. Coffee and alcohol
3. Meat
4. Sugar and white flour

There are individual differences in how people respond to various foods. The best thing to do is to keep a food diary in which you record what you've eaten and how your joints feel shortly thereafter. This will give you information on your own unique reaction to various foods. You don't want to avoid your favorite things if you don't have to. You don't have to totally avoid joint-enemy foods. Just know how they affect your joints, and refrain from eating them when their impact on your joints is inconvenient or undesirable.

Oligomeric Proanthocyanidins (OPCs)

OPCs are foods which contain flavonoids. They restore the level of vitamin E and prevent damage to cartilage, thus alleviating the pain of arthritis. Some of the foods that contain flavonoids are grapes, blueberries, cranberries, and cherries. If you're into more bitter tastes, you can eat orange peels or lemon peels to get your flavonoids. The necessary dose is 40 - 120 mg daily.

Weight

Your joints have to support your body weight. The more you weigh, the harder it is on your joints. So, the best thing you can do for yourself is to attain and maintain ideal body weight. If you lose a significant amount of weight, you'll be amazed at how much better your joints feel. You'll find movement much more fluid and effortless, also.

Vitamin and Mineral Options

Glucosamine

Glucosamine is the most popular alternative and complementary product for the pain and inflammation of arthritis. It's a nutritional supplement rather than an herb. It promotes and maintains the function of *cartilage* in the joints. Cartilage is what flakes off the joints and into the space surrounding the joint, creating the "rust" and impaired mobility.[1]

Glucosamine is available in three forms: glucosamine hydrochloride, glucosamine sulfate, and N-acetyl-glucosamine. The most popular formulation for arthritis is glucosamine sulfate.[1]

The only side effects that have been reported for glucosamine are mild. They include heartburn, stomach ache, and diarrhea.[1]

The usual dose of glucosamine for arthritis is 1500 mg daily. The capsules are available in 500 mg portions, and it's better to take one 500 mg capsule three times daily than it is to take them all at once.[1]

Chondroitin Sulfate

Chondroitin sulfate is a substance found in fish and shark cartilage, as well as in human cartilage. It's also a nutritional supplement that promotes the production and maintenance of cartilage.[2]

The side effects of chondroitin sulfate are similar to those of glucosamine. They include mild stomach ache, nausea, and diarrhea.[2]

The recommended dose for arthritis is 1200 mg daily in divided doses. Since the tablets contain 400 mg, it is best to take one 400 mg tablet three times daily.[2]

Glucosamine Chondroitin Sulfate

This combination is the most popular nutritional supplement for arthritis. That's because it combines the tremendously beneficial effects of both glucosamine and chondroitin, while exhibiting only a few, if any, mild side effects.[2]

There are many formulations of this supplement. Be sure to read the labels to determine the amount of each substance. Buy the one that has 500 mg glucosamine and 400 mg chondroitin per tablet. Then take one tablet three times daily.[2]

Methylsulfonylmethane (MSM)

There are some claims that MSM is beneficial for arthritis, but there is no credible research to support those claims. So, for now, there is little to say about this supplement.[2]

S-Adenosyl-L-Methionine (SAMe)

SAMe is a natural substance found in the cells of the human body. It's a metabolite of the amino acid L-methionine. It has the ability to penetrate into the fluid that exists between the joints, called synovial fluid. Once there, it functions in the support of joint health, and increases mobility and comfort of the joints.

The side effects include mild stomach ache, nausea, diarrhea, and gas. Anxiety, insomnia, and overactive muscles have also been reported. However, when these side effects occur, they often diminish over time or resolve with a lower dose.

SAMe is most frequently available in 200 mg tablets. The daily dose for joint health is 200 – 1200 mg in divided doses. You should always take SAMe on an empty stomach (either one hour before a meal or two hours after a meal). Once you see improvement in your joints, you may cut the dose in half. Most people begin to notice a positive result within two weeks of starting SAMe.

Botanical and Herbal Options

Feverfew (Tanacetum parthenium)

Feverfew has anti-inflammatory properties that make it useful in the treatment of joint inflammation. Since arthritis and other forms of joint stiffness usually involve swelling or inflammation, it can be of benefit.[1]

One of the ways that Feverfew exerts its effect is to thin the blood, so it's important to refrain from using aspirin at the same time. Also, be sure to mention this to your doctor as a medication you're using. You need to stop this herb three weeks before having any surgery. Another side effect to be aware of is that it can cause extreme sensitivity if a non-topical form comes into contact with your skin.[1]

Feverfew preparations are available in both topical and ingestible forms. The dosages are as follows:

Capsules: 200 – 250 mg daily
  (There are capsules of varying mg dosages.)
Tablets: Two 12 mg tablets daily
Fresh leaf: 1 – 3 leaves (25 – 75 mg) once or twice daily[1]

Aloe (Aloe vera)

Aloe has anti-inflammatory properties that make it useful for arthritis. While it certainly isn't one of the most popular herbs used for this disease, it's widely available and generally beneficial.[1]

The most prominent side effect of Aloe is softening of the stool to the extent that it's marketed as a remedy for constipation. This side effect makes it dangerous if you use excessive amounts, because it can create an imbalance in electrolytes.[1]

The available dosages follow. The appropriate dosages for arthritis are unknown.

Capsules: 250 mg, 470 mg
Gel: 99% and 72%
Softgel tablets: 1000 mg[1]

Hormonal Medication Options

As I mentioned earlier, estrogen acts as a joint lubricant. Therefore, while estrogen isn't an actual medication for joints, it certainly makes your joints less stiff and painful. Any form of **estrogen**, either alone or in combination with progesterone or testosterone, will have a positive effect on your joints.

Non-hormonal Medication Options

The medical therapies for osteoarthritis focus on reducing inflammation. There are no medications available to stop the progress of arthritis, and there is no cure. So, the medications focus on decreasing the pain of arthritis by lessening the extent of inflammation. The enzyme that creates pain in arthritis is called cyclooxygenase (COX). It's easiest to just refer to this as "COX."

There are two forms of the COX enzyme. COX-1 exists in the gastrointestinal tract, while COX-2 exists anywhere there is inflammation. So, in this discussion on arthritis, we're primarily interested in COX-2.

Acetominophen

Acetominophen is the active ingredient in Tylenol. It reduces pain, but doesn't reduce inflammation. It has a weak and reversible ability to inhibit both COX-1 and COX-2. Acetominophen is effective in relieving the pain of arthritis, especially in the knees. The total daily dose in adults with normal liver function should not exceed 4 gm. You should take it in divided doses, every four hours throughout the day.[3]

Nonsteroidal Anti-Inflammatory Drugs (NSAIDs)

There are 26 NSAIDs available in the United States alone. They fall into two categories.[3]

The nonselective NSAIDs inhibit both COX-1 and COX-2. These include ibuprofen and naproxen (Advil, Aleve, Motrin).[3]

The selective NSAIDs have 50 times more selectivity for COX-2 than they do for COX-1. They include celecoxib (Celebrex), rofecoxib (Vioxx), and valdecoxib (Bextra).[3]

The pain relieving and anti-inflammatory effects of both the nonselective NSAIDs and the COX-2 selective NSAIDs are similar.

However, the nonselective NSAIDS relieve *pain* with lower doses, and require higher doses to reduce *inflammation*. If you fail to respond to one NSAID, it doesn't mean you won't respond to another. So, you may want to try a few. Over time, the effectiveness of one drug may decrease and you may find more relief by changing to another.[3]

The side effects of these agents include stomach aches and stomach irritation. These symptoms may be severe enough to warrant discontinuing the drug.[3]

The dosages of these medications are variable depending on your personal situation.[3]

As you may know, both rofecoxib (Vioxx) and valdecoxib (Bextra) have been removed from the market due to an association with strokes and heart attacks. Celecoxib (Celebrex) is still available. Who knows whether the strokes and heart attacks are a direct result of these drugs or whether the patients using them were already at high risk for these diseases? Face it; people with arthritis tend to be sedentary, and therefore overweight and physically unfit. That alone makes them high risk for both strokes and heart attacks.

The message is that you have to weigh benefits and risks individually. If you're a thin, fit, active person and you consume a low fat diet, don't smoke, and don't have any risks for stroke or heart attack, you may be a good candidate for a medication of this type for your arthritis.

Steroids

Sometimes, an injection of steroids into the joint itself serves to reduce inflammation and improve function of the joint. This is usually a last resort before more invasive options, like surgery, become necessary.[3] If you require steroids by mouth rather than by injection into the joint itself, beware of the fact that they cause significant weight gain. They also tend to increase your risk of osteoporosis.

Chapter 19: Dry Skin

Description

As a female, estrogen has made your skin softer and smoother than that of a male. But when you start losing estrogen during perimenopause, you may notice that your skin becomes dry and itchy. You may notice that you need more lotion and moisturizer than you did previously.

Skin Anatomy

Your skin consists of three layers. The outer layer of dead skin undergoes constant replacement by new, moist cells from the lower layers. Now, I know this sounds more like snake skin than it does human skin, but, believe it or not, we do slough our skin. As we age, the efficiency with which we accomplish this sloughing process decreases, leaving skin more dry and scaly.

Beneath the outer layer, there is a layer of collagen. Collagen gives your skin its taught, elastic tone. The aging process involves loss of collagen, leaving skin more lax. Additionally, the moisturizing oils of your skin decrease, leaving your skin dry. Skin damage, in the form of sun exposure, smoking, and pollution causes collagen to break down, also. The result is that your skin wrinkles.

The lowermost layer of skin is the basal layer. Think of it as the foundation for the skin. It contains fat, which increases in some areas of your body, and decreases in others.

The layer that causes your skin changes at the time of menopause is the middle layer. The collagen decides to "let go," which you see as wrinkles. The interesting thing is that it seems to happen all of a sudden. It's as if the collagen provides support and tone for your skin, and then, one day, just can't take it anymore, and gives up.

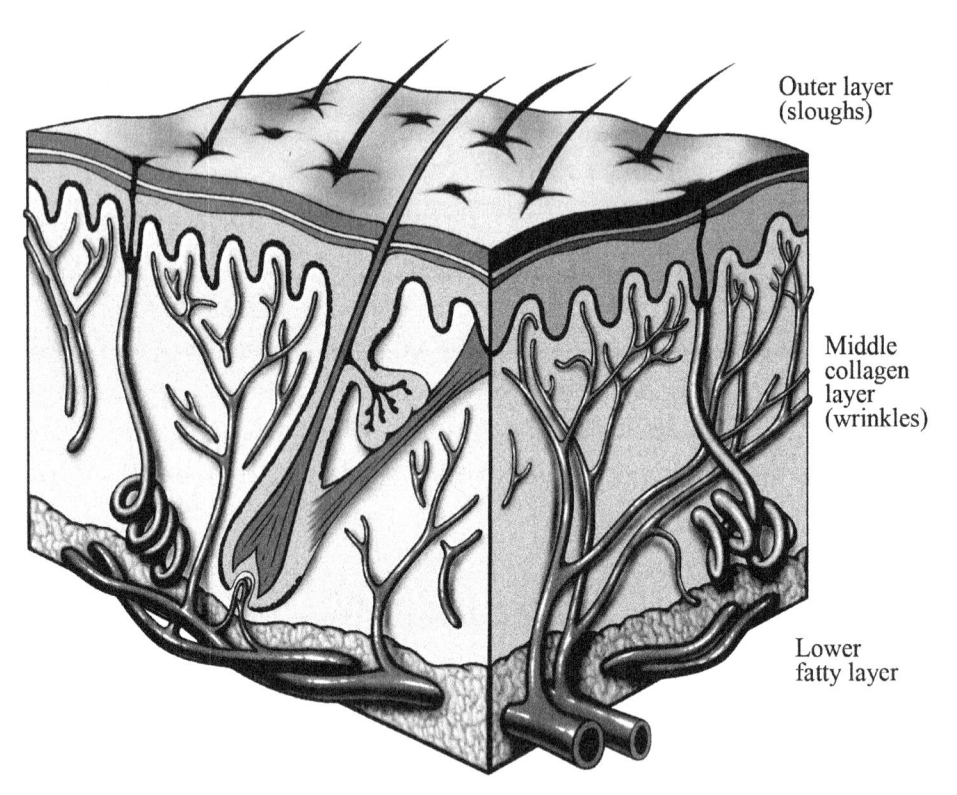

Figure 8: Layers of the skin

So, if you add up all the effects of dry skin due to lack of estrogen, inefficient sloughing, loss of collagen, and wrinkling, you notice a lot of changes in your skin. It all makes sense, but you probably don't care about how sensible it is. You want soft, unwrinkled skin.

Management Options

Diet and Lifestyle Options

Sun Protection

Avoiding sun exposure is one of the best things you can do to preserve your skin in its moist, well-supported, unwrinkled state. While sunscreen is a good practice, it's even better to simply cover your skin with thin, light clothing to avoid sun exposure. You should use sunscreen on your face, neck and hands every day.

Some exposure to the sun is healthy, and provides you with vitamin D. The best times of day to get sun exposure are early in the morning and late in the afternoon. All you need is 20 minutes. And you only need to expose your hands and arms to get adequate quantities of vitamin D.

Sun affects your skin by causing two types of changes in your skin. First, it makes your skin very thick, like leather; second, it causes your skin to wrinkle, forming deep crevices. Neither change is attractive. If you were a sun goddess at an early age, you'll see the effects of sun damage more prominently as you reach menopause.

Skin is elastic, and it ages in a strange manner. It holds its tone and shape for years, and then, all of a sudden, it just lets go and begins to sag. The more sun exposure it's had over the years, the earlier it loses its tone. Sun exposure is a guaranteed way to get your skin to sag sooner. So, avoid it.

Water

Did you know that your body is composed of cells that consist primarily of water? That's right: 75% of your muscle and 25% of your fat are water. On average, 65% of the human body is water. And, did you know that the largest organ in the human body is your skin? Nothing is more beneficial to your skin than supplying it with more of its main constitutional substance. The first step in the process of wrinkling and thickening is loss of moisture. That's why the most important thing for your skin is water. You should drink *at least* eight 8 oz glasses of water daily. This is the *minimal* requirement. More is better. The best way to drink an adequate quantity of water is to carry a water bottle with you everywhere you go and just take a sip every few minutes. Don't worry; you won't look strange because this has become a fashionable thing to do.

Try this simple experiment. Drink loads of water daily for two weeks. Drink enough to make your urine practically clear every time you urinate. That's all you have to do. Then, pay attention to what people say about your skin. No doubt, you'll get some questions as to what you're using on your skin or what you've had done to your skin. It's impressive.

Diet

Fiber is an important factor for skin. Most people don't eat nearly enough fiber. You can get adequate fiber by consuming 1 tsp - 1 tbsp flaxseed daily if your diet doesn't provide adequate amounts. Sprinkle it on salads, in cereals, or eat it plain. It's necessary to crush it first. Of course, there are a multitude of other sources of fiber, also. Fruit, vegetables, grains, and beans are good choices.

Fatty fish (salmon and sardines) provides omega 3 fatty acids that are important for skin. Fish two to three times weekly is ideal. I guess it seems ironic that fatty fish have scaly skin even though they have such high quantities of omega 3 fatty acids in their own bodies. It would make more sense for them to have soft, smooth skin. Nevertheless, the omega 3 fatty acids in fish make *your* skin look great. They make it smooth and supple, and give it a special glow.

Lotion

Lotion, lotion, lotion. Replenishing the moisture in your skin requires large quantities of lotion. You should apply lotion, from your head to your toes, daily after bathing. Use a thick, rich lotion rather than a thin runny one. Alternatively, you may use massage oil. You may also need to use paraffin occasionally to seal moisture in your skin.

Remember to reapply moisturizer throughout the day if it gets rinsed off or if you sweat.

Vitamin and Mineral Options

Antioxidant Vitamins

Antioxidant vitamins are the ones of interest with regard to the skin. **Vitamins C**, **E**, and **A** are the antioxidant vitamins. Vitamins C and E are especially good for your skin. They stimulate collagen and can actually reverse the appearance of sun-damaged skin. Dosages are as follows:

Vitamin C: 200 mg daily
Vitamin E: 1000 IU daily
Vitamin A: 3333 IU daily

Additionally, **Coenzyme Q10 (CoQ10)**, **Alpha Lipoic Acid (ALA)**, and **Proanthocyanidins** are also essential for skin health. Here are the dosages:

Coenzyme Q10: 30 – 100 mg daily
Alpha Lipoic Acid: 300 mg daily
Proanthocyanidins: 40 – 120 mg daily

Botanical and Herbal Options

Green Tea (Camellia sinensis)

Green tea is a wonderful antioxidant herb. It inhibits the negative effects of ultraviolet light, thus preventing skin damage. A cup a day can work wonders in keeping skin youthful. One cup of green tea contains 50 – 100 mg of polyphenols, which are the skin-enhancing ingredients. If you prefer, you may take it in the form of a capsule or tablet in a dose of 100 mg daily.

Hormonal Medication Options

Estrogen

Topical estrogen increases the thickness of collagen, increases moisture of your skin, and decreases the size of skin pores. The dose is 1 gm (containing 0.01% estradiol and 0.3% estriol) daily. Direct application in the form of a cream isn't the only route to soft, smooth skin. You can take estrogen in any of its other forms and improve the moisture of your skin, also.

Progesterone

Topical progesterone possibly improves skin. It's not as effective as estrogen, but suffices for some women. The dose is nonspecific. Just rub a small amount of 2% progesterone into your skin.

Chapter 20: Hair Loss on the Scalp

Hair Phases

Hair has three phases: (1) A growth phase (anagen) lasting about seven years, when your hair gets longer; (2) A resting phase (telogen) of about two to four months, when your hair just takes a break from all activity; and (3) A falling out phase (catagen), when you lose hair. Normally, there are hairs in each of these three phases at all times so that one phase is not greatly dominant over the others. Under such conditions, you don't notice significant changes in your hair. The duration of each phase varies from one body location to another.

Anything that synchronizes the hairs, so that a majority of them are all in the same phase, will create a situation in which you notice changes in your hair. Hormones just happen to have such an effect. Many women comment about the fact that their hair changed when they were pregnant. It may have gotten straighter, curlier, thicker, or thinner. That's because the high levels of hormones during pregnancy synchronized their hairs to an extent that created a noticeable difference overall.

During the process of peri-menopause, the loss of estrogen has a tendency to place more hairs in the falling out phase, which you perceive as hair loss. The effect is different in various parts of your body, so hair loss in some locations is more apparent than in others.

Male hormones (androgens) also have an effect on hair. At menopause, the male to female hormone ratio changes, and there is a predominance of male hormones. Androgens act on scalp hair to shorten the growth phase of scalp hair.

I know you're thinking that I'm building up to something here. And I am. So, hang on to your wig!

For the majority of women, the most common pattern of hair loss during peri-menopause is male pattern baldness. You know, thinning on the top of your head. This is common for 37% of peri- menopausal women. I know, I know, ugh! If you're thinking, "This is really getting bad," read on. Remember, I'll be giving you solutions for all these things.

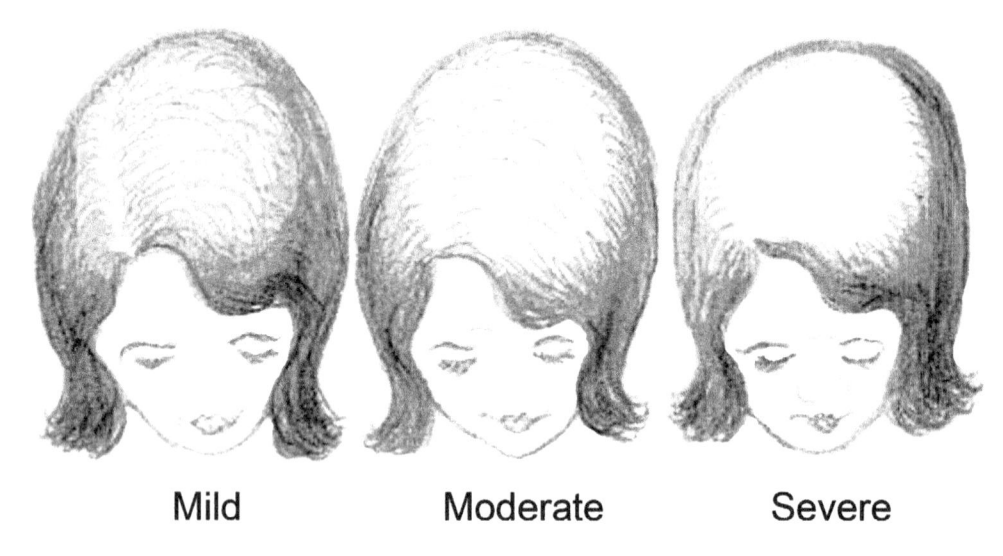

Mild **Moderate** **Severe**

Figure 9: Male pattern baldness

Management Options

Diet and Lifestyle Options

Weight Control

Weight control is important in limiting hair loss because fat cells produce extra androgens, which stimulate male pattern baldness. So, use a safe, reasonable method to attain and maintain your ideal body weight.

Reduce Hair Manipulation

You may have experimented with or adopted a routine of manipulating your hair in some way over the years. It may look great, but it may also make your hair fall out more easily. Unfortunately, it doesn't take a lot to induce hair loss. Something as simple as too much brushing can do it. Then there's curling, straightening, blow drying, highlighting, low lighting, dying, and extending. It's amazing how much stuff we do to our hair! Maybe just being more gentle with your hair will make a difference.

Vitamin and Mineral Options

Multivitamin

A well-balanced, multiple vitamin supplement, designed specifically for women, is a great idea here. Not only will it help provide all the necessary vitamins and minerals for maintenance of hair growth, but it will also have an overall beneficial effect on your well-being.

Hair Growth Vitamins and Minerals

Most health food stores and nutrition centers have various brands of products that are specifically designed to enhance hair growth and hair strength. Most contain an array of vitamins and minerals for healthy hair, skin, and nails. They're harmless as long as you're aware of the total daily intake of the vitamins that are duplicated in any other vitamin and mineral preparations you consume.

These products usually contain the following ingredients:

Vitamin B1 (Thiamine)
Vitamin B2 (Riboflavin)
Vitamin C
Niacinamide
Folate (Vitamin B9)
Biotin
Vitamin B5 (Pantothenic Acid)
Horsetail silica

MSM (Methylsulfonylmethane)
Choline
PABA (Para Aminobutyric Acid)
L-cysteine
Zinc

Botanical and Herbal Options

Wu Pian is a Chinese herb that has shown good results in inducing hair growth and reducing grey hair.[1] You might have difficulty finding much literature on this one, though. I did.

Hormonal Medication Options

Estrogen

Any form of estrogen, alone or in combination with progesterone or testosterone, will have an effect on improving hair loss. It does so by increasing the ratio of estrogen to other hormones in the body.

Birth Control Pills

Birth control pills serve to balance the ratio of androgen to estrogen, decreasing the hair follicle's susceptibility to the effects of the androgen. Thus, the male pattern of baldness doesn't have an opportunity to establish itself.

Non-hormonal Medication Options

Dexamethasone

Dexamethasone is a powerful steroid that suppresses androgen production. It has the typical significant side effects of most steroids, including a reduction in the body's ability to fight infection, an increase in the risk of bone loss (osteoporosis), and an increased risk of diabetes.

Spironolactone

Spironolactone is an androgen inhibitor that serves to decrease testosterone. It's most valuable in the form of a pill taken orally for purposes of preventing hair loss on your scalp.

Minoxidil (Rogaine)

Minoxidil is a medication for high blood pressure that has the convenient side effect of causing hair growth. It's available in the form of a spray or liquid that you can apply directly to your scalp in the areas needing more hair growth. It's approved by the FDA (Food and Drug Administration) for use in inducing hair growth, and doesn't require a prescription. It is sometimes combined with Tretinoin (Retin A), with excellent results. Side effects are rare and mild, consisting of possible skin irritation and mild, temporary increase in heart rate.

Chapter 21: Hair Growth in Undesirable Locations

Description

Now isn't it ironic that you would have loss of hair in *desirable* locations at the same time that you have growth of hair in *undesirable* locations? It just seems like Mother Nature is confused. It certainly isn't nature at its best!

The reason for hair growth in undesirable places is similar to the reason for hair loss. The hair growth that is characteristic of perimenopause involves growth of thick, coarse, mostly dark hair. "Oh great," you say? Well just wait until you discover *where* this hair typically grows! It appears on your *face* of all places. Can you believe that? Many women notice the presence of thick, coarse, dark hair on their chin and upper lip as they approach menopause. These "whiskers" are a result of an increase in the amount of male hormone (testosterone) relative to the amount of female hormone (estrogen).

This imbalance in the ratio of androgens to estrogens also contributes to the loss of hair that I described in the previous section. It induces the shortening of the growth phase, causing the hair on your head to become finer and thinner. It wouldn't be so bad if the hair growth on your face were fine and thin. But, no, it's thick and coarse where you want it to be fine and thin, and fine and thin where you want it to be thick and coarse.

Male pattern balding and growth of whiskers is the same hair pattern of loss and growth that are normal for men. Males have both estrogen and testosterone, but the ratio between the two favors baldness and facial hair. The hormone shifts of menopause bring your ratio of male to female hormones closer to that of a male. That's why you notice balding and whiskers. All this, just when you needed something to make you feel *more* attractive and sexy, not less!

Management Options

Mechanical Options

Waxing

Waxing is a readily available, mildly uncomfortable procedure with which most women have either personal or indirect familiarity. It's quick, and results in regrowth of hair that's thinner and lighter in color. You need to allow the hair to grow back before repeating the waxing procedure, so you wax infrequently and notice recurrent hair growth in between waxes. Immediately after waxing, and for a few days afterwards, the area is entirely hair-free.

Electrolysis

Electrolysis consists of directing an electric current into the hair follicle through a needle. This is done one hair at a time, so it takes a while to remove the hair from hairy areas. It's not the most comfortable procedure, so you may choose to do only a few hairs in a single session. Another consideration is to apply a topical anesthetic cream an hour before the procedure. You wouldn't want to use electrolysis in large areas of hair growth. It would be too painful and take a very long time.

Electrolysis is available at salons designed specifically for the procedure. It's also a common service at spas. You'll find that you will require multiple treatments, usually on a monthly basis. So, I vote for going to a spa, having the electrolysis, and coupling it with some luxurious treatments while you're there. It'll ease the pain a bit, I'm certain.

Laser

Laser hair removal is a more technical, evolving practice. You should consult a physician who specializes in laser hair removal if you choose this route. It's painful enough to warrant a topical anesthetic cream, and may be more permanent than electrolysis.

Hormonal Medication Options

Estrogen

Any form of estrogen, alone or in combination with progesterone or testosterone, will have an effect on reducing hair growth in undesirable locations. It does so by increasing the ratio of estrogen to other hormones in the body.

Birth Control Pills

Birth control pills decrease or inhibit hair growth by decreasing the effect of androgen on the hair follicle. This usually results in thinner, lighter hair. It's possible for birth control pills to inhibit hair growth altogether.

Non-hormonal Medication Options

Spironolactone

Spironolactone counteracts the effects of male hormones. Thus, it's an anti-androgen. For purposes of hair removal, it's best to apply it topically, so that it targets the hair follicle directly and limits the amount of androgen that affects the hair follicle.

Dexamethasone

Dexamethasone actually suppresses the production of androgens. It's a very powerful steroid. It increases the amount of hair on your head, while decreasing the amount of hair on your face. It has significant side effects, however. These include an increased susceptibility to infection, an increase in the risk of bone loss (osteoporosis), and an increase in the risk of diabetes.

Eflornithine Hydrochloride (Vaniqa Cream)

Vaniqa is a cream that reduces unwanted hair on your face. It requires a prescription. It doesn't cause the hair on your face to fall out, and it doesn't prevent it from growing in the first place. It works by slowing the growth of hair on your face. You'll probably still have to do some of the other things listed here to get things under control. Vaniqa will help you in the long term, but not in the short term.

You use Vaniqa by applying a thin layer of the cream to the areas of your face that have unwanted hair. Also cover the areas closest to the hairy ones. Leave it on for at least four hours. Do this twice a day, separated by at least eight hours. The results aren't immediate. It takes time to affect the growth of hair. Use it for at least six months in order to see a real difference.[1]

Chapter 22: Vaginal Dryness

Vaginal Anatomy

An understanding as to why vaginal dryness plays a part in perimenopause requires a basic review of vaginal anatomy and physiology. Here are the basics in just a few sentences.

The vagina is a hollow tube. However, the sidewalls of the vagina are not smooth. They're extremely wrinkled. Envision a stretchy tube-top that you can bunch up and wear as a midriff, or stretch out and wear down to your hips. The wrinkles in a tube-top allow you to change its size and shape. That's what the wrinkles in the vagina do, too. These wrinkles in the vaginal walls are called **vaginal rugae**. The purpose of the wrinkles is to allow the vagina to stretch. Because of these wrinkles, the vagina can lengthen, as it does during intercourse, and it can widen, as it does during childbirth.

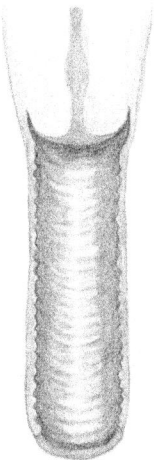

Figure 10: Vaginal rugae (folds)

These vaginal wrinkles make the walls of the vagina quite thick. Thick vaginal walls are necessary for the vagina to withstand the friction that's produced during intercourse. Estrogen is the substance that keeps the vaginal walls thick. It's also the substance that keeps the vagina moist. At this point, you can probably see where we're going with all of this.

In the absence of estrogen during peri- and post-menopause, the vaginal walls become very thin, dry, and fragile. There's no estrogen to keep them thick and healthy. It's no different than dry skin that needs lotion to keep it thick and moist. Because it's so dry, the vagina becomes itchy. Just think of estrogen as the vagina's favorite lotion. Without it, the vagina becomes itchy, just as dry skin does. Additionally, intercourse becomes uncomfortable, even painful, due to the thin vaginal walls. The term for these thin, fragile vaginal walls is **vaginal atrophy**.

Because of these changes in the vagina, many symptoms are possible, including itching, dryness, pressure, tenderness, burning, unusual-smelling discharge, lack of lubrication, and painful intercourse.

The vagina is very selfish in its need for estrogen. It needs estrogen more than many other part of the body. Some women require estrogen to keep the vagina happy even if they don't require estrogen for any other reason. Some women who are not estrogen deficient or who take estrogen supplementation still require local application of additional estrogen to the vagina.

There are estrogen creams, both pharmaceutical and non-pharmaceutical, for this purpose.

Management Options

Diet and Lifestyle Options

Sexual Activity

Sexual activity works wonders to maintain vaginal health during and after menopause.[1] Masturbation may also help in maintaining vaginal secretions and elasticity.[1] Now see, there *are* some management options that are just plain fun. It's just the opposite of adolescence. Then, you were *discouraged* from having sex; now, you're *encouraged* to have it.

The reason sexual intercourse and masturbation keep your vagina in good shape is because they both prevent vaginal atrophy. You know how muscles atrophy if you don't use them? Well, the vagina is similar. Vaginal atrophy refers to a thinning and drying out of your vaginal walls. It loses all the wrinkles that made it able to endure the friction of intercourse. It stops producing the lubrication that kept it moist. So, if you keep up the sexual activity, your vagina won't atrophy. It's a "use it or lose it" phenomenon.

Diet

Soy

Soy-based foods, including tofu and tempeh, contain estrogen in the form of phytoestrogens. This has the same effect as natural estrogen in providing vaginal lubrication. However, it requires a tremendous amount of soy because phytoestrogens are a lot weaker than human or pharmaceutical estrogen.

Mechanical Options

Lubricants

The most basic, non-medical means of managing vaginal dryness is to apply vaginal lubricants to the vagina. They constitute temporary measures for relief of vaginal dryness during intercourse.[2] They consist of a combination of thickening agents and skin protectants in a water-soluble base.[2] They have a short duration of action, such that they are not a long-term solution to the problem of vaginal dryness. You can use lubricants in anticipation of intercourse only, or at all times.

The most widely available lubricant is K-Y Jelly, which is water soluble. Sylk is another lubricant that is an extract of kiwi fruit. There are also some herbal lubricants, such as Emerita's Personal Lubricant. Health food stores have a variety of products from which to choose.

Moisturizers

Moisturizes tend to provide more than transient lubrication. The most popular moisturizer is Replens. It's an adhesive that holds water in place against the vaginal surface until it sloughs off, which is usually after 24 hours or more.[2] It requires only one to two applications a week, and doesn't require reapplication prior to sexual intercourse.[2] It lowers the pH (acid – base balance) of the vagina, which improves all the vaginal symptoms of menopause. Replens does result in a clumpy, residual discharge, so it's wise to wear a panty liner to avoid soiling your clothes.[2]

Vitamin and Mineral Options

Vitamin E

Vitamin E has some mild vaginal lubricating effects. This is mostly due to the fact that it has a moisturizing effect on skin in general.

Botanical and Herbal Options

A number of the herbal therapies that are useful for the management of menopause have the ability to provide vaginal lubrication and resolve the discomfort of vaginal dryness. These herbs include **phytoestrogens, Black Cohosh, Dong Quai, Chasteberry, Joyful Change,** and **Wild Yam.** None of these herbs has a specific indication for vaginal dryness. They're all commonly promoted for management of menopause in general, and their ability to reduce vaginal dryness is due to their estrogen-like effect.

Hormonal Medication Options

Estrogen

All forms of estrogen have the effect of providing vaginal lubrication. Estrogen helps maintain the normal acidity (pH) of the vagina so that bacteria don't grow. Without estrogen, the vagina becomes less acidic. That results in a discharge and an odor.

Vaginal Dryness

Local therapy in the form of <u>estrogen cream</u> is easy to use. Most creams undergo minimal absorption into the blood stream. Estradiol vaginal cream is quite popular. The dosage is 0.5 mg twice a day for one week, then two to three times weekly thereafter.

<u>Estrogen vaginal tablets</u> are also effective. Dosage is one tablet in the vagina every other day for two weeks, followed by one tablet twice weekly.

<u>Estrogen vaginal suppositories</u> are similar to tablets. The dose is 0.5 mg every night for two weeks, and then twice weekly thereafter.[2]

An <u>estrogen vaginal ring</u> is also available. This is a flexible silicone ring that remains in your vagina for 12 weeks. It delivers estrogen in a daily dose that depends on the total amount of estrogen in the ring.[2] The ring distributes estrogen throughout your body.

<u>Estrogen skin patches</u> provide adequate estrogen for all aspects of menopause if the dose is appropriate. The advantage of patches over pills is that absorption through your skin eliminates the need for the estrogen to travel through your digestive system (especially the liver) before reaching the blood stream. Skin patches allow the medication to permeate your skin and go directly into your blood stream. The Estraderm, Alora, Ecslim, Vivelle and Vivelle-Dot patches are designed for twice weekly application. The Climara patch only requires once weekly application.[2]

Estrogen therapy has the effect of restoring vaginal cells, increasing vaginal secretions, increasing thickness of the vaginal walls, increasing blood flow to the vagina, and restoring the bacterial flora to one resembling pre-menopause.[1]

Note: <u>SERMs</u> (Selective Estrogen Receptor Modulators) have some of the properties of estrogen, but, unfortunately, don't have anything to offer in the realm of improving vaginal dryness.[2] In fact, they tend to *increase* vaginal dryness.

Testosterone

Testosterone is also effective in treating vaginal dryness. The dose is 0.5 - 1 mg daily or every third day for either the vaginal cream or the skin patch. The benefit of testosterone is that some of it turns into estrogen and helps with some of the other symptoms of menopause (hot flashes and night sweats). It doesn't result in excessively high estrogen levels.[3]

Tibolone

Tibolone is a synthetic hormone product with weak properties similar to estrogen, progesterone, and testosterone.[2] It is effective in improving vaginal dryness and painful intercourse due to vaginal dryness. It does *not* increase the risk of uterine cancer.[2]

Chapter 23:
Urinary Problems

Anatomy

Normal Anatomy

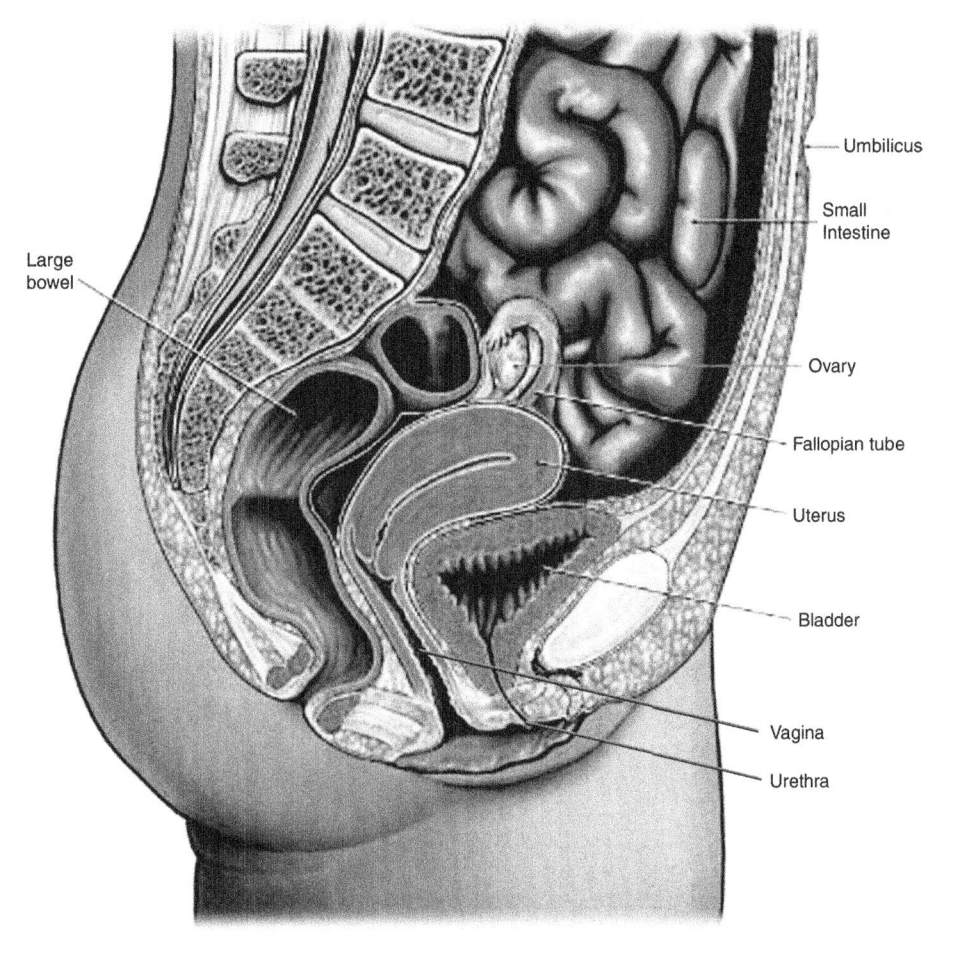

Sagittal view
Medical Illustration Copyright © 2008 Nucleus Medical Art, All rights reserved

Figure 11: Anatomy of the female reproductive tract

Here's a picture of the female reproductive anatomy. It represents what your internal organs look like if you sliced a body in half and looked at it from the side. It will be your reference illustration for this section, and I'll refer to it repeatedly.

Urinary problems are fairly common during the phases of menopause. This is primarily due to the fact that the vagina and the urinary system are located in the same general area. Urine leaves your body through a tube called the **urethra**. Now, I don't know if you've ever attempted to identify your urethra, but if you tried, you would discover that it's located up in between your labia, near the opening of your vagina, and it's difficult to identify on your own body.

Look at the figure above. Do you see that thin tube extending downward from the bladder? That's the urethra. It's only a few millimeters from the vagina, which is the tube just to the left of the urethra, and extending down from the uterus. Pay attention to the fact that the urethra is pretty small and frail compared to the other structures nearby.

At menopause, loss of estrogen starves the vagina and urethra of their hormonal support. This loss of support presents itself in the form of loss of muscle tone in the pelvic region.

In the previous section, I mentioned the fact that the vagina needs a lot of estrogen. As you might expect, because the urethra is in the vaginal area, it also needs a lot of estrogen. Without estrogen, the urethra becomes very angry. It manifests that anger in a number of ways, most notably, urinary tract infections and urinary incontinence (leakage).

Urinary Tract Infections (UTIs)

Cause

One urinary symptom of menopause is frequent urinary tract infections. These occur because the tissue at the opening of the urethra is dependent on estrogen to keep the cells functioning in their ability to ward off bacteria. Without estrogen, bacteria are able to get into the urethra and travel to the bladder, creating a urinary tract infection. This manifests as burning during urination, blood in the urine, and cramping in the area of the bladder.

The acid-base balance (designated as pH) of the vagina has a lot to do with the development of vaginal and urinary infections. Before perimenopause begins, the pH of the vagina is 3.5 – 4.5. This is in the low (acidic) range of pH values. This acidic environment discourages the growth of bacteria.[1] After menopause ensues, the acidic environment becomes more basic in pH, with values greater than five. This allows more bacteria to grow. The result is that you're more prone to infections.

Symptoms

A urinary tract infection is quite obvious. It really gets your attention, even if you're not paying much attention to your urinary system. Typically, you'll notice severe burning during urination. It's painful enough to make you stop your urinary stream, and to cringe when you start it again. Another common sign is blood in your urine. This indicates a more severe infection, and usually occurs with the burning sensation I described above. Bladder cramping is also possible. It feels like a dull, achy sensation that persists whether or not you're urinating. Almost any woman who's had a urinary tract infection can describe it to you in accurate detail.

Management Options

Diet and Lifestyle Options

Any obstetrician/gynecologist can tell you that Saturday and Sunday mornings are notorious for numerous calls from patients with urinary tract infections. That's because weekend evenings are hazardous to urinary health. The typical behaviors that create the weekend morning urinary tract infection go something like this:

The evening activities involve alcohol, and plenty of it. And, because you are busy drinking alcohol, you have no time or interest in drinking water. So, you become dehydrated from the alcohol and fail to have any desire to urinate. After all this excessive alcohol consumption and non-water drinking, you end up significantly dehydrated. There's really not much urine in your bladder, and the little bit that's there is highly concentrated. Then you indulge in sexual intercourse, which does a wonderful job of thrusting bacteria into your urethral opening. Once there, the bacteria migrate up your urethra and into your bladder. Since there's no urine in your bladder to induce you to urinate and flush out the bacteria, and since you're so relaxed from the alcohol, you just fall asleep after intercourse. The bacteria just love the highly concentrated urine in your bladder, and use it to breed and replicate throughout the night. They reproduce into a huge army of bacteria, and, voila! You wake up with severe burning upon urination.

The scenario above is the absolute best way to guarantee that you'll get a massive urinary tract infection. It works every time.

The lessons to learn from that little vignette follow. Keep these in mind in an effort to prevent urinary tract infections.

Drink plenty of water. It fills the bladder; it dilutes any bacteria that reside there; and it causes you to urinate frequently. Drink a minimum of 12 ounces of water for every alcoholic beverage you consume. Cranberry juice is also a good alternative drink because its acidity makes it difficult for bacteria to adhere to the bladder wall, and ultimately prevents urinary tract infections.

Urinate very frequently, ideally once every one to two hours. You should be drinking enough water to send you to the bathroom at least every two hours. And, your urine should be dilute. It should be clear to slightly yellow-tinged. It shouldn't be deep yellow in color.

Always, always urinate after intercourse. In the figure above, did you notice how close the opening of the urethra is to the opening of the vagina? Well, the fact that the urethra and the vagina are so close to one another has special significance when it comes to urinary tract infections. The bottom line is this: There's *no way* you can have intercourse without pushing bacteria into your urethra. It doesn't matter what position you assume for intercourse, or whether you use condoms, or what you attempt to do to avoid it. It's simply unavoidable! Mere insertion of the penis into the vagina deposits bacteria into the urethra, and the thrusting actions of intercourse only augment the process. The bacteria creep up the urethra and into the bladder. Once there, they find the perfect environment to have a big party and to replicate rapidly. (I guess you could say they have an orgy!)

So, it's your job to flush the bacteria out of your bladder and urethra after intercourse. You can do this simply by urinating after intercourse. I mean *immediately* after intercourse. Even a little dribble of urine can flush out large numbers of bacteria from the bladder and urethra. This may not seem romantic, but neither is a burning urethra the following morning. Train your partner to literally force you to go to the bathroom to urinate after intercourse. Believe me, it's no fun for him when you have a urinary tract infection, either.

Practice good pelvic hygiene. Let me clarify something about the term "pelvic hygiene." It means keeping your genital region clean by means of regular bathing. It *doesn't* mean that you should douche!

Douching is actually *detrimental* to your vaginal and urinary health. It's what women used to do ages ago when water was unavailable for bathing. Douching was their only option. It was better than not bathing at all. That's no longer the case for women living outside third world countries.

Douching *increases* your risk of urinary tract infections and vaginal yeast infections because it flushes away all the good bacteria which keep your vaginal environment healthy. It changes the pH (acid – base) balance to one which allows bacteria and yeast to grow more readily.

Finally, **don't ingest things that make your urine concentrated, like caffeine and soft drinks.** If you do, be sure to balance them with plenty of water to dilute it again.

Urinary Incontinence

Incidence

Another symptom of the menopausal process is leaking of your urine. The term for this is **urinary incontinence**. This is one of those entities that is really common, yet no one talks about it. Don't hesitate to mention it to your healthcare provider. It's amazing how many women fail to mention it and suffer in silence. Speak up! Urinary incontinence is a problem for 15% to 35% of menopausal women. You're incontinent if you used to be able to control your urine, and later notice difficulty in doing so. This occurs as a result of many things.

Causes

The most significant contributor to urinary incontinence is pregnancy. Once again, refer to the figure above. Do you see where the uterus is? *It's smack dab on top of the bladder!* During pregnancy, your uterus increases by *1000 times*. It becomes huge and heavy, and it remains on top of your poor little bladder for the entire pregnancy. It's not easy for your bladder to support the weight of a huge uterus. And if it's difficult for the bladder, just think how difficult it must be for your frail little urethra. The process of pregnancy involves carrying a heavy uterus, which contains a baby, a placenta, and lots of amniotic fluid, all resting on your bladder for months and months.

After months of sustaining all this extra weight, your tired bladder and urethra then must endure the pushing required to deliver the baby. Did you think that they just stayed in place and ignored all the forces of pushing out a baby? Of course not! When you push to deliver a baby, your bladder and urethra get "bent out of shape" so to speak. They move downward over and over again.

All these months of pregnancy, along with all the hours it takes to push out a baby, add up. Eventually, your bladder and urethra just can't take it anymore! As a response to supporting all the weight and forces of pregnancy, your bladder and urethra lose some of their muscle tone. It's similar to the difference between a buff, tone, muscular body and an overweight, non-muscular body. The tissues of your body have a certain amount of elasticity. For a time, they'll spring back into their tone, taught state. But, not forever. Eventually, they lose their elasticity, and they become slack. Continued pressure or stretching results in loss of your tissues' ability to return to their taut, well-supported state. At some point, your tissues give up and become lax.

In the urinary system, the urethra has muscle surrounding it. After a few pregnancies, repeated sessions of pushing, and the aging process itself, that muscle becomes weak. This is the very muscle which has to contract in order to hold your urine and prevent leakage. It's the same muscle that you tighten when you hold your urine until you find a toilet. The process of menopause adds the absence of estrogen to the lax muscle surrounding the urethra. It's as if estrogen nourished the muscle to keep it strong enough to at least hold urine. In the absence of estrogen, the muscle loses its sustenance and its strength. Once that happens, you begin to leak urine.

Types of Incontinence

Stress Urinary Incontinence (SUI)

You may notice incontinence primarily when you cough, sneeze, laugh, lift something heavy, or exercise. This is because all of these events place sudden extra pressure on the bladder, forcing urine into the urethra. It's difficult for the weak muscle surrounding the urethra to tighten in order to prevent leakage. The pressure constitutes stress on the bladder and urethra, so we call this type of urinary incontinence "Stress Urinary Incontinence." We use the acronym SUI to refer to this phenomenon.

Urge Incontinence

Alternatively, you may notice incontinence before your bladder becomes full, without any form of stress to make your urine leak. Your bladder may contract spontaneously and involuntarily, creating a sudden overwhelming urge to urinate. The result is that there is a sensation that the urine will begin to leak. Sometimes it does leak. We call this phenomenon "Urge Incontinence." Urge incontinence has much more of an impact on your quality of life because it's so unpredictable, and the leaks can be huge gushes of urine that you just can't control.

Incontinence of any kind can be a distracting and demoralizing problem.[2] Surprisingly, many women fail to tell their healthcare provider that they are experiencing incontinence. They find it embarrassing and humiliating to volunteer such information. Unfortunately, many healthcare providers fail to inquire about it. As a result, this is a very common, often unaddressed problem for many women. If you have incontinence, simply say so. Saying, "I leak" is enough to get the discussion started. Then specify the circumstances that cause you to leak. Don't be embarrassed. It's a common problem, but it isn't normal. You don't have to live with it. There are plenty of ways to help you.

Management Options

Diet and Lifestyle Options

Kegel Exercises

Kegel exercises are strengthening exercises for the muscles which surround the urethra. The urethra is the tube through which your urine travels to exit your body. There are muscles at its base which have the effect of creating a sphincter (or closure) to inhibit the flow of urine out of the urethra. Think of the muscles around your urethra as if they're the drawstring on a cloth bag. If you open the bag, the strings relax, allowing the bag to remain open. If you tighten the drawstrings, the bag closes, and keeps its contents from spilling out. That's how the muscles around your urethra work. You can tighten them to keep urine in or you can relax them to let urine out.

Kegel exercises entail tightening the same muscle that you contract to stop a stream of urine. These drills require that you hold the contraction for ten seconds, relax for five seconds, and repeat the process five times. You should do these exercises five times daily. Because no one can tell you're doing them, feel free to perform Kegels anywhere. They may be the only exercise you can do without sweating, raising your heart rate, or making it obvious that you're exercising at all.

Kegels are multi-purpose in that, in addition to strengthening the urethral muscles, they strengthen your pelvic muscles. The muscles surrounding your vagina get a great workout, and become stronger. As a result, they serve to improve both incontinence and sexual function. That's efficient! You improve two things with the same exercise. You tighten the muscles around your vagina as well as the muscles around your urethra. Your partner will love it if you have strong vaginal muscles, because they enhance his excitement during intercourse. He'll wonder how you developed such tight vaginal muscles when he never even saw you working out.

Dietary Habits

There are many dietary influences on the bladder. Here are some of the dietary measures which can improve incontinence:

1. Increase the **protein** in your diet. Protein increases muscle fibers and increases the speed of muscle contraction, including the bladder muscle.[2]
2. Take **calcium** supplements. Inadequate calcium can interfere with normal nerve function and muscle contraction.[2]
3. **Avoid bladder irritants**. They can lead to bladder pain and bladder spasm. These include: caffeine, chocolate, spices, alcohol, acidic foods, and aspartame (the artificial sweetener).[2]

Avoidance of bladder stimulants, such as caffeine, is very helpful in controlling incontinence. Caffeine is an offensive agent because it causes the bladder to spasm much more strongly than other liquids. Caffeine is a diuretic, which means that it speeds urine formation. Non-diuretic liquids fill the bladder slowly, and don't cause bladder spasm the way diuretics do.

Stop Smoking

Recall my description of what your bladder and urethra go through when you push to deliver a baby. I said that you put pressure on your bladder and urethra over and over again. With each push, your bladder and urethra descend under the weight created by the pushing. The same thing happens when you cough. You press on your bladder and urethra with each and every cough. Now, you don't have the weight of a heavy uterus and its contents, but repeated coughing can add up to a lot of extra pressure on your bladder and urethra over time. I'll bet you never thought of how much your bladder and urethra go through. So, coughing is one of the things that puts pressure on the bladder and causes urine to leak. Well, what's the most common habit that leads to coughing? If you guessed smoking, you're right on track. If you're a smoker, you're off track, so quit. It's fairly simple to understand this. The less you smoke, the less you cough. The less you cough, the less you leak.

Weight Reduction

If you've got a heavy belly, and it sits right on top of your bladder, pressing on it, you're going to end up with leakage of urine. Recall the description I gave you above for the pregnant uterus sitting on top of your bladder. Do you think your bladder knows the difference between weight from a pregnant uterus and weight from a heavy belly? Of course not! Weight is weight. And the bladder and urethra respond to all weight in the same manner. Each five unit increase in body mass index (BMI) is associated with a 60% to 100% increase in the risk of incontinence.[2] It's the same phenomenon that pregnant women experience. Their heavy uterus sits on their bladder and they have to urinate often. They leak sometimes, too.

Behavior Modification

Behavior modification techniques are economical, have no side effects, and produce excellent results. They require a motivated, attentive, coherent woman who is able to get to a toilet. There are a variety of techniques available for incontinence. While it may seem strange to think in terms of training your bladder, it's no different than the potty training you mastered when you were a toddler. The fact is that the bladder responds very well to training. This is just another example of the recurring cycles we see throughout life. Some aspects of menopause resemble adolescents and others resemble toddlers.

Prompted voiding simply involves voiding at regular intervals. The medical community uses the word "void" to mean urinate, or empty your bladder, or pee, or pee pee, or tinkle. Take your pick. I guess it would sound weird to call this behavior modification "prompted peeing." In any case, prompted voiding is only effective during active practice of the technique. Once you stop, it has no long-term benefits.[3]

Timed voiding involves adhering to a fixed voiding schedule. This is very easy to implement and remember, and you can design your own schedule. Usually, it involves voiding every two hours.[3]

Habit retraining attempts to modify behavior in order to achieve long-term results. At first, you have a voiding interval, and you urinate only at those designated times. If you need to urinate at other times, do so, but record all urinations. Then modify the intervals to suit your own habits. Over time, attempt to lengthen the intervals between voiding by suppressing the urge to void at undesirable times. This allows voluntary reprogramming of your bladder clock.[3]

Bladder drills are the most formal and the most popular of the behavioral modification techniques. With this technique, you set a voiding interval that's slightly shorter than your normal, desirable interval. Thus, you void just before you'd have the urge to do so. Then, increase the interval progressively over the next weeks or months. Keep records indicating when you cannot adhere to the schedule. This trains your bladder and allows you to regain control.

Vitamin and Mineral Options

Vitamin C and **zinc** supplementation improve the quality of connective tissue, and thus the efficiency of muscle contraction.[2]

Vitamin B12 enhances your awareness of bladder fullness.[2]

Hormonal Medication Options

Estrogen

Both urge and stress incontinence respond to local application of estrogen in the vaginal area. Direct application of estrogen in the form of a cream is more effective than any other form of estrogen because it goes directly to the source of the problem. It isn't absorbed into the blood stream and distributed throughout the body to the same extent as other sources of estrogen. Thus, even if you don't wish to take estrogen for any other reason, you may still benefit from estrogen cream in your vagina.

Non-hormonal Medication Options

Urge incontinence responds to medical therapy. This is in contrast to stress urinary incontinence, which usually requires either a mechanical method or surgery. The drugs that are effective for urge incontinence prevent bladder contractions, which is what causes urge incontinence in the first place.

Tolterodine (Detrol)

Tolterodine (trade name Detrol) is the most popular medication for urge incontinence. It's available in immediate release and long-acting formulations. Unfortunately, this drug has some significant bothersome side effects, including dry mouth, dry eyes, constipation, headache, and indigestion.

Anticholinergics

Drugs in this category include propantheline bromide, methanteline bromide, and emepronium bromide. Just call this the bromide group. These are only effective in half of the women who try them, primarily because of their side effects. They cause dry mouth, constipation, blurred vision, rapid heart rate, and (get this) urinary retention. You aren't a candidate for use of these drugs if you have narrow angle glaucoma because it causes the glaucoma to get a lot worse.[3]

Antispasmodics

The antispasmodics include dicyclomine hydrochloride, oxybutynin chloride, and flavoxate hydrochloride (the chloride group). Oxybutynin (Ditropan) has been the gold standard for urge incontinence. It blocks bladder contractility. Oxybutynin is quite popular and very effective.[3] It's available in immediate release, extended release, and skin patch forms.

The antispasmodics are limited by side effects of dry mouth, blurred vision, rapid heart rate, dizziness, drowsiness, stomach upset, and constipation.

Tropsium chloride is the newest agent in this class. It has fewer side effects, but requires an empty stomach for adequate absorption. That means you have to take it one hour before, or two to three hours after, meals. The dose is 20 mg twice daily.

Tricyclic Antidepressants

This group of antidepressants has the effect of inhibiting overactivity of the bladder. The primary drug of interest is imipramine hydrochloride (Tofranil). Side effects include dry mouth, constipation, blurred vision, headache, rapid heart rate, and hallucinations. You aren't eligible for this drug if you have high blood pressure or heart disease.[3]

SSRI Antidepressants

The most significant antidepressant in this category for stress incontinence is Doloxetine. It also has some significant side effects, including nausea, dry mouth, constipation dizziness, fatigue, increased sweating, and drowsiness.

Incontinence Devices

Incontinence devices are useful if you have stress incontinence only with specific activities for which you can insert a device over your urethra to seal it off temporarily. These devices constitute mechanical measures which help with *stress* urinary incontinence only. There's really no place for these in the treatment of urge incontinence. Some of these devices are the following:

CapSure Shield and Fem-Assist are both made of silicone. They come with an ointment that creates a vacuum to close the urethra. You must remove them to urinate and then reinsert them. They're disposable after one week's use.

Reliance Urinary Control Insert is a small balloon catheter that inserts into the urethral opening. You have to remove it to urinate. Because it goes in the urethra, it increases your risk of urinary tract infections.

Impress Softpatch is an adhesive-coated single use patch that covers the urethra. You remove it when you urinate, and then toss it. You then put a new one over your urethra. So, you need to carry a few of these with you everywhere you go.

Devices that change the angle of the urethra to prevent urine leakage include Introl's Bladder Neck Support Prosthesis, the Incontinence Ring, and the Incontinence Dish.

Injectable Substances

These are substances, such as collagen or fat, which increase the volume and density of tissue surrounding and supporting the urethra. The injection is done with local anesthesia in the office setting. While more than one injection is often necessary, the results are very effective, with an 82% to 95% rate of immediate improvement.[4]

Surgical Procedures

There are a variety of surgical procedures for *stress* urinary incontinence in particular. The most appropriate one for any individual woman depends on her particular circumstance, and requires evaluation by a gynecologic or urologic surgeon. In general, they all serve to elevate the neck of the bladder and change the angle of the urethra.

Electrical Stimulation Techniques

Stimulation of the pelvis through the vagina or the anus is effective in controlling spontaneous bladder contractions.[3] This entails using an electrical current to cause a vibration in the cells of the tissues surrounding the bladder. Think of it as a vibrator for the bladder. Use of low frequency energy (< 10 Hz) causes the most profound effect. Many women are able to suppress bladder overactivity with a single treatment. Tampon-like devices for insertion into the vagina are available for convenient, easy application. There are no side effects with this therapy.[3]

Acupuncture

Acupuncture involves identifying areas of disruption in the flow of vital energy (qi) of the body, and then stimulating these areas with needles. Areas over the lower back (sacrum and coccyx) are specific acupuncture points which regulate and activate the kidneys and bladder.[2]

Some studies have shown complete or partial resolution of incontinence with acupuncture. It can be as effective as medications, without the side effects.[2]

Hypnosis

Although there is little data to support hypnosis for incontinence, it may be a successful form of management. This could be due to psychological factors which play a role in how the bladder functions.[2] Regardless of the reasons, it doesn't hurt to give it a try. And if it works, hooray!

Chapter 24: Weight Gain

Cause

Unfortunately, just as puberty is associated with weight gain in the form of breast development, formation of round hips, and an increase in height, menopause is associated with weight gain of a different character, most notably, an increase in width. As you transition from pre-menopause, through peri-menopause, and into post-menopause, your metabolic rate slows. This means that your body stores more calories as fat than it used to.

As you enter post-menopause, your estrogen falls by 90%. Before this happens, the major estrogen in your body is a form called estradiol. Once it's gone, it's replaced by another form of estrogen called estrone, which your fat cells produce. In response to the shift in the type of estrogen, your body fat gets redistributed. The most common location for storage of this fat is the abdominal area. So, you notice that your waistline enlarges, and that hourglass shape becomes a non-hourglass shape.

The solution to this phenomenon is to first realize that weight gain during the menopausal transition is a normal physiologic process. That said, the response you choose will determine whether this process will become a problem for you or not. The simple fact is that you'll have to eat less or exercise more to offset the change in metabolism. Some women need only change the content, rather than the amount, of their dietary intake to prevent weight gain. Once again, no two women are alike. Each one of us must find the solution that best suits our needs.

One of the most common misconceptions about hormone replacement for menopause is that the hormones cause massive weight gain. Not true! Birth control pills may cause you to gain about two or three pounds. Hormone replacement therapy is only capable of doing the same or less than that. In fact, the quantity of hormones in the hormone replacement drugs for menopause is only a fraction of that in birth control pills. So, try to refrain from blaming hormone replacement for the weight gain of menopause. Instead, place the blame on sweet Mother Nature, just as you did during puberty.

Body Mass Index (BMI)

One of the most common measures for analyzing the body for obesity is Body Mass Index (BMI). It utilizes both height and weight to determine whether you're underweight, normal, overweight, obese, or morbidly obese. Calculating your BMI is easy, and you can do it using either the Metric System or the Imperial System. The formulas for each are as follows:

Metric using kilograms and meters:

$$BMI = \frac{\text{Weight in kilograms}}{(\text{Height in meters})^2}$$

Imperial using pounds and inches:

$$BMI = \frac{\text{Weight in pounds} \times 703}{(\text{Height in inches})^2}$$

Now, here's how you interpret your BMI:

BMI	Weight Status
Below 18.5	Underweight
18.5 – 24.9	Normal
25.0 – 29.9	Overweight
30.0 – 39.9	Obese
40 and above	Morbidly obese

It's a good idea for you to calculate your BMI now, and keep the result handy. You'll need to refer to it a number of times as you progress through the remainder of this book.

Management Options

Diet and Lifestyle Options

Diet

The word is **diet**, *not dieting*. What this means is that you need to adopt a permanent way of eating that meets your needs and desires. It's a *permanent* change, not a temporary one. Any diet that has a beginning and an end will never produce lasting results because you'll return to your former eating pattern once it's over. And it's the *former* eating pattern that gave you reason to lose weight in the first place. So, *no* diet*ing*.

The basic principle to understand for purposes of menopause focuses on how quickly or slowly your body metabolizes food. So, we're talking about metabolism. Your metabolic rate slows as you age. And, unfortunately, menopause itself results in a slower metabolism. Your metabolic rate also depends on how *frequently* you eat. Your goal is to do what you can to speed up your metabolism.

Let's go back to basics. How do babies eat? They eat every couple of hours, right? How do animals eat? The ones that can eat frequently do so. And, they aren't fat. So, there's something about eating frequently that's consistent with Mother Nature's plan. The only reason humans have modified the plan to one that involves eating less frequently is to accommodate our social schedules and work schedules.

What you need to understand is this: Your metabolic rate adjusts to how frequently you feed your body. If you eat *frequently*, your body learns to metabolize food *quickly*, store very little as fat, and anticipate food again very soon. Alternatively, if you eat *infrequently*, your body learns to *slow* its metabolism, store as much as possible in the form of fat, and anticipate the need to rely on itself until the next meal, which it isn't going to receive for a long time. Face it: Your body is a fine-tuned machine. Its most basic goal is survival. So, it does whatever it has to do to provide itself with adequate food reserves. If you don't feed it, it will store its own reserves and burn as little energy and as few calories as possible.

Think about that. It explains why skinny people are always eating. They've trained their body to metabolize food as quickly as they consume it. It also explains why obese people swear that they only eat once a day. They do! And their bodies are very efficient at storing that huge meal as fat.

My message to you is this: First, eat breakfast! It jump starts your metabolism. Many women *lose* weight simply by adding breakfast to their daily routine. Then, eat frequent, small meals throughout the day. You'll find that you don't get very hungry between meals. That will prevent you from pigging out when you do eat. You'll also eat lighter foods that don't have to "stick to your ribs." You'll feel better all day, and you'll function more efficiently because you won't have sugar highs and lows throughout the day. You'll probably notice that you don't crave sweets, either.

As for the contents of your diet, you've heard it all before. Eat a high protein, low fat diet, with plenty of fruits and vegetables, lots of fiber, and limited refined carbohydrates. Pass on the fast food and the sweets. Oh, and do you know how much weight you can lose by simply limiting or omitting alcohol? A lot! Alcohol has a lot of calories, and usually you're not counting calories or anything else very well when you're drinking. Try drinking a lot of water instead. It's miraculous at helping you lose weight.

Exercise

You already know that exercise burns calories. Thus, it leaves fewer calories to be stored as fat. The other thing that exercise does is increase your metabolic rate. You need two types of exercise to gain maximal benefit: aerobic exercise and resistance training.

Aerobic exercise is the kind of exercise that raises your heart rate. This is the calorie burning and heart healthy stuff. It's like erasing some of the calories you've eaten. To really make a difference in your metabolic rate, you need at least 30 minutes of *continuous* aerobic exercise sufficient enough to increase your heart rate on a daily basis. So, all the *intermittent* moving you do at work, separated by a few minutes here and there at your desk, doesn't qualify.

<u>Resistance training</u> refers to anything that builds muscle. It includes lifting weights, using an elastic band, or doing isometric exercises in which you use muscle strength to hold a position for an extended period of time. Resistance exercises involve using muscular strength to overcome resistance. The great thing about building muscle is that muscle burns calories even at rest. The more muscle you have, the higher your metabolic rate. That's why muscular people eat mass quantities of food and still look great. Muscle also gives you that toned, sculpted look. Be aware that muscle weighs more than fat, so you may not notice a decrease in actual body weight, but you'll notice a reshaping of your body. Don't focus on the scale. Focus on how your clothes fit and how you feel. Focus on those compliments from other people, too.

Let's talk about the *quantity* of exercise for a minute. You've probably heard or read that you need "20 minutes of exercise three times a week." Well, let me qualify that. There's a difference in the quantity of exercise necessary to prevent a heart attack and the quantity of exercise necessary to *maintain* your current weight. And there's an even greater difference in the quantity of exercise necessary to *lose* weight. The "20 minutes three times a week" you've heard about pertains to heart health. It may suffice to prevent a heart attack, but it won't stabilize your waistline or accomplish weight loss.

To *maintain* your current weight and simply avoid weight gain, you'll need to exercise *daily*. Weight maintenance has to do with utilizing your total calorie intake. You eat every day, don't you? Well, if you put calories in every day, you have to burn them off every day. Input has to balance output.

If it's weight *loss* you're after, it takes burning 3500 calories *more* than you consume to accomplish weight loss of a single pound. So, if you burn 500 more calories per day than you consume, you'll lose one pound in seven days.

Non-hormonal Medication Options

Sorry. There are no safe, magic medicines for weight loss. Of course, there are commercials and testimonials all around you, but that's not the answer. Remember, you're shooting for permanent lifestyle changes here, not quick fixes.

And finally, I have a plea. You've probably heard someone justify smoking to avoid weight gain. While I understand that you can't chew and inhale smoke at the same time, it's a lame excuse for smoking. Find something to keep your hands busy so that you can't use them to raise cigarettes *or* food to your mouth all day. Don't trade one health risk for another. Substitute a bad habit with a good habit or a positive improvement in your life. Turn your negatives into positives!

Chapter 25:
Decreased or Increased Sex Drive

Description

Some women experience a decrease in their sex drive (libido) at the time of peri-menopause and/or post-menopause. This refers to the psychological interest in sex. Others find that stimulation of their genitalia fails to excite them anymore, and they have difficulty achieving orgasm. This is different than the physical disinterest that may arise due to dryness of the vagina or from fatigue. There's a very simple, logical, physiologic reason for this change in sex drive.

Your sex drive, or lack thereof, is all about *testosterone*!

You already know that the ovaries produce eggs and estrogen. What you may not know is that the ovaries also produce *testosterone*. Testosterone is the male hormone. It's also the hormone that contributes to sex drive in both males and females. In the process of transition into menopause, the ovaries stop producing testosterone, just as they stop producing eggs and estrogen. It's as if the ovaries go on strike with regard to all of their functions. They completely shut down and refuse to cooperate.

The good news is that Mother Nature provided us with testosterone from someplace else, in addition to the ovaries. The adrenal glands, located just above the kidneys, also produce testosterone. That's the reason that only some, rather than all, women experience a decrease in their sex drive. That's also the reason that most women experience a decrease, rather than a complete loss, of sex drive (loss of libido). And because the adrenal glands *continue* to produce testosterone, while the ovaries *discontinue* producing estrogen, some women actually experience an *increase* in their sex drive. *Testosterone* is the main determinant of sex drive. If there's more testosterone in your body than there is estrogen, you'll have an increased sex drive. It all depends on the relative amounts of estrogen to testosterone.

As I've explained, peri-menopause is a process rather than a sudden change. During the course of this process, there are a variety of sexual changes that may take place for you individually. I began this section with the most common change in sexual function at the time of menopause. However, there are many ramifications and variations of the possibilities. The key word is change. It is a *change* in sexual function that you should focus on. Here's a list of some of the possible changes you may notice:

1. Decreased frequency of sexual activity
2. Vaginal dryness
3. Vaginal itching
4. Pain or burning with intercourse
5. Decreased or increased sensitivity of the clitoris
6. Decreased or increased response to sexual stimulation
7. Decreased or increased number of orgasms
8. Decreased or increased intensity of orgasm
9. Decreased or increased sexual desire[5]

Notice that most of these changes have a range of possibilities. Realize also that most of these features are relative to the pre-menopausal state, meaning that the change is compared to how it was for you before peri-menopause began. Decreased libido is usually associated with a blood estrogen (estradiol) level of less than 50 pmol/l or a salivary estrogen (estradiol) level of less than 1 pg/ml. While these laboratory values are really just academic, you may find them helpful.

Sex actually gets *better* for some women with menopause. This may be due to their testosterone level, or it may be due to their comfort level. They're more experienced, less inhibited, and have more freedom with their time and space at home. Women who have frequent sex during menopause have fewer sexual problems than those who don't.[1]

Categories

In general, there are two components of sex drive in females. The first is the <u>mental aspect</u>. This includes interest in sex, the perception of having the energy for sex, and the desire for sex (lust). You might want to refer to this one as "sex on the brain." You know, thinking about sex, having sexual thoughts that distract you from concentrating on other things, looking forward to sex, or planning for sex. It's the one that's missing when your partner wants to have sex and you tell him you have a headache. You may actually have a headache, or you may just have no interest in sex.

The second component is the <u>physical (genital) aspect</u>. This refers to the sensitivity of your genitalia to stimulation, the level of pleasure from genital stimulation, the extent of vaginal lubrication, and your ability to have an orgasm. This is working just fine if you have the urge to masturbate and you orgasm readily, even if it takes you a long time to reach orgasm. It's missing or impaired when you are really interested in having sex, but your body doesn't cooperate with your interests. So, you may not get excited with fondling. Or you may not be able to reach orgasm.

It's very important to make a distinction between these two components of the sexual response because the therapeutic options for the two differ. It's also important to understand that the two aren't necessarily connected. Either one may occur in isolation, without the other. So, you may have a mental interest in sex, but be unable to lubricate enough or get stimulated enough to have an orgasm. Alternatively, you may have no interest in sex and still be able to lubricate or have an orgasm.

Decreased sex drive is a common side effect of certain medications. Unfortunately, all of the antidepressant medications (SSRIs, monoamine oxidase inhibitors, and tricyclics) have sexual side effects that include inhibited orgasm and loss of sex drive.[2]

Management Options

Diet and Lifestyle Options

Make Sex Exciting

It may be that your sex life has become somewhat routine or predictable. Maybe all you need to do is spice things up a little with some new, unexpected surprises. It'll excite both you and your partner.

Sexy lingerie may be all it takes to create a whole new interest in sex. If you're thinking that you don't look good in sexy lingerie, then just stop thinking. It's not about what *you* think. It's about what your *partner* thinks when it comes to wearing that stuff to enhance your sex life. Men just love it. The mere act of putting it on shows that you have confidence in yourself, and that's sexy. Be playful in it. Lingerie goes a long way! For one thing, it lasts forever, given the fact you never keep it on for more than about three minutes. You can get a whole wardrobe of outfits, from bunny costumes to, belly dancer costumes, to thongs. Chances are, they'll help you and your partner form lasting memories of some really good times.

Adding candles, incense, or music to make things romantic may do the trick. It may even take getting away from home to change the atmosphere and get things going.

The message here is to be creative. Use your imagination, and put a little energy into it. Have fun anticipating the surprise and excitement it'll create and the memories you'll share as a result. Go to a sex shop and see what they have. Most sex shops have a lot of normal stuff with a touch of flare, as well as plenty of sex toys.

Botanical and Herbal Options

Cayenne (Capsicum species)

Cayenne is a female orgasm stimulant. It's available as a cream, and the active ingredient is capsaicin (0.25% - 0.75%). It tends to cause burning, stinging, and redness of the skin, so you have to use it according to instructions. You apply it for two consecutive days and wait two weeks before using it again. Use in excess of two days can result in blisters and ulceration, neither of which can possibly enhance your sex life.

Damiana (Turnera diffusa)

Damiana increases sexual function. It's available in a variety of dosages, ranging from 380 mg – 450 mg. You may find various products for menopause containing Damiana. Use of Damiana as an aphrodisiac and for sexual enhancement is one of its unproven uses. The studies on it have involved rats, not women.

Cubeb (Piper cubeba)

Cubeb is a less well-proven sex drive stimulator, but it isn't associated with any heath risks. You'll find it in powder, exract, and tincture forms.

Chasteberry (Vitex agnus-castus)

Chasteberry is also known as Chaste Tree, Monk's Pepper, Angus Castus, Indian Spice, Sage Tree Hemp, and Tree Wild Pepper. It contains hormone-like substances which reduce libido (sex drive) in males, and may enhance libido in females.

Hormonal Medication Options

Estrogen

Declining estrogen levels affect sex drive and sexual response. That's because estrogen affects sexual arousal, the sensitivity of your clitoris, and orgasm. Estrogen levels also have an effect on the blood flow to your sexual organs. Thus, you may successfully treat your decrease in libido with estrogen. Some of the options are as follows:

Estrogen skin patch 0.1 mg weekly
Oral estrogen tablet (0.5 or 1 mg) twice daily.

Vaginal estrogen in a dose of 25–50 mg one hour before intercourse

Some women notice significant *worsening* of their sex drive with estrogen pills, patches, or creams in the dosages adequate for overall management of menopause. That's because the increase in estrogen dilutes the effect of testosterone. Thus, while estrogen may improve other symptoms of menopause, it may exacerbate the decrease in libido.[2]

A combination of estrogen and testosterone in appropriate proportions is the most popular method for addressing decreased sex drive. The best known product is called Estratest HS (half strength) or Estratest (full strength). They're both formulated for a single daily dose.

Testosterone

As I mentioned earlier, male hormones are responsible for sex drive. Androgens are the category of male hormones that are pertinent in menopause, and testosterone is the specific male hormone that pertains to sex drive. The laboratory test for evaluating sex drive is free testosterone. Normal free testosterone levels in pre-menopausal women vary from 50 – 100 ng/dl. The level is considered low if it is less than 20 ng/dl. After surgical removal of the ovaries (Bilateral Oophorectomy), the value is usually less than 10 ng/dl.[3]

Replacing testosterone can improve mood, well-being, motivation, memory, sex drive, desire to masturbate, sexual fantasies, nipple sensitivity, and sensitivity of the clitoris.[2]

If you have decreased sex drive that manifests as a disinterest in sex, the most beneficial option is a pill containing both estrogen and testosterone.[3] That's because there are no isolated oral testosterone therapies that are approved by the Food and Drug Administration (FDA) for women.[3] The only one that is FDA approved is a combination of estrogen and testosterone (Estratest HS [half strength] and Estratest). Bioidentical testosterone is available in the form of a capsule or a vaginal cream. The dosage is 1 - 2 mg every other day, and increasing as needed.

DECREASED OR INCREASED SEX DRIVE

Other, less effective or less available methods of testosterone replacement are DHEA, testosterone skin patches, and testosterone gel.[3] The dose of DHEA is 5 - 10 mg once or twice daily. Not all women are able to convert DHEA to testosterone, so DHEA won't work for them. For those women, testosterone is a better choice.[4]

If you have decreased sex drive due to lack of sensitivity to genital stimulation, there's a topical form of testosterone. It's an ointment or cream that you apply to your clitoris and vagina.[3] So far, there are no data on the safety or effectiveness of this product.[3]

There is some evidence that testosterone can decrease hot flashes.[3] That's because androgens are converted to estrogens in the body. So, some women notice a decrease in their hot flashes when they use testosterone cream. However, you wouldn't use testosterone cream specifically for hot flashes.

Androgens also have beneficial effects on bone.[3] They help preserve bone mass and thus decrease osteoporosis.[3] Testosterone has a positive effect on the heart, with lowering of cholesterol.[3] It may decrease healthy HDL, however.[2] There is no known harmful effect of low dose testosterone on the uterus.[2]

Side effects of testosterone are acne and unwanted hair growth on the chin and chest. These resolve when testosterone use is discontinued.[3]

Some of the varieties of testosterone are listed below:

1. Methyl Testosterone sublingual (under the tongue) pills 0.5 mg daily
2. Testosterone vaginal cream 2% applied topically to the vagina and clitoris (available from compounding pharmacies)
3. Androgel topical gel 0.35 mg daily applied to the hairless skin anywhere on the body
   (The effect lasts 24 hours. This may cause throbbing of the vagina within 30 minutes of application.)[2]

Progesterone

The effect of progesterone on sex drive is primarily one of preventing loss of sex drive and maintaining an already existing sex drive. It can't create a sex drive that is nonexistent. So, progesterone may prevent a decline in your sex drive, but it won't restore your sex drive once it has waned.

Non-hormonal Medication Options

I'm sure you've heard of Viagra and other drugs that abound for the benefit of ensuring that men enjoy their sex lives to the fullest. Well, none of the drug companies has made a similar drug for women yet. So, what are we to do? Use the ones they make for the guys, of course! They do the trick for men by increasing blood flow to the penis. And, they can do the same thing for you by increasing the blood flow to your clitoris. You may have to request these medications because some doctors may not have ever thought to offer them to women, and they aren't FDA approved for women. Therefore, some physicians may refuse to prescribe them for you. But, there's no harm in asking for them, and I know of no harm in using them. Here are the names:

1. Sildenafil (Viagra) 25-50 mg one hour before intercourse
2. Tadalafil (Cialis) 10 mg one hour before intercourse
3. Vardenafil (Levitra) 10 mg one hour before intercourse

If you try one of these medications, you'll probably need less stimulation to have an orgasm, you'll orgasm more quickly, you'll feel more aroused, and you'll enjoy your orgasms more.

Each of these drugs may cause side effects that include headache, flushing, bad taste in your mouth, or nasal congestion.

Chapter 26: Acne

Sequence of Events

Can you believe this one? It isn't enough that you have to revisit the unstable emotional issues of puberty again with menopause. To make matters worse, you may notice a resurgence of facial acne. Yuck!

Just as in adolescence, the acne which occurs at the time of menopause is *hormonal* in nature. This means that hormones cause the acne rather than bacteria. The acne of menopause is *not* a result of poor hygiene.

Following is the sequence of events which result in hormonal acne:

Increased absolute or relative levels of male hormones (androgens), such as testosterone and DHEA, induce the sweat glands to produce more oil.
The extra oil makes the skin slough faster.
The rapid slough process clogs the pores and hair follicles with dead skin cells and oil.
The bacteria which normally exist on the skin attack the oil, breaking it down into fatty acids.
The fatty acids induce an inflammatory response which forms a blackhead or pimple, and that's what you see.[1]

The short version of this sequence is that male hormones produce oil which clogs your pores.

Management Options

Diet and Lifestyle Options

Diet

Diet is an important factor in the development and prevention of acne. It's no different than when you were an adolescent. Which foods caused your acne then? The same foods will probably contribute to acne now. In general, an anti-acne diet is one that's high in fiber and low in sugar. Finally, I can't stress the importance of water, water, water. Remember the emphasis on water in the section on dry skin? It's important for acne, too.

Ideal Body Weight

Achieving and maintaining ideal body weight actually decreases acne due to the fact that fat cells produce excess androgens. Androgens are the male hormones which induce excess oil production from your sweat glands.

If you reduce your body weight, you'll also reduce the number of fat cells you have, right? Well, it's the fat cells that initiate the process of acne-forming androgen production.

Think back to high school. Which group of students had the most acne, the fat teens or the skinny teens? The heavier ones did. And that was because they had higher levels of androgens. What about the boys versus the girls? The boys had more acne didn't they? Androgens were to blame.

These examples illustrate the fact that maintaining ideal body weight can reduce your tendency to have acne and maintain a clear complexion by lowering your androgen levels.

Hygiene

Hygiene measures contribute to prevention of acne. These include regular facials (how nice), and thorough, but gentle, face cleansing morning and night. Good hygiene helps to unclog those pores. While it's not really a hygiene issue, use of makeup that is appropriate for your skin type (dry, oily, etc.) can help you avoid acne, also. That's because your skin will react to makeup that has too much or too little oil in it for your skin type.

Vitamin and Mineral Options

Vitamin supplements to ensure adequate intake of **vitamin C** and the **B vitamins**, as well as mineral supplements to ensure adequate **zinc**, will do much to lessen acne.

Botanical and Herbal Options

Tea Tree Oil (Medaleuca alternifolia)

Tea Tree Oil is a natural antibacterial that provides many women with the remedy they need for the acne of menopause. Apply it directly to your pimples at night.

Hormonal Medication Options

Birth Control Pills

Birth control pills work wonders to reduce acne in adolescents. Likewise, they may be just as effective during menopause. They target the source of the problem, which is an imbalance of hormones. Be sure that you use very low dose pills. Remember, you're not a candidate for birth control pills if you smoke, even occasionally.

Estrogen

Any form of estrogen may improve acne, simply by changing the ratio of estrogen to testosterone in your body. Don't expect it to work as well as birth control pills do. But, it should help somewhat.

Non-hormonal Medication Options

Vitamin A Formulations

Vitamin A products are very effective in the treatment and prevention of acne. These include Tretinoin (Retin-A and Renova) and Isotretinoin (Accutane). The tretinoins are topical medications which require a prescription. They act by allowing rapid sloughing of the cells, but increase the speed of oil release so that it doesn't clog the pores and hair follicles. Accutane is a pill taken by mouth, and it's very irritating to skin. Therefore, it is only for severe acne. It acts by inhibiting oil production by your skin, and also by inhibiting growth of bacteria on your skin.

Benzoyl Peroxide

Benzoyl Peroxide products serve to dry the skin and kill bacteria. They are available in many forms, including creams, gels, lotions, and pads.

Antibiotics

Antibiotics may be effective in menopausal acne, but are less desirable than any of the other medical options. That's because the acne of menopause isn't brought on by bacteria. So, antibiotics don't address the source of the problem. Rather, antibiotics simply kill the normal bacteria on your skin, and may change the flora of normal bacteria in other parts of your body as well. For many women, they create a vaginal yeast infection.

Chapter 27: Headaches

Description

Headaches are a problem for some women at the time of peri-menopause. They're actually quite common during pre-menopause, too. If you notice a pattern of headaches that coincides with a particular time in your menstrual cycle, they're usually hormonal in nature. That means the headache is brought on by hormonal changes. It usually happens just before your period begins, and coincides with a drop in both estrogen and progesterone.

During peri-menopause, when estrogen and progesterone are fluctuating, headaches may be an exaggeration of previous hormonal headaches, or they may appear for the first time.

Sometimes, hormonal headaches are actually <u>migraine headaches</u>. Migraines are much more common in women than they are in men. They result from blood vessels which dilate, possibly in response to certain triggers. Some of the things that may trigger a migraine include stress, sugar, chocolate, and MSG (monosodium glutamate). Stress probably plays the largest and most consistent role in causing migraines for most women.

Women who experience natural menopause (as opposed to surgical menopause) have a favorable headache outcome, with 66% of them reporting improvement in their migraines. The opposite is true for women who experience surgical menopause; 66% of them have a worsening of their migraines.[1]

There are a variety of headache types, and there are further subvarieties of the individual categories of headaches. Since headaches aren't unique to menopause, and since they can result from many significant medical conditions, it's important to see a headache specialist any time headaches are severe, frequent, or persistent.

Management Options

Diet and Lifestyle Options

Stress Reduction

Stress reduction works wonders to avoid and manage headaches. That's true whether or not your headaches are hormonal in nature. Think about how often a stressful event gives you a headache. Stress and headaches just go together! We all have our own individual ways of reducing stress. So, whether that means napping, resting, deep breathing, doing yoga, getting a massage, or exercising, do what works for you.

Diet

Soy

Because it's a phytoestrogen, soy has the effect of regulating the amount of estrogen in your body. It reduces headaches, possibly by reducing blood pressure slightly. Of course, there are a variety of other benefits from soy, so it's good for you even if you don't have headaches.

Botanical and Herbal Options

Feverfew (Tanacetum parthenium)

Feverfew thins the blood and prevents spasm of blood vessels. Both of these actions serve to reduce the number and severity of migraine headaches.

Hormonal Medication Options

Birth Control Pills or Patch

If you're still having periods, you may want to consider using a low dose birth control pill or patch for your headaches. They balance your estrogen and progesterone levels, and prevent the hormonal fluctuations that lead to headaches. Of course, you have to be a non-smoker to take advantage of this option.

Warning: You may not take birth control pills or patches if you have migraine headaches with *aura*.

Cyclic or Continuous Hormone Replacement Therapy

These medications are the lower dose combinations of estrogen and progesterone (HRT) for menopause, rather than for pregnancy prevention. They still balance estrogen and progesterone levels, so they may still help with your headaches. Most hormonal headaches result from too little progesterone or too much estrogen. Hormone replacement therapy balances the two and flattens out the fluctuations that cause hormonal headaches.

Progesterone

Progesterone is the hormone that seems to work the best for headaches, especially hormonal headaches and migraine headaches. If you're having periods still, you can apply ¼ - ½ tsp of 2% progesterone cream to your skin daily during the two weeks before your period. If you're not having periods any longer, you can apply the same amount daily three weeks out of the month. If you're already using progesterone cream daily for other reasons, just continue to do so. It'll help your headaches, also.

Non-hormonal Medication Options

Nonsteroidal Anti-Inflammatory Drugs (NSAIDs)

These are the medications with which you're probably already familiar for headaches. They include ibuprofen and naproxen (Advil, Aleve, Motrin). They function by reducing inflammation. In the case of a headache, the blood vessels are inflamed. So, these medications reduce or prevent inflammation of the blood vessels in your head.

Antihypertensive Agents

If you have frequent, severe migraines, it may be reasonable to take a medication designed to prevent migraines from recurring. There are a few medications indicated for high blood pressure which actually function well in preventing migraines. They belong to a category of drugs called Beta-blockers. Of course, you'd have to see your doctor about this. And if you're having frequent, severe headaches, you'd need an evaluation anyway to ensure that nothing more serious is going on.

Vasoconstrictors

Vasoconstrictors constrict blood vessels. Constriction is the opposite of dilation, and since dilation is what causes pain when you have a headache, they work wonders. There are a variety of medications in this category. So, see your doctor to determine which one is best for you.

WORKSHEET TIMEOUT:
Answer question # 4 on your worksheet.
Circle all your symptoms of menopause.

Okay. Thus far in this section, we've discussed all the signs and symptoms of menopause. It's the stuff you'll need to recognize and manage during your transition into post-menopause (and possibly thereafter). Much of it will be temporary, and affect you for only a few years. None of it represents a life-threatening situation.

Headaches

Now we're going to discuss the *diseases* pertinent to how you manage your menopause. This is the stuff that will affect you *for the rest of your life*. I give seminars based on this book. What I've discovered in the seminars is this: The material you're about to encounter is *much* more impactful than the material you've already covered. I find that to be especially true for *post*-menopausal women. I'll be teaching you about diseases, helping you determine the diseases for which you are at risk, and giving you numerous options for lowering your risks. The post-menopausal women in my seminars can't believe that no one has ever informed them about these things. They realize that they could have managed their menopause in ways that reduced their risks for a variety of diseases. Whatever your age, and wherever you are in your journey towards the menopausal phase of your life, the information you're about to learn could save your life.

CHAPTER 28: HEART ATTACK

Statistics

Heart attack is the ***leading killer*** of postmenopausal women. I know this may surprise you. Most people have the misconception that cancer is the leading killer of women. Not so. Heart attacks kill twice as many women as all forms of cancer combined. To be even more specific, heart attack kills *one out of every two women,* while breast cancer kills one out of every 29 women.[1]

Another misconception is the belief that heart attack is more common in men than in women. The fact is that heart attack is the number one killer of *both* men and women. In fact, one out of every two individuals dies from a heart attack. Within ten years of becoming postmenopausal, a woman's risk of having a heart attack is equal to that of a man ten years younger.[2] But, women are more likely to be disabled or die from a heart attack than men.[3] Therefore, in any discussion of menopause, as with any discussion of aging in general, we must address the issue of heart attack. Closely related to heart attacks are strokes and blood clots (thrombi).

Causes

Heart attacks are a result of fat accumulation in blood vessels. Fat just seems to cause problems any time it accumulates. The term for fat in heart attack lingo is "lipids." These lipids clog blood vessels, restricting or prohibiting blood flow to the organ the vessel serves. Think of the lipid build-up as a "road block." Since blood cells carry oxygen, the organ beyond the road block suffers from oxygen deprivation, and either dies or becomes damaged. Death or damage to the heart constitutes a heart attack. Heart attacks, strokes, and blood clots are all the same phenomenon in different locations. They're all just road blocks which prevent the ability of oxygen-carrying blood to travel to its destination, which is either the heart (heart attack), the brain (stroke), or an extremity (blood clot).

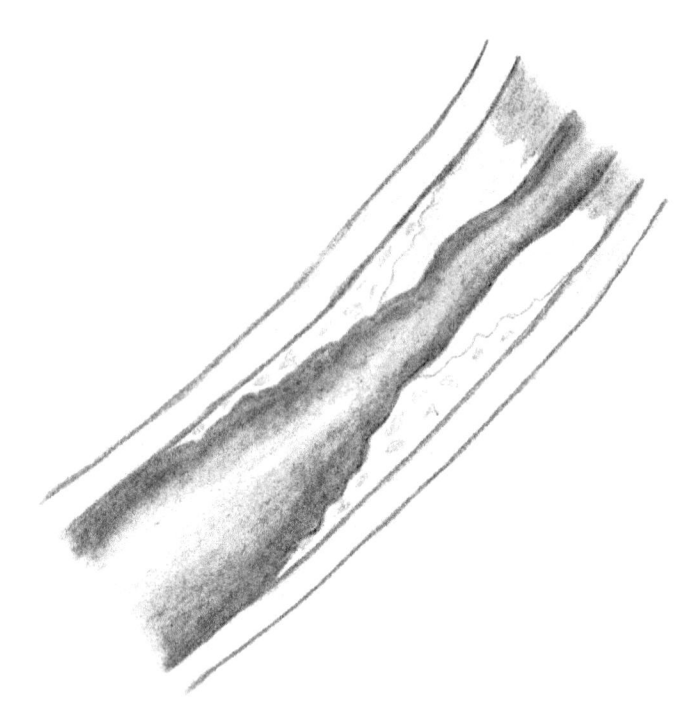

Figure 12: Artery with cholesterol build-up, creating a "road block"

Lipids are fatty substances in the blood which have an effect on the development of heart disease. There are a variety of lipids in the blood. Some of them increase the risk of heart attack and others decrease the risk. At least some fats are good. The lipids that are important with regard to heart disease are cholesterol, triglycerides, high density lipoproteins (HDL), and low density lipoproteins (LDL). HDL is a good lipid, while LDL is a bad lipid. So that you don't have difficulty remembering which is which, I'll refer to them as "healthy HDL" and "lousy LDL." Unfortunately, menopause causes a *decrease* in healthy HDL and an *increase* in lousy LDL.[4] Of course, this is the opposite of the desired effect. For every 1% decrease in lousy LDL, the risk of heart attack decreases by 1%.

Now, while the absolute values of total cholesterol, healthy HDL, lousy LDL, and triglycerides are important, it's the ratio of total cholesterol to healthy HDL that's most important in determining your risk of heart attack. It's sort of like the ratio of height to weight being more important than just weight alone. If your total cholesterol divided by healthy HDL cholesterol is less than or equal to four, you're at low risk. If it's greater than four, you're at high risk.

$$\frac{\text{Total Cholesterol}}{\text{Healthy HDL}} \quad < \text{ or } = 4 \quad \text{Low Risk}$$

$$\frac{\text{Total Cholesterol}}{\text{Healthy HDL}} \quad > 4 \quad \text{High Risk}$$

Symptoms

You're probably familiar with the symptoms of a heart attack in males. Most people have at least a vague idea. What you may not know is that the symptoms of a heart attack differ in males and females. In males, a heart attack is characterized by chest pain beginning beneath the ribs at the location of the heart, and it's a heavy, crushing sensation. The pain radiates into the left arm. This is the classic, familiar, and typical description of heart attack in males.

Such is not the case for females, in whom the "pain" of a heart attack usually involves the *neck, jaw, or back (between the shoulder blades)*.[3] If they have any "chest pain" at all, it's in the *upper chest*, well above the level of the heart. Indeed, some women do not have *any* chest pain when they experience a heart attack. If they do, they may describe it as *tightness, aching, or pressure* rather than as pain. Others describe a heart attack as nothing more than a feeling of *indigestion*. Finally, some women have a silent heart attack, with no symptoms at all. They simply have changes on their electrocardiogram (EKG).

One of the symptoms of *menopause* is a change in heart rate, or racing of the heart. The medical term for this sensation is "heart palpitations." Palpitations are due to hormonal changes. They are not indicative of a heart attack, but they sometimes mislead women, and cause them to ignore other signs that may indeed be indicative of a heart attack.

Symptoms of Heart Attack in Males and Females

	Males	**Females**
Descriptive words	Chest *"heaviness"*	Chest *"tightness"* Chest *"aching"* Chest *"pressure"*
Location of "pain"	*Chest* pain	*Neck* pain *Jaw* pain *Back* pain *No* pain (silent)
Other symptoms	*Radiation* to the left arm	*Indigestion*

Risk Factors

There are many factors which contribute to an increased risk of heart attack. Here's a list of them:

1. **Previous heart attack**
2. **Smoking**, past or present
3. **Lousy LDL cholesterol that is high** (greater than 130 mg/dl)
4. **Healthy HDL cholesterol that is low** (less than 46 mg/dl)
5. **Ratio of total cholesterol to healthy HDL greater than 4**
6. **High triglycerides** (greater than 200 mg/dl)
7. **Obesity** (body weight > 25% over ideal, or body mass index greater than 25)
8. **Fat accumulation in the abdominal region** (truncal obesity, defined as waist to hip ratio of > 0.8, or a waist measurement > 35 in or 63.5 cm)
9. **High blood pressure** (greater than 130/85)
10. **Diabetes** (especially type 2, or adult onset)
11. **Sedentary lifestyle**
12. **Gum disease**

13. **High levels of the amino acid homocysteine in the blood**
14. **Depression**
15. **Family history of heart attacks**

Genetics plays a large role in this, so your family history for heart attacks is also important. If you have a family history of heart attacks, you should weigh this factor heavily in making management decisions for menopause. I have listed it last, however, because it's the factor over which you have no control. Use it to balance your priorities, but don't view it as your destiny. Despite a family history of heart attacks, you can do a great deal to change your risk.

Besides genetics, though, there are three risk factors with a much greater impact on women than on men.[3] The first of these is type 2 diabetes. The risk of heart attack is increased by three to seven times in women with type 2 diabetes, but only by two to three times in men with type 2 diabetes.[3] The second is high triglycerides, and the third is low healthy HDL. If you have a combination of these risk factors, your risk increases greatly.

Years ago, the medical profession espoused the belief that estrogen prevented heart attacks. This was based primarily on the fact that, until the age of menopause, women have a much lower rate of heart attack than men. After menopause, the rate of heart attack in women increases dramatically. Additionally, numerous studies confirmed that women who took estrogen after menopause continued to have lower rates of heart attack than men, whereas women who didn't take estrogen demonstrated a heart attack rate equal to that of men. More recent studies have challenged the assertion that estrogen has a protective effect on the heart, while others have indicated progesterone as the offending agent, and estrogen as a harmless one. The chapter entitled "What About the Research Studies" gives you a lot more information on this.

WORKSHEET TIMEOUT:
Answer question # 5 on your worksheet.
Circle all your risk factors for a heart attack.

Management Options

Diet and Lifestyle Options

The most significant risk factors for heart attack are based on lifestyle. That's a good thing, because it means that you have control over them by the choices you make. Lifestyle refers to diet, exercise habits, weight control, smoking, and alcohol consumption. These lifestyle changes decrease your risk of heart attack, stroke, blood clots, high cholesterol, and diabetes. So, a few changes in lifestyle go a long way in improving and extending your life. Some habits actually affect the timing of menopause. For instance, smoking can cause menopause to occur two years earlier than it would otherwise.[5]

Diet

Awareness of dietary measures which serve to decrease your risk of heart attack is probably not new to you; however, putting them into action may be. A low fat, low cholesterol diet is one of the most important habits you can adopt to reduce your risk of heart attack. Remember, heart attack is the number one killer of both males and females. It's well worth your effort to make a commitment to maintain a low fat, low cholesterol diet. We're fortunate to have nutrition information on food products, making it quite simple to make wise choices. You probably have to exercise a bit more caution when dining out. In either case, you're doing yourself a huge favor if you lower your intake of fat and cholesterol.

To elaborate just a bit on fats, you need to distinguish between saturated and unsaturated fats. It's the *saturated* fats that are most harmful. Most food labels specifically indicate the amount of saturated fat in the food. Use food labels to see how much of each type of fat is in the foods you eat. Limit your saturated fat intake to less than 75 kcal/day.

Now, although fat intake is the primary focus in a discussion of heart attack, you need to realize that sugar and refined carbohydrates also play a significant role in causing heart attack. That's because refined carbohydrates are converted into sugar. Sugar induces insulin release from the pancreas, which serves to convert the sugar into energy. The catch is that insulin also has a role in storing fat. That's because insulin makes the liver produce lousy LDL. So, an overabundance of sugar or refined carbohydrates gets stored as fat, which has the same effect on clogging the arteries as fat in its original form.

The best diet for heart health is one that consists of lean meats, reduced fat dairy products, high fiber grains, fruit, and vegetables. The best fruits and vegetables are those that are high in antioxidants (blueberries, strawberries, greens, spinach). Soy products, such as tofu, tempeh, and soy dairy substitutes also serve to decrease total cholesterol, lousy LDL cholesterol, and triglycerides. So, enjoy the soy. There's an inverse relationship between intake of soy products and heart attacks. That explains why Asian diets, which are high in soy, are associated with very low rates of heart attack. Other important foods for heart health include fish, garlic, and green tea.

Exercise

This isn't a book on exercise, I promise. I realize that this recommendation keeps coming up over and over. That should mean something, and it does. In the case of menopause, regular exercise has many benefits other than the usual ones of cardiovascular health. It helps curb the weight gain inherent in the process of menopause; it decreases stress; it increases metabolism; it reduces hot flashes; it improves sleep. There is simply no good reason to omit exercise. It can make a major difference in your menopausal experience. I know, you probably think you don't have time. Well, you need to make time or else you'll run out of time. You must make exercise a *priority*. If you don't, you won't make time for it.

One of the ways exercise benefits heart health is by increasing the circulation of lymph. Lymph is the waste, or sewer, system in the body. The more efficiently the lymph rids your body of waste, the less likely waste will build up to pollute your body. Lymph has a special role in preventing heart attack in that it helps clear lousy LDL cholesterol out of your arteries.

It doesn't take excessive exercise to prevent a heart attack. As little as 20 minutes three times per week of an activity that adequately raises your heart rate for the full 20 minutes suffices. Maintenance of an increased heart rate is the key to heart health. You need to attain and maintain a certain heart rate for 20 consecutive minutes. We call this your "target heart rate." There are charts to guide you in knowing what your target heart rate should be. Target heart rates vary according to age.

Weight Control

I've isolated weight control as a separate discussion because there are some issues specific to menopause to which you should pay particular attention. Of course, maintenance of ideal body weight is the best preventive measure to avoid heart attack. However, with regard to obesity, the *location* of excess fat is critical to whether or not it increases your risk of heart attack.

As you know, we each have a tendency to gain weight in some regions of our body more readily than others. Some women store excess weight in the hips and thighs. We refer to these women as having a pear shape. Other women store excess weight in their abdominal region. They have a large belly, and we refer to them as having an apple shape.

Menopause is associated with weight accumulation in the *abdominal* area. The waistline seems to disappear, and is replaced with a "spare tire." This is unfortunate. It's another instance in which you want to just roll your eyes and wonder how much more difficulty this adds to the whole experience of menopause.

Even more unfortunate is the fact that heart attacks are associated with excess weight in the abdominal region. In medical terminology, we refer to a fat belly or fat torso as "*truncal obesity.*" Truncal obesity is defined as having any of the following:

(1) A waist to hip ratio of greater than 0.8;
(2) A waist measurement of more than 35 in or 63.5 cm; or
(3) An apple-shaped body (rather than a pear-shaped body).

Heart Attack

If you read literature on heart attack, you will see that there is a very strong relationship between truncal obesity and heart attack. Once again, Mother Nature has created a twist that seems unfair. Nevertheless, you really need to take this seriously. Doing so could save your life.

The quantity and level of exercise necessary to prevent or lose excess abdominal weight is significantly more than that needed for basic heart health.

No Smoking

Here we are again, discussing smoking! What can I say? It's the worst thing you can do for your heart, lungs, skin, breast, and circulation. Smoking significantly increases *all* the health risks for menopause. It also increases all the side effects of therapy for menopause. You can reduce your symptoms and inconveniences of menopause immensely by simply discontinuing smoking.

Smoking causes more than half the deaths due to heart attacks in women under the age of 65. Smoking actually lowers the age of menopause by approximately two years. The more you smoke, the earlier you'll experience menopause.

So how much mileage will you get from throwing out the cigarettes? A lot! After just one year of not smoking, you will have decreased your risk of heart attack by 50%.[6] After three years of not smoking, you will have nearly erased your increased risk of a heart attack.[6] Now that's a good return on your investment in yourself, don't you think? And just imagine how much money you'll save!

Now, let's pause for a moment and put things into perspective. Thus far, we've only discussed four things that you can do to prevent a heart attack. How much of a difference do you think those four basic things can make? The answer is ... a tremendous difference! Get this: Women who eat a heart healthy diet, exercise regularly, maintain an appropriate body weight, *and* don't smoke have an **84%** lower risk for a heart attack than other women. Adopting *all four* of these lifestyle habits lowers your risk of heart attack immensely. Here's the sad part: Only **3%** of the female population actually does all four of these things.[1]

Limited Alcohol

Studies have shown that a *single* alcoholic drink daily is beneficial for the heart.[7] That's because one drink a day increases your healthy HDL.[6] But, drinking more than two drinks per day, even with two alcohol-free days per week, is associated with an increased risk of heart attack.[5] And that's because it raises your blood pressure.[6] These statistics are only for women, and are specific for heart health in women. The data for men are different. The data for other diseases in women are different, too.

For example, the data for breast cancer contradict this magical one a day limit. That same single alcoholic drink daily increases your risk of breast cancer. So, you have to take into account your own risk status for each of these diseases. You need to tailor this information to your own personal situation and use this information to your advantage. Remember, there are many ways to improve heart health without having to rely on alcohol if you have concerns regarding both heart attack and breast cancer.

Dental Hygiene

Gum disease is significantly related to heart attacks. (Go figure!) This includes gum infection, gum inflammation, and bleeding gums. The exact mechanism of association of gum disease to heart attacks is unclear, but there's a definite increase in heart attacks among people with gum disease.

Treatment of gum disease entails proper brushing, daily flossing, and dental hygiene appointments for cleaning every six months. While these are habits that all people should observe throughout their lifetimes, now is most certainly the time to begin if you haven't already done so.

Vitamin and Mineral Options

Calcium and Magnesium

I address the two of these together because the body uses them together. It's as if they're attached at the hip in terms of how they interact in the heart. They function in regulating the electrical activity of the heart. It's important to balance them so that the ratio of calcium to magnesium is 1:1 or 2:1. Take these minerals with meals for proper absorption.

The necessary dose of calcium is 400 – 1200 mg daily. The majority of menopausal women need as much as 1500 mg daily. Few women get more than 400 mg of calcium in their diet.

The necessary dose of magnesium is 400 – 1000 mg daily. It's really not that difficult to get enough magnesium, but it's surprising how many women are actually deficient in magnesium. Foods rich in magnesium include unpolished grains, nuts, and green vegetables. The leafy green vegetables are the best vegetable sources of magnesium. Milk, meat, and starchy foods have small amounts of magnesium, and processed foods have almost none. Magnesium deficiency is common due to all the processed foods we eat. Another source of inadequate magnesium is frequent use of antacids for indigestion or heartburn, such as cimetidine (Tagamet) and ranitidine (Zantac).

Potassium and Sodium

Increasing the potassium and decreasing the sodium in your diet will go a long way in preventing heart attacks and strokes. The desirable ratio of potassium to sodium is 5:1. The typical, average diet has a ratio of 1:2. As you can see, most people are way off balance on this. Why? Because we rely on fast foods and processed foods, both of which have lots of salt in them. In addition, we neglect to ensure adequate intake of fresh fruits, vegetables, and whole grains. Check food labels. They list both the actual amount and the percent of daily requirements for potassium and sodium in the food product.

Vitamins B6, B12, and B9

High levels of vitamins B6, B12, and B9 (folate) are associated with a decreased risk of heart attack. It's best to take all of these together in the form of a B complex vitamin or multivitamin. The necessary dosages are as follows:

Vitamin B6: 40 – 80 mg daily
Vitamin B12: 20 mcg daily
Folate: 400 – 800 mcg daily

If you wish to use foods as a source of the B vitamins, the best foods are dark green leafy vegetables, breakfast cereals, whole grains, beans, and citrus fruit.

Vitamin C

Vitamin C serves to help prevent fat from adhering to the blood vessels, and increases the absorption of calcium and magnesium. Of course, citrus fruits are rich in vitamin C, and supplements come in many forms, such as pills, fizzy tablets, and powders. The recommended dose is 1000 – 3000 mg daily.

Vitamin E

Vitamin E decreases the risk of blood clots. You may think of it as the anti-aging vitamin. The required dose is 200 – 800 IU daily. The best formulations are either d-alpha–tocopherol or mixed tocopherol.

Natural vitamin E exists in plants, animals, and some types of algae. The richest sources of vitamin E are vegetable oils such as sunflower oil, safflower oil, canola oil, cottonseed oil, wheat germ oil, and olive oil. All of these have an abundance of alpha-tocopherol, which is the active ingredient in vitamin E. The fatty parts of meat also contain vitamin E, as do fruit, nuts, and unrefined grainy cereals.

Vitamin B3

Vitamin B3 (niacin) improves all the different types of lipids in your body. It raises your healthy HDL, and lowers cholesterol, triglycerides, and lousy LDL.[6]

The problem with niacin is that the necessary dose to achieve all these great effects on your heart is 1.5 – 3 gm per day, which causes side effects.[6] The most common side effects are flushing, possible harm to your liver, increased blood glucose levels, and aggravation of gout.[6] So, be careful to adhere to the recommended dosages, and don't take it if you have any kind of liver disease.[6]

Coenzyme Q10

Coenzyme Q10 is a fat soluble substance that is present in the cells of your body. Your body actually makes its own CoQ10 unless the process for doing so is impaired. CoQ10 improves your heart's ability to pump blood. Unfortunately, the statin drugs for decreasing cholesterol also decrease coenzyme Q10. They do this by blocking an enzyme which produces both cholesterol and CoQ10.

The necessary dose of CoQ10 is a minimum of 30 mg daily. For women at high risk of heart attack, it's 60 – 90 mg daily, and even higher doses are appropriate for women with significant heart disease. Because it's fat soluble, it's best to take CoQ10 with a meal that contains some fat.

Foods which contain generous quantities of CoQ10 are organ meats (liver), sardines, mackerel, and peanuts.

You can measure your CoQ10 levels with a blood test. The normal level is 0.8 – 1.2 mcg/ml of blood. The therapeutic level for purposes of preventing heart attack is 2.5 – 3.5 mcg/ml of blood.

L-Carnitine

L-Carnitine does many things to improve heart health, including suppressing triglycerides, increasing healthy HDL, and regulating heart rate. The dose is 250 – 500 mg daily.

Alpha Lipoic Acid (ALA)

Alpha Lipoic Acid helps to maintain levels of vitamin C and vitamin E. Additionally, it assists in insulin metabolism. The recommended dose is 50 – 200 mg daily.

Homocysteine

Homocysteine is an amino acid found in animal protein. Elevated levels of this amino acid are associated with a high risk of heart attack. While at least 10% of the population has a genetic predisposition for high homocysteine levels, the majority of people have elevated levels due to a diet high in animal fat.

Women have a significant increase in homocysteine levels after age 55. Levels greater than 15 mcmol/l are considered high risk. A major cause is dietary deficiency of vitamins B6, B12, and folate.

A simple blood test can give you information on your homocysteine level. It's wise to get a baseline level at the time of menopause. You can then repeat the test as needed if it's elevated.

It is well worth decreasing a high homocysteine level. Doing so can decrease your risk of heart attack by 20%, decrease your risk of stroke by 40%, and decrease your risk of blood clots by 60%. That's a lot of mileage from a simple change.

One of the means by which you can decrease your homocysteine level is to take supplemental vitamin B6, vitamin B12, and folate. Of course, the most significant reductions in homocysteine levels will occur by reducing your intake of animal protein. Vegetarians have a definite advantage here, especially vegans, who omit dairy products as well as red meat, poultry, and seafood from their diets.

Botanical and Herbal Options

Hawthorne

Hawthorne is an herb that lowers the risk of a heart attack. It also has the ability to allow a decrease in the dose of statin drugs for high cholesterol. There are many forms of Hawthorne, including berries, tea, and pills. The recommended dose is 100 – 250 mg three times daily if you use pills. The desirable pill formula is 10% proanthocyanidins or 1.8% vitexin-4-rhamnoside.[8]

Phytoestrogens

Soy intake is associated with favorable changes in your lipid profile. If you consume 50 gm of soy protein in combination with a low fat diet (less than 30% of daily calories) and low cholesterol intake (less than 300 mg daily), you can expect a 12% decrease in your cholesterol level and an 11.5% decrease in lousy LDL levels.[9]

Hormonal Medication Options

Years ago, the medical profession believed that hormone therapy for menopause had a protective effect on the heart. Since then, a study has shown that hormone replacement for menopause *does not* protect the heart against heart attack, and in fact may increase the risk for some women. The study that I'm referring to is the Women's Health Initiative, or WHI. It presented results as they pertain to the population as a whole. It did *not* individualize the information. This means that you must take this new information into consideration, but it does not mean that you should automatically avoid hormones for management of menopause. The basic message is that you shouldn't take hormone replacement with the primary goal of protecting against a heart attack. You should institute the measures that I've discussed above for that purpose.

With regard to the risk of a first heart attack, the overall long-term results of the Women's Health Initiative (WHI) show that hormone therapy ***does not*** pose a significant risk of heart attack in women who have been postmenopausal for *less than ten years*.[10] The number of blocked arteries you have when you become post-menopausal depends partly on your estrogen exposure in your pre-menopausal years.[11] Once you are no longer exposed to estrogen, your risk for blocked arteries increases. So, as the time since menopause increases, the risk of heart attack increases.[10] If you begin taking estrogen *early* in your post-menopausal years, it doesn't increase your risk of heart attack. But if you begin taking it late in your post-menopausal years, it does.[11] In fact, estrogen appears to actually protect against a heart attack in pre-, peri-, and early post-menopause.[12]

Compared to women who have never used hormone therapy for menopause, there's an initial increase in the risk of a second heart attack in women who have had one in the past. However, as the duration of hormone use increases, the risk of a second heart attack becomes lower than in women who have never used hormones at all.[13]

Estrogen

Here are the facts about estrogen on the heart: It helps the vessels of the heart dilate, lowers lousy LDL, raises healthy HDL, and lowers cholesterol. On the flip side, it increases triglycerides. It works better alone than it does with progesterone. It doesn't increase the risk in women who don't have heart disease; nor does it decrease the risk of heart attack in women who already have heart disease.

Both the oral (pill) form of estrogen and the skin patch form of estrogen increase healthy HDL, but the oral form does so to a much greater degree. Likewise, the oral form decreases lousy LDL to a greater degree than the skin patch.[14] The patch has the benefit of lowering triglycerides. Oral estrogens increase the risk of blood clots because they travel through the liver. (Do you see how different forms of estrogen differ in their positive and negative features?)

Timing is key to the effect of estrogen on the heart. If you begin taking estrogen with or without progesterone *early* in your post-menopausal years, it does *not* increase your risk of heart attack. But, if you begin taking estrogen with or without progesterone *late* in your post-menopausal years, it *does.*

Progesterone

One of the management options that is associated with the best effect on lipids is natural micronized progesterone.[4] This is a tablet that's available from a compounding pharmacy or as a pharmaceutical product called Prometrium.[4] While *synthetic* progesterone has demonstrated a negative effect on the heart, natural progesterone in the form of a *bioidentical* hormone has not. So, your heart likes bioidentical progesterone more than it likes synthetic progesterone. This is an example of the variability we see with progesterone. The type of progesterone matters with regard to your heart.

Non-hormonal Medication Options

Some women benefit from lipid-lowering medications in addition to dietary modifications. You should have blood tests to determine your levels of lipids (fats) and cholesterol. If you have elevated values of lipids, you need to repeat your blood tests twice a year until they're normal, and then continue to check them annually.[4]

Statins

Cholesterol-lowering drugs are available if you have high cholesterol levels and, either can't accomplish the lifestyle changes above, or have seen no change in cholesterol despite lifestyle changes. The category of drugs that reduces cholesterol is called "statin drugs." Some of the more familiar statin drugs are pravastatin (Pravachol), lovastatin (Mevacor), atorvastatin (Lipitor), and simvastatin (Zocor). Because statin drugs are so popular, there are new brands appearing rapidly.

Overall, the statins reduce heart attacks by 24% to 38%. They also decrease strokes. Most statins have the negative side effect of interfering with liver function.

Aspirin

Aspirin thins the blood, decreasing the likelihood of blood clots. One baby aspirin or one adult aspirin daily produces the best results. Possible side effects are stomach upset and gastrointestinal bleeding. You shouldn't take aspirin if you're taking: (1) other blood thinners; (2) any type of SSRI antidepressant, such as fluoxetine (Prozac), sertraline (Zoloft), or paroxetine (Paxil); or (3) any type of nonsteroidal anti-inflammatory agent (NSAID), such as naproxen sodium (Anaprox) or ibuprofen (Motrin, Advil).

Remember to inform your healthcare provider about any botanical/ herbal, or alternative medicines you use, because many of them thin blood in the same way aspirin does. Be sure to inform the anesthesiologist before surgery, also. You don't want to have surgery with a bunch of blood thinners on board.

Final Note

Despite the fact that I discuss each of these options in isolation, please be aware of the fact that the best choice may be a combination of options. Take note of the options that continue to repeat themselves as beneficial for multiple aspects of menopause.

Stroke

A stroke is a roadblock in the arteries which supply the brain with blood. It's the same thing as a heart attack, but the brain is the affected organ rather than the heart. The process is the same, though, with the brain, rather than the heart, incurring damage from lack of blood and oxygen. Everything I've said about management options for preventing heart attack pertains to strokes.

Blood Clots (Thrombosis)

Here again, the information in the section on heart attack applies. A blood clot is the same phenomenon occurring in a vessel that supplies an organ other than the heart or the brain. In this case, a blood clot, rather than an accumulation of lipids, causes the road block.

Chapter 29: Osteoporosis

Definition

Did you know that your bones are always undergoing remodeling and reconstruction? Your skeleton adds and removes bone cells constantly. Estrogen plays a huge role in the process of bone composition in that it regulates the process of bone turnover. Before menopause, bone loss is balanced by bone formation, so that your overall quantity of bone is stable. When estrogen practically disappears at the time of menopause, it creates an imbalance in the process of bone turnover, such that bone loss outpaces bone formation. New bone no longer replaces lost bone. Thus, bone becomes fragile, and the risk of fracture increases. This is one of the more familiar aspects of menopause.

Osteoporosis is a process through which we lose bone. It results from either inability to form new bone or reabsorption of old bone.[1] Normal bone is very thick and strong, with tiny holes in it. The best way to get an idea of what normal bone looks like is to visualize a sponge containing little tiny holes. Osteoporosis is a loss of bone such that the tiny holes in bone grow much larger. This leaves the bone looking more like Swiss cheese than like a sponge. Bone that is osteoporotic is less dense, and therefore, weak and brittle. It is prone to easy breakage.

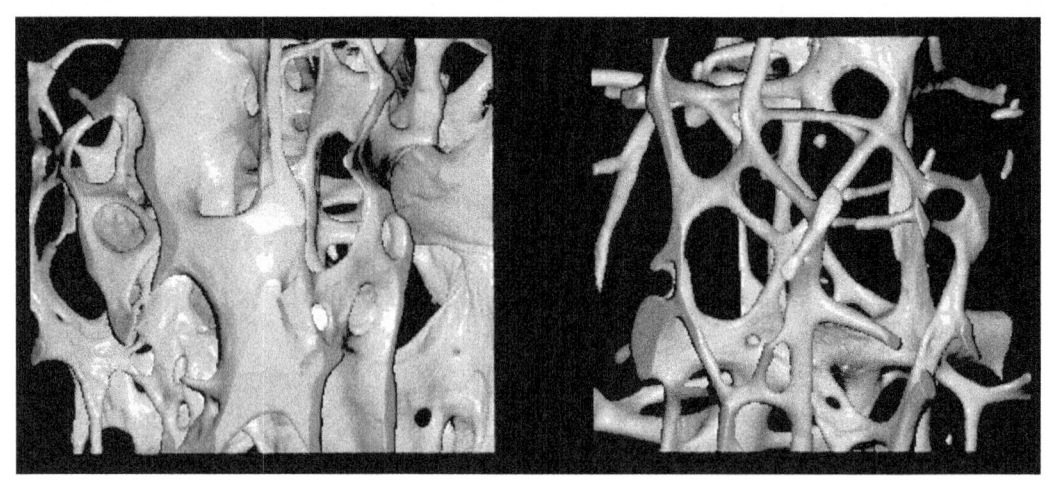

© Copyright Photo researchers, Inc.
Figure 13: Normal bone (left) versus osteoporotic bone (right)

Puberty is the time when we have peak amounts of calcium deposition in bone.[1] Anything that inhibits the process of calcium deposition at the time of puberty can sabotage the ability of the bone to achieve peak bone mass. Thus, anorexia, bulimia, excessive exercise, low body weight, and inadequate hormone levels during puberty are all possible inhibitors.[1] Once again we have a developmental process that involves puberty at one end and menopause at the other.

Rates of Loss

Now here's the kicker: Bone mass decreases by 2% each year for the first five years of post-menopause. After that, there is a steady 1% loss of bone mass every year for the rest of your life.[1] If you live for another 50 years, that's a lot of bone loss. Over time, the loss of bone mass significantly increases your risk of bone fracture. Thus, a 50 year old woman has a 40% lifetime risk of hip, spine, or wrist fracture.[1]

Symptoms

Fortunately or unfortunately, osteoporosis does **not** produce any symptoms. For most women with osteoporosis, the very first sign is bone fracture or breakage, oftentimes from minimal trauma. I tend to view this as an unfortunate circumstance. If there were early symptoms, you would have a warning before a disastrous event. However, some of the signs that may indicate *advanced* osteoporosis include decreasing height, back pain, curvature of the back, or fracture resulting from minimal trauma.[2] The hip and the spine are the most common sites of fracture or breakage due to osteoporosis, both of which produce devastating results. The third most common site is the wrist.

Epidemiology and Prognosis

The effects of osteoporosis go much deeper than bone. In fact, it's a fatal disease. Approximately 25% of menopausal women suffer a hip fracture due to osteoporosis. A full 20% of these will die from the complications of that fracture. Of those who survive, 50% will require assisted living or home health care. These women may never regain the ability to walk or to live alone again. Fractures of the spine are equally devastating. They result in chronic back pain, humpback curvature in the upper back, and loss of height. They can restrict movement in multiple ways. Even a fracture of the wrist can result in pain, disfigurement, and disability.[3] I'm not trying to frighten you. This is reality.

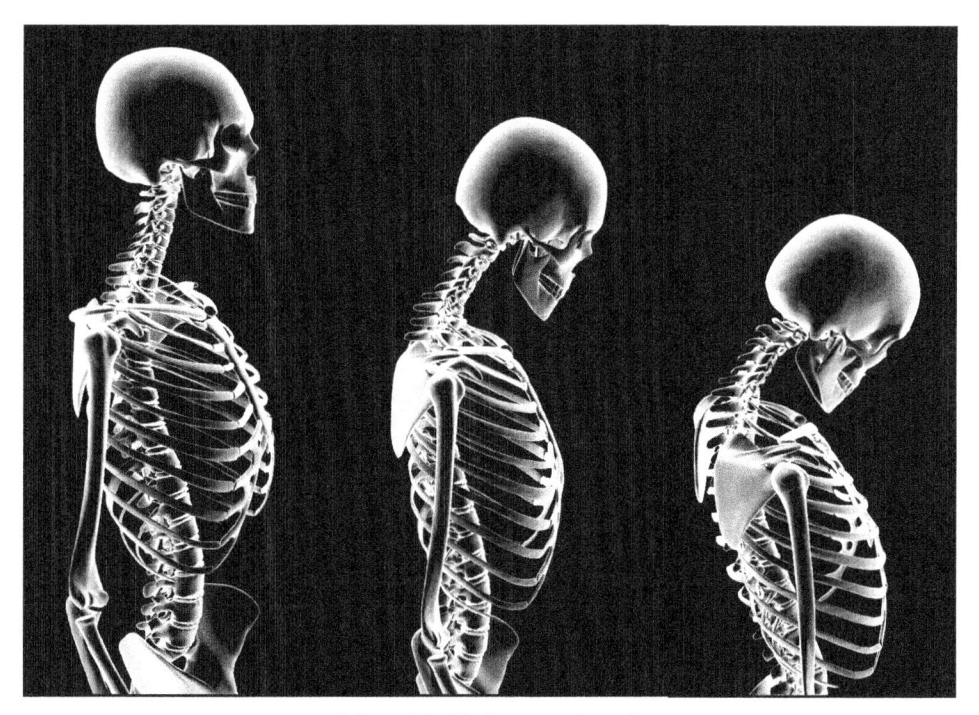

© Copyright Photo researchers, Inc.

Figure 14: Postural changes as a result of osteoporosis

Bone Architecture

There are two kinds of bone in your body. This is important because one kind is more prone to osteoporosis than the other. The type of bone that is susceptible to fracture is called **trabecular bone**. It's porous, loosely packed, and has a large surface area. It's also weaker and contains lower levels of calcium. As a matter of fact, the word "osteoporosis" literally means porous bone (Osteo = bone, Porosis = porous). Only 20% of the bone in your body consists of trabecular bone. Examples of trabecular bone are the spine (vertebrae) and the hip.

The other 80% of your bone is called **cortical bone**. Cortical bone is harder, stronger, more densely packed, and contains more calcium than trabecular bone. It has a smaller surface area. Thus, it is less inclined to fracture. Examples of cortical bone are the long bones of the legs and arms. Some trabecular bone is surrounded by the stronger cortical bone. Over the course of a lifetime, a woman loses about 35% of her cortical bone and 50% of her trabecular bone.[4]

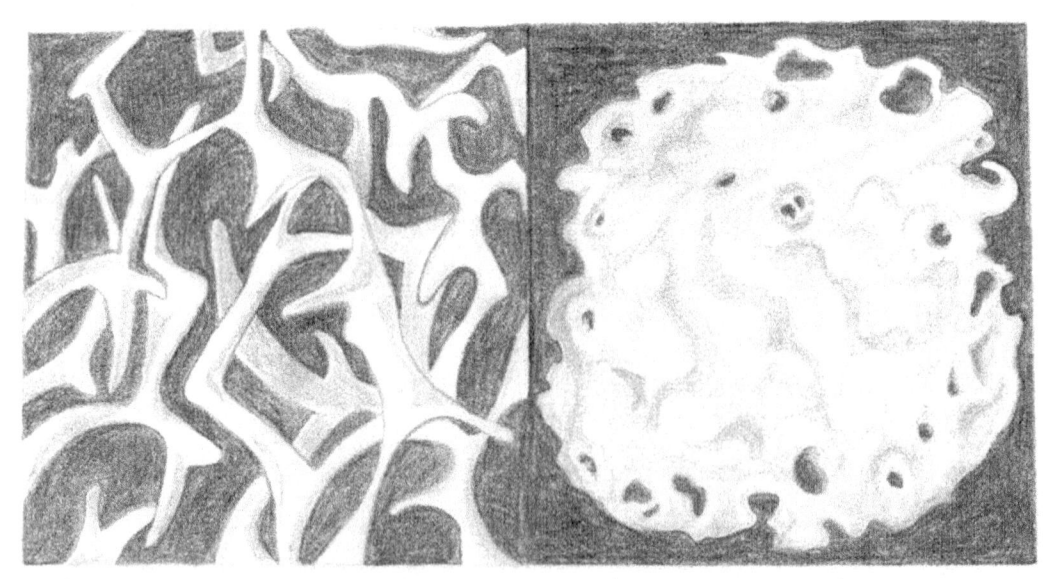

Figure 15: Trabecular bone (left) and cortical bone (right)

The best way to envision the difference between trabecular and cortical bone is to think about knitting. You've probably seen a variety of knitted garments in your lifetime. Maybe you even knit yourself. Well, some knitted garments are loosely knit. They have a lot of space between the strands of yarn. You can see through them, and you can stretch them easily. They aren't very strong. This loosely knit pattern is representative of trabecular bone. Alternatively, tightly knit garments have no space between the strands of yarn. You can't see through them, nor stretch them easily. They're quite strong. The tightly knit pattern is representative of cortical bone.

Risk Factors

Some women are naturally at higher risk of osteoporosis than others. Genetic factors play a role in determining peak bone mass, but physiologic, environmental, and lifestyle factors are also significant.[1] If you're at high risk of osteoporosis, you'll need greater surveillance and you'll need to know what your choices are for protecting yourself against bone injury. Here's a list of the things that place you at high risk of osteoporosis. Put a check next to the ones that apply to you.

1. **Caucasian race**
2. **Naturally blonde hair color** (not dyed)
3. **Thin body habitus**, with small frame or less than 18% body fat
4. **Family members with osteoporosis or fractures**
5. **Premature menopause** (before the age of 40 without adequate hormone replacement)
6. **Anything that increases your risk of falling**
   The risk of falling requires some elaboration. Some of the things that place you at a higher risk of falling may surprise you. Even if they don't surprise you, it's important to call your attention to them. The list is long, so brace yourself.

   a. Having a history of falling or fracture in the past
   b. Tendency to faint
   c. Dizziness
   d. Loss of consciousness
   e. Difficulty with balance
   f. Poor coordination
   g. Arthritis
   h. Impaired vision

i. Muscle weakness
j. Use of multiple medications (especially for depression, seizures, high blood pressure, sedation, and pain relief)

7. **Sedentary lifestyle**
8. **Tobacco use** (cigarette smoking)
9. **Diet high in caffeine** (more than 16 oz daily of coffee or 60 oz daily of cola)
10. **Excessive alcohol consumption**
    (In general, this means more than one drink daily. More specifically, it means more than 25 gm daily, which includes more than 24 oz of beer, more than 8 oz of wine, or more than 3 oz of an 80 proof alcoholic beverage each day.)
11. **Chronic excessive exercise**
12. **History of anorexia or bulimia**
13. **Diabetes**
14. **History of thyroid disease** (hyperthyroidism or hypothyroidism)
15. **Vitamin D deficiency or lack of sun exposure**
16. **Use of medications for thyroid disease**
17. **Use of steroids** (cortisol, dexamethasone, prednisone, etc.)
18. **Regular use of various medications**, such as:
    a) Any medication for convulsions
    b) Diazepam (Valium)
    c) Chlordiazepoxide (Librium), or lorazepam (Ativan)
    d) Lithium
    e) Blood thinners
    f) Tamoxifen (before menopause)
    g) Immunosuppressants

If you have two or more of these factors, you should weigh the osteoporosis element heavily in your decision-making process for managing menopause.

The propensity for osteoporosis is greatly dependent on race. Caucasian (white) women are at greatest risk, followed by Mongoloid (Asian) women. Negroid (black) women have the lowest risk due to the fact that they have more pigment in their skin. This pigment (called melanin) is associated with a stronger foundation for bone. The lifetime risk of hip fracture for a 50 year old is 14% for a Caucasian woman and 6% for a Negroid woman.[2] So, you may be more or less at risk by virtue of your race alone. Of course, that's a factor you can't change.

Males have a lower risk of osteoporosis than females do because of their larger frames and their higher levels of testosterone.[3] It just isn't fair.

Some of the factors which contribute to poor bone quality are steroids, nutritional deficiencies, anorexia or bulimia, and lack of exercise. More than 50% of osteoporosis in peri-menopausal women may be due to causes other than hormonal factors.[1] This gives you many options for preventing osteoporosis.

Once osteoporosis develops in bone, it's very difficult, but not impossible, to replace or reverse the bone loss that has already occurred. It's sort of like trying to reverse the effects of aging without plastic surgery. This is critical to our discussion of menopause because women achieve their maximal quantity of bone at the age of 20. Most women maintain their peak bone mass until the age of 30. And then it's downhill. Thereafter, natural bone loss occurs very slowly as we age. Of significance is the fact that bone loss is maximal in the first post-menopausal years.[5] Because of this, you are in greatest need of protection against osteoporosis in your immediate post-menopausal years.[5]

In females, bone density is greatly dependent on the hormone estrogen. I bet you guessed that. Women experience a drastic increase in bone loss with estrogen cessation at the time of menopause. Left untreated, you'll lose at least *1%* of your bone *per year* after menopause. This statistic is important due to the simple fact that our life expectancy has increased to the point that we are now spending one third to one half of our lives in the post-menopausal state.

You really can't discuss menopause without including the subject of osteoporosis. The two are inextricably linked because osteoporosis is the *only* menopausal issue for some women. You may not have any *symptoms* of menopause that concern you in the least. But osteoporosis doesn't produce symptoms. It results as a consequence of estrogen loss. So, it's critical for you to know about it. There are a number of alternatives from which to choose in addressing the issue of osteoporosis. Some involve hormones; some don't. Some don't require any medicine at all.

WORKSHEET TIMEOUT:
Answer question # 6 on your worksheet.
Circle all your risk factors for osteoporosis.

Calcium

Calcium is one of those things which is fraught with misconceptions and assumptions. You may have been led to believe that calcium alone can prevent osteoporosis. Wrong! Osteoporosis is the result of bone *loss* due to inadequate estrogen levels. The loss of bone ultimately results in weakened bone simply because there is less bone mass present. Calcium, on the other hand, serves the purpose of only **strengthening** bone. Calcium doesn't prevent bone loss. Calcium doesn't do the same thing for bone that estrogen does. Osteoporosis can occur in strong bone or in weak bone. Think of it like this: Estrogen addresses the *quantity* of bone, while calcium addresses the *quality* of bone. Inadequate estrogen results in a smaller *quantity* of bone. Inadequate calcium results in a lower *quality* of bone.

Visualize this: Bone consists of many bridges connecting one area of bone to another. The more bridges there are, the higher the *quantity* of bone. In other words, the more bridges there are, the more bone there is. And the stronger the bridges are, the higher the *quality* of the bone. Calcium can only strengthen the bridges. It can't build new bridges like estrogen can.

Calcium	**Estrogen**
Strengthens bone	*Maintains* bone
Prevents bone *weakening*	Prevents bone *loss*
Improves *quality* of bone	Improves *quantity* of bone

If you take plenty of calcium, but have no estrogen, you'll have high quality bone, but not enough of it. You can still lose high quality bone. You need both quality and quantity. So, you need to preserve your bone (compensate for estrogen loss) and strengthen it (take calcium). Calcium alone isn't sufficient to prevent bone loss in the peri-menopausal period.[5] And by the way, exercise strengthens bone also.

I'm not trying to belittle calcium's value. It's very important in bone health. I'm just making sure you understand the differences between inadequate estrogen and inadequate calcium as far as your bones are concerned. In fact, peri-menopausal and post-menopausal women need to consume 1500 mgs of calcium daily. Most women only consume approximately 400 mgs of calcium per day in their diet. So, calcium supplementation is important. If you take calcium, be sure to take vitamin D also, because vitamin D is necessary for your body to absorb the calcium. The recommended amount of vitamin D is 400 - 800 IU per day. Many calcium preparations already contain vitamin D. Check the label to be sure.

Bone Density

Bone Density Tests

The test for measuring bone mass to determine if you have osteoporosis is called a *"bone density test."* It measures the quantity of mineral in your bone. It *doesn't* measure bone strength or bone structure. In essence, it tells you how much bone you have, but not how well formed or how strong it is.

There are many varieties of bone density tests. Some evaluate your hip and your entire spine. Some evaluate just your heel. Others evaluate your index finger or your forearm. Some use ultrasound. Others use some form of radiation. Some take only seconds to complete, while others are more of a production. You should definitely have a bone density test when you enter peri- or post-menopause. This will provide a baseline bone density value for later comparison.

I think it's wise to use whichever method you find desirable or accessible for your first bone density test. You may want to use one of those quick, nifty instruments that just tests your finger or heel. They're great for screening, and many doctors have them in their offices. However, if your result reveals anything other than a perfectly normal value, I recommend that you proceed to a more thorough test, such as the one that actually measures your hip and spine. Dual Energy X-ray Absorption (DEXA) is the most thorough bone density testing device currently available. It measures your hip and your entire spine, and it's the gold standard for measurement.

Here are some general principles to keep in mind: Spine fractures are more common in women younger than age 65, so DEXA of your spine is the preferable site if you're younger than 65. On the other hand, hip fractures are more common in women over age 65, so DEXA of your hip is the preferable site if you're over 65. DEXA is also preferable over alternative techniques that measure sites other than the hip and spine if you have multiple risk factors.[2] As you might predict, measurement at two sites rather than one increases the accuracy of the results.[2] DEXA is the only method that is valid for serial measurements from one year to the next.[2] That's important if you have signs of bone loss on your scan. It's not as critical if your bone density is normal. Fortunately, the radiation exposure from DEXA is extremely small, and equals that of normal daily background radiation.[6]

Low bone density at any skeletal site predicts the likelihood of fractures at any location, but most accurately predicts the specific site of the test.[6] So, if you test only your hip, the result is more accurate for determining your risk of hip fracture than it is for spine fracture.

The quality and density of your bones are not the only things that determine your risk of bone fracture. It's also important to recognize that how frail you are and how likely you are to fall are potent predictors of bone fracture. If you're a very small-boned thin woman, you're at higher risk than if you're a big-boned, muscular woman. If you have trouble maintaining your balance or have inflexible joints which limit your mobility, you're more likely to fall, and your joints are less likely to bend in a way that keeps bones from breaking. If you have a visual impairment or get confused easily, you're more likely to trip over things or bump into things. Thus, balance, mobility, visual impairment, and mental clarity are all important factors to consider in addressing whether or not you need to give special attention to preventing osteoporosis.[6]

Guidelines for Bone Density Testing

So, what are the guidelines for bone density testing? In other words, who should have the testing and when? The answer depends on whom you ask, and their answer depends on which set of guidelines they consult. You see, there are multiple societies, foundations, task forces, and organizations which have formulated guidelines for bone density testing. In essence, they tend to target age 65 as the mandatory age, and to include anyone with certain risk factors. They take cost into account as it pertains to the percentage of healthcare dollars dedicated to bone density testing. By and large, they are *economic guidelines*. Because fractures from osteoporosis occur most commonly in women over the age of 65, and because this is the age group for which intervention has proved most beneficial, the guidelines have been designed to reflect this.

The word "economic" means that these are the guidelines for the population at large from a monetary standpoint. It's as if the economists put together some rules to address bone density testing that also save the most money. They're more focused on treatment than they are on prevention. That's because it's worth it to spend money on treatment, while it may be a waste of money to spend it on prevention. Medicare even has a list of "eligible patients" for whom they will pay for bone density testing.

The other feature of the guideline mentality is that it caters to the *population at large*. There is no individualization. Of course, you're not interested in the population at large. You're interested in prevention and peace of mind for yourself. And none of the guidelines talks about those things.

You'll find a variety of guidelines as to when you should have a bone density test. Discrepancies abound. If you want to know what your status is at the beginning of your menopausal transition, it's imperative that you have a bone density test at the time you become post-menopausal to determine your baseline value of bone density, and thus your risk of osteoporosis. Thereafter, it's necessary to repeat the bone density test on a regular basis (annually or biannually) to remain aware of the status of your bone. So, as soon as you've gone without a period for 12 consecutive months, get your bone density tested. Of course, you may do so sooner, but remember that the most important time is in the first year of post-menopause.

All therapies for preventing bone loss are most effective when they are started soon after the onset of menopause. So, it's absolutely more reasonable and justifiable for you to have an assessment for osteoporosis at the time you become post-menopausal, regardless of age, regardless of the guidelines, and regardless of large scale economics. Remember, you're unique, and the guidelines are population-wide rather than individual, and economic rather than preventive. They're designed to balance the likelihood of detecting osteoporosis with the cost of testing for it in the population at large. Don't ever let guidelines allow you to become complacent or exercise a lower level of diligence than common sense dictates. Don't allow such limitations to inhibit you if you have even the slightest desire or need to evaluate your bone density. I believe in knowledge and peace of mind, so my recommendation differs from the standard population-wide economic guidelines you'll encounter elsewhere. Remember, you must detect osteoporosis early in order to intervene in its progress.

T Score

The measurement for bone density is a value called the "*T score.*" The T score compares your bone density to that of an average healthy 30 year old woman. A value equal to or above that of an average healthy 30 year old woman is normal. A value lower than that of an average healthy 30 year old woman is abnormal. Why age 30? Age 30 is the reference age because it's the oldest age at which we maintain our maximum bone density.

In terms of actual values, a T score value of 0 or above is normal, indicating an absence of osteoporosis. A value between -1 and -2.4 is borderline. The term used for borderline bone density is **"osteopenia."** This means that the bone density is less than normal, but not abnormal enough to qualify for osteoporosis. It is a precursor to osteoporosis.

Osteoporosis

If you have osteopenia and you do nothing to treat it, you'll probably develop osteoporosis. Think of a T score indicating osteopenia as a huge warning signal. Finally, a T score of -2.5 and lower represents full blown osteoporosis. If you have a value this low, you need to take this information very seriously and become diligent about preventing progression of this disease.

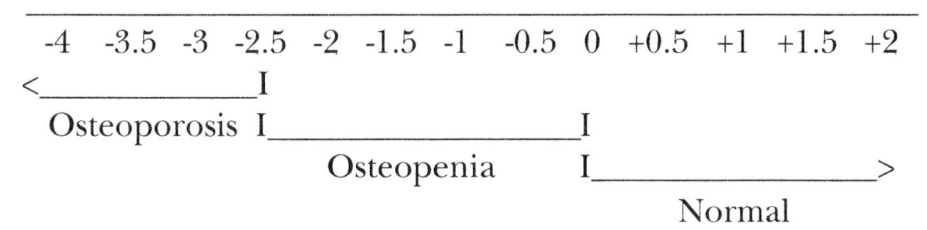

```
 -4  -3.5  -3  -2.5  -2  -1.5  -1   -0.5  0  +0.5  +1  +1.5  +2
<_____I
   Osteoporosis  I_____I
                    Osteopenia          I_____>
                                            Normal
```

To review, here's a summary of T scores and their significance:

T Score	Meaning	Recommendation
Greater than or equal to 0	Normal	Jump for joy
-2.4 – -0.1	Osteopenia	Measure hip/spine bone density Begin treatment
Less than or equal to -2.5	Osteoporosis	Begin treatment

Here are some startling facts: For each *whole number* difference in bone density, there is a *doubling* of the risk of fracture.[2] So, if your T score is -1, you're is twice as likely to suffer a fracture than you are if your T score is 0. If your T score is -2, you're four times as likely to suffer a fracture than if your T score is 0. Here's another way think about it: For every whole number decrease in T score, you will have a *10% to 15%* decrease in your bone mass. And for every whole number decrease in T score, your risk of fracture increases by an amount that is equal to *10 to 13 years* of normal aging. Yikes!

If you've obtained T score measurements on different parts of your body or you've used different bone density devices, use the lowest score to determine your risk of osteoporosis.[2] Individual women with the same T score will have different risks at various ages. For instance, a 70 year old with a T score of -3 has a 5.5% risk of hip fracture over the next five years, whereas an 80 year old with the same T score has a 9% risk. This is due to decreasing bone quality, decreasing muscle strength, and decreasing balance with age.[2]

Z Score

Another scoring value for bone density is the "*Z score.*" The Z score compares your bone density to a woman of *your age and ethnicity*. So, instead of using ideal bone density as a standard like the T score did, it uses the average bone density of women in your own age and ethnic group as a standard. In essence, it tells you whether or not your bone density is appropriate for the normal aging process. Thus, you may have a low T score, but an average Z score. For a young adult woman, the T score and the Z score should be the same.

With regard to assessing the presence or absence of osteoporosis, it's the *T score* on which you want to focus. You want to compare your bone density to the best value your bone density can be. Remember, everything in life is relative. If you compare yourself to the average, you may look pretty good, but you really want to look good when you compare yourself to the best. Deciding that a normal Z score is acceptable when it is lower than your T score is like deciding that a "C" is an acceptable grade, and an "A" isn't worth the effort. Never settle for mediocrity! Always try to be the best you can be!

Now, although the T score is extremely important, you don't want to base all decisions solely on the T score. That's because even though bone density may account for 70% of your bone's value, there are other characteristics of bone that count for something. Bone quality, rate of bone turnover, and bone structure also play a role in the development of osteoporosis.[2]

Urine Testing

If you go back to our discussion of normal bone, you'll recall that bone turns over. This means that new bone forms while old bone breaks down and gets absorbed. Urine testing for osteoporosis takes advantage of the breakdown process. Since the overall rate of bone remodeling is important in determining bone quality, the products of bone breakdown are useful in assessing the presence of osteoporosis.[2]

Urine testing of collagen fragments is a nifty way to monitor bone breakdown. This is possible because bone breakdown is accompanied by release of collagen fragments into your urine. Consider this a test that can give you daily information about bone loss rather than having to wait months in between bone density tests. Fortunately, the test comes in the form of a kit that doesn't even require a prescription. While this testing method may be convenient, it's not as representative of the big picture. Knowing how much collagen exists in your urine each day doesn't translate into knowing your bone density.

Management Options

If you're at increased risk of osteoporosis, it's imperative that you consider the multiple options available to avoid or arrest bone loss. There are enough options to serve your needs and still honor your preferences. The key to osteoporosis is prevention. The goal is to prevent fracture by: (1) slowing or preventing bone loss; (2) maintaining bone strength; and (3) minimizing or eliminating things that contribute to falling and injuring yourself. Please don't wait until you have a change in bone density to begin adopting behaviors and utilizing agents to prevent bone loss.

Diet and Lifestyle Options

Prevent Falls

When you were young, you hurt yourself by engaging in sports or other physical activities. As you age, you're more likely to hurt yourself doing basic, simple things. The last thing you want to do is to break a bone doing normal, non-physical things in your own home. You can actually ***fall-proof your home*** to prevent injury to yourself just as you child-proof your home to protect a toddler. It's really simple to do, and it makes a huge difference in your tendency to fall. Here's a list of fool-proof, fall-proof measures:

1. <u>Proof your floors</u>.[7] Use floor cleaners and floor waxes that aren't slippery in the non-carpeted areas. If you have any throw rugs, area rugs, or runners, make sure they don't skid. Buy some of those non-skid mats that fit under the rug if necessary.
2. <u>Make sure all your rooms are well lit</u>.[7] The best thing to do is to get those lights that turn on automatically when the sensor detects motion. That way, the lights will turn on as you enter a room rather than your having to enter in the dark and find the light switch. Put runway lights along your stairwell. Just buy some white holiday lights and string them along the sides of the steps. It will actually look quite decorative.
3. <u>Pick up after yourself</u>.[7] Don't leave things lying around the house on the floor. You might forget that there's something on the floor and trip over it. Train your family to pick up things, also.
4. <u>Rearrange your furniture</u>.[7] Arrange it so that there's plenty of walking space in the rooms of your home.
5. <u>Fall-proof your bathrooms</u>.[7] Put non-skid rubber mats in the tub and shower. If you have trouble standing in the shower, put a chair in it to sit on while you bathe. You can also put bars next to the tub, shower, and toilet so that you have something to grab onto when you move from place to place. Remember, your tub and shower may not be very slippery…until you're using soap, shampoo, and hair conditioner.
6. <u>Check your stairways and floors for defects</u>.[7] Make sure you repair anything that appears broken, loose, or weak.
7. <u>Adjust the heights of household items</u>.[7] Situate them so that you don't have to climb onto stools to reach things. Check the height of your furniture, also. If your chairs are too high or too low, adjust them. Do the same with your bed.

Exercise

There are two categories of exercise that serve the purpose of strengthening and building bone. The first is weight-bearing exercise, and the second is resistance exercise.[8]

<u>Weight-bearing exercise</u> includes any activity that places weight on the joints. That means any activity which requires you to bear and support your weight as you work against gravity. Walking, running, dancing, step aerobics, climbing stairs, and using the elliptical machine are all weight-bearing exercises. Most sports fall into this category, also. This includes tennis, racquet ball, roller skating or roller blading, baseball, basketball, football, and skiing. Some aspects of yoga and Pilates also qualify as weight-bearing exercise. Swimming doesn't, because the water removes the impact of your body weight on your bones. It's still a great aerobic activity for heart health and weight loss. Regardless of your risk of osteoporosis, and regardless of the choices you make for management of your own menopause, you really should incorporate weight-bearing exercise into your regimen.

<u>Resistance exercises</u> involve the use of your muscle strength to overcome resistance. Lifting free weights, using the weight machines, and working out with resistance bands are all great ways to do resistance exercises. You only need to do these two to four times each week. Be sure to give your muscles a break between workouts. Do this by limiting your resistance training to every other day at most. Don't try to do resistance exercises two days in a row. You increase the likelihood that you'll hurt yourself. Also note that you don't have to use heavy weights to gain the benefits of resistance exercises. You can do a lot of repetitions with light weights instead of a few with heavy weights, and you'll be in good shape. I mean that both literally and figuratively.

Balance is Key

When was the last time you walked along the curb, balancing on it the way you did when you were a kid? When did you last stand on one leg and try to do a task without supporting yourself by holding on to something? When was the last time you tried to close your eyes and do something just for fun? Do you see what I'm getting at? We tend to fall as we age because we lose our balance. And we tend to lose our balance simply because we don't test it or practice balancing. We don't "have fun" trying things the way we did when we were children. If you want to maintain your balance well into your elder years, you have to challenge yourself a bit. Go to the gym and try to balance on some of the equipment there. Try working out with one of those big stability balls. Or try doing your weights standing on one leg or on an unstable surface (like a BOSU), or both. Have a trainer show you how to do some exercises safely. You'll be amazed at how quickly you progress from wobbling all over the place to finding it easy to balance. Before you know it, you'll be asking that trainer for some more difficult balancing acts. Other people will come join you, also. We all had fun doing these things as kids, and we really haven't changed our tendency to enjoy such things that much.

Two other great ways to work on your balance are by doing yoga or Pilates. Yoga includes some standing poses that require you to balance yourself in some interesting positions. No matter how good you get, there's usually another step with which you can challenge yourself as you progress. Pilates involves the use of "core balance." That's the central balancing force you use in the base of your gut. It helps you achieve better posture and use your muscles to maintain your balance.

<u>Smoking Cessation</u>

Protection of your bones is just another great reason to quit smoking. Remember the risk factors for osteoporosis? Smoking was one of the biggies. Obviously, if smoking is a factor that puts you at higher risk for the disease in the first place, quitting reduces the likelihood of developing osteoporosis.

Osteoporosis is another one of those diseases for which you have so much control over some of the risk factors (smoking, alcohol, sedentary lifestyle, diet) and no control over others (genetics, race, natural hair color, medical problems, and necessary medications). So why not take advantage of your ability to do something about the ones you *can* control.

Sun Exposure

Sun exposure provides vitamin D, which is necessary for your bones to absorb calcium. Sun exposure is the preferable way to ensure adequate vitamin D because the vitamin D that your body manufactures is superior to vitamin D supplements in assisting with calcium absorption.

Intense sun exposure is unnecessary, because your body has the ability to store vitamin D for use over time. Thus, exposing your hands and arms for 20 minutes, four to five times weekly, for only four to five months per year will do the trick.[3] Full body exposure for only 15 minutes provides the equivalent of 10,000 IU of a vitamin D supplement. Dark skin and aging impose a requirement of more sun exposure for adequate vitamin D.

Now, I'm not saying here that you need to be a sun goddess. In fact, it's extremely important to avoid sun exposure due to the risk of skin cancer. I'm not promoting tanning or sun burning. The best time of day to achieve sun exposure is early morning or early evening, when the sun is mild in intensity. At all other times, wear sunscreen at the very least. Better yet, cover your skin with clothing.

Diet

Limit Caffeine

Caffeine consumption may have an effect on calcium loss and bone density. Excessive amounts of caffeine may interfere with your body's ability to absorb and use calcium. Studies have shown an increase in calcium excretion in the urine after consuming caffeine.[9] You don't have to omit caffeine altogether. Just limit your intake. Don't be dependent on it to wake up in the morning, stay focused during the day, or avoid falling asleep before bedtime. Enjoy it in moderation.

Limit Alcohol

Alcohol consumption and its relationship to bone loss are confusing. Long-term alcoholism increases the frequency of bone fractures.[9] More than seven drinks per week is definitely a risk factor for osteoporosis.[9] That means you benefit yourself most by having far less than seven drinks per week. If you contrast this with the beneficial quantity of alcohol for your heart, though, you'll realize that what's good for your heart isn't so good for your bones. The "moderate" alcohol intake of only one drink per day that's beneficial for *heart* health seems to be borderline or "excessive" for *bone* health. This is a perfect example of why it's important to figure out what your risks are and to tailor your management to **your** areas of greatest concern. As with many other things in life, some choices may benefit you in some ways and not in others.

So, once again, drink alcohol in moderation. It's not the most critical factor in bone health, but it certainly plays an important role.

Soy

Soy-based foods, such as tofu, soy beans, soy milk, etc. are all full of phytoestrogens. Regular consumption of soy protein can protect bone to the same extent as estrogen. Soy protein has a greater effect on porous, loose, trabecular bone than it does on hard, dense, cortical bone.[9] It tends to provide greater protection from osteoporosis in the spine than it does in the hip.

Get this: Even though Asian women have lower bone density than Black or White women, they have a lower incidence of hip fractures than the other two groups.[10] This represents strong evidence of the effect soy has on increasing bone density. Studies have shown that postmenopausal women with the highest consumption of soy products have the highest bone density at the hip (6.4% greater) and spine (8.4% greater).[10]

Flaxseed

Flaxseed is another potent source of phytoestrogens. Eating flaxseeds is like eating soy in seed form. They have a nice nutty taste. You can just eat a few spoonful alone or you can sprinkle them in just about any kind of food. They're especially good in salads. Grind them up before eating them so that they don't go through you whole. The grinding exposes all the nutrients and enables you to absorb them.

Protein

Protein is an important substance in supporting bone health. Previous suspicions that protein contributed to osteoporosis are unfounded. The same amount of protein that is necessary for overall health is appropriate for bone health. So, use the standard dietary guidelines for the new food pyramid. Notice that it doesn't call for nearly as much protein as most people eat. However, increased quantities of protein are necessary for women who are physically active. Animal protein may be less desirable than vegetable protein because it causes an increase in the excretion of calcium in the urine.[9]

No Soft Drinks

Soft drinks contain high concentrations of phosphorous, which moves calcium out of bones. Thus, high concentrations of phosphorous-containing foods or beverages increase osteoporosis. The more soft drinks you consume, the lower your blood calcium level and the higher your risk of osteoporosis. So, limit, or preferably, eliminate soft drinks. They have absolutely no nutritional value, anyway. Try satisfying your thirst with good old water.

Vitamin D Foods

Vitamin D-rich foods include egg yolks, liver, salt water fish, and cod liver oil. Vitamin D fortified milk and cereals are also good sources of vitamin D. Why vitamin D? Because vitamin D is necessary for your bones to absorb calcium. If your vitamin D levels are deficient, you can only absorb 10% to 15% of your calcium intake.

Calcium-Rich Foods

You can get a lot of calcium from your diet, but most women don't. In fact, most women get only 400 of the 1500 daily recommended milligrams of calcium from their diet. Some of the foods that are highest in calcium content are dairy products, raisins, spinach, sardines, and broccoli. If you do get significant amounts of calcium from your diet, just add enough in the form of supplements to get the full 1500 mg.

Vitamin and Mineral Options

Calcium

Calcium has a helping role in the prevention of osteoporosis. This means that it makes bone stronger, and it enhances all of the other modalities available for bone health. Adequate calcium intake enhances the positive effects of exercise and other therapies on bone mass.

To reiterate what you learned earlier, don't make the mistake of assuming that calcium alone can prevent or treat osteoporosis. All it can do is make whatever bone you have stronger. It can't keep you from losing bone. It's important, but it's not a substitute for the things that *prevent* bone loss. You need both strong bone and large quantities of bone.

Calcium is available in many forms. The ones that allow maximal absorption from the digestive system are calcium citrate, calcium malate, or a mixture of calcium ascorbate, calcium succinate, calcium tartrate, and calcium fumarate. I know this is technical, and I only mention these by name because they're the names you'll see on the calcium products you buy in stores. Don't focus on the names too much. Just know that you can use any of them.

Taking an adequate amount of calcium is one thing. Ensuring that it gets absorbed into your blood stream is another. And there are a couple of things that tend to interfere with the absorption process. Absorption of calcium is greatest when taken with food. It's also best when the stomach's acidity is greatest (low pH). Absorption also increases at night. It's best to divide doses of calcium rather than taking large quantities all at once, because adults are only able to absorb 30% to 50% of a calcium load. This means that the most you'll actually use is 50% of the dose of calcium you take at any one time. So, to get the recommended daily dose, you have to take calcium more than once a day. That's not the only thing for which you have to compensate, though. The acidity of your stomach decreases with age (in other words, the pH increases). Since low acidity decreases the amount of calcium you absorb, the extent of calcium absorption decreases as you age, too.[11] Fortunately, estrogen has the effect of increasing absorption of calcium.

Magnesium

It's important to take calcium and magnesium together in a ratio of 2:1. Magnesium has the effect of improving the absorption of calcium. Plus, it has a major influence on the type of calcium crystals that are present in bone.[9] Some women with decreased bone density don't have an increased fracture rate because they have better bone *structure* as a result of high levels of magnesium.[9]

Vitamin D

Vitamin D supplementation is necessary if it's not possible to get adequate sun exposure. This may be because of immobility, lack of windows, or living in a place with little sunshine. Because greater amounts of vitamin D are necessary as you age, the dosages of vitamin D vary based on age. Below age 65, the dose is 400 – 800 IU daily. Above age 65, the dose is 800 – 1200 IU daily.

A blood test for vitamin D can give you information about your need for supplementation. The normal range is 75 – 250 nmol/l. A level of 20 – 25 nmol/l is indicative of severe vitamin D deficiency.

Vitamin B9

Vitamin B9 (folate) reduces the level of homocysteine. Homocysteine increases your risk of osteoporosis. Most multivitamins have adequate folate to decrease high homocysteine levels. You can get folate from green, leafy vegetables and from fortified grain products. But, the amount of folate absorbed from food differs from the amount absorbed from a supplement in the form of a pill. You absorb 50% of the folate in *unfortified* foods, and 85% of the folate in *fortified* foods. But you absorb nearly all of the folate in a *supplement*. This means that, when it comes to folate, you're better off getting it from a supplement than you are from foods.

Other Vitamins

Three other vitamins that have minor roles in bone health deserve brief mention. They include vitamins B6, C, and K. **Vitamin B6** decreases the level of homocysteine. **Vitamin C** promotes the structural proteins that form bone. And **vitamin K** assists in drawing calcium to bone.

Trace Minerals

Trace minerals that are important in building and maintaining healthy bones include **manganese, boron, zinc, copper,** and **silicon.**[9] You can maintain adequate levels of all of these by taking a multivitamin daily.

Botanical and Herbal Options

Phytoestrogens

Phytoestrogens can reduce your risk of osteoporosis. While most studies examining the effect of phytoestrogens on bone have been performed on animals, a human study has shown that 40 gm of soy protein daily for a six month period of time increased bone density by 2.2%.[12]

Remember that phytoestrogens are essentially low dose estrogen in the form of food. If you shop around, you'll see that there are soy protein substitutes for nearly every type of animal product. It's really easy to eat soy these days. If you don't like the soy products in isolation, mix them with other foods, and you can still get adequate quantities to really make a difference in your bone health.

Green Tea (Camellia sinensis)

Green tea contains antioxidants that are beneficial in maintaining bone health. Just one cup of green tea a day is adequate. Of course, you may have as much as you desire.

Hormonal Medication Options

Estrogen

Estrogen is the mainstay of therapies that are available to prevent osteoporosis. As such, estrogen in any form will do the trick. Pills, skin patches, vaginal rings, shots, and gels are all effective.

In using any form of estrogen to avoid or arrest osteoporosis, it's critical for you to realize that there is a minimal adequate dose to accomplish that goal. If you take less than the minimal adequate dose, you'll fall short of the desired results. For years, the medical profession thought that the minimal adequate dose was 0.625 mg of conjugated equine estrogen or its equivalent. Now, there's evidence that even a lower dose may prevent bone loss, especially in older women. However, some women need a higher dose. So, be sure to monitor your bone density to ensure that the dose you take is protecting your bones. This is not a "one dose suffices for all women" matter. A particular dose of estrogen may serve to alleviate your symptoms of menopause, but that doesn't mean that it's adequate to prevent osteoporosis.

It's also important to realize that, even though you may be taking the minimal adequate dose of estrogen for the average woman, it may not be enough for you individually. That's because, simply put, women aren't carbon copies of one another. We're all different. We have varying body sizes, bone structures, fat stores, and rates of bone loss. The dose of estrogen that prevents bone loss for your friend may not be enough to do the same for you. Regardless of whether or not you're consuming the minimal adequate dose to prevent osteoporosis, it's imperative that you have your bone density checked on a regular basis to ensure that you're not falsely secure in your management technique.

Estrogen replacement provides protection of bone only *while* you're actually taking it. If you discontinue estrogen, the beneficial effects on bone will cease, and bone loss will begin to occur.

Testosterone

Testosterone is beneficial in avoiding osteoporosis because it makes bone more dense. Recall that men have lower rates of osteoporosis because of their higher levels of testosterone. Androgen therapy provides the same effect in women. Of course, there are side effects to androgen therapy, such as oily skin, acne, and growth of coarse whiskers on your face.

Progesterone

Progesterone, in the form of either a 2% skin cream or a pill, is also capable of stimulating bone growth in an effort to prevent or reverse osteoporosis.

Calcitonin (Miacalcin, Fortical)

Calcitonin is analogous to the hormone calcitonin that comes from your parathyroid gland. It's a hormone that regulates calcium metabolism in your body. This drug is available in injectable and nasal spray forms. It decreases the loss of calcium in your urine, and thus decreases your risk of bone fracture. It also significantly reduces the pain associated with spinal fractures.[1] Side effects include flushing, runny nose, back pain, night time urination, joint pain, and nausea. It decreases second spine fractures, but only with a dose of 200 IU daily.[2]

Calcitonin is a form of calcium that's available for purposes of strengthening bone. It is *not,* however, a first line therapy for the prevention or the treatment of osteoporosis.[13] It is recommended only for women who are at least five years post-menopausal.

Teriparatide

Teriparatide (Forteo) is a pharmaceutical preparation of parathyroid hormone. Parathyroid hormone acts to increase bone absorption that's inhibited because of low calcium levels.[2] So, if your calcium falls below the normal range, it brings it back up. In essence, it's the only therapy that prevents bone loss by *building* bone rather than by preventing its breakdown. In intermittent doses, parathyroid hormone has a positive effect on bone density, and that's how teriparatide exerts its effect.[2] It works by stimulating the formation of new bone.

It is recommended for women with severe osteoporosis (T score < -3) or a history of fractures, especially if they've failed other treatments. It's really a last resort medication. It requires a daily injection, and it's expensive. It's worth both the pain of an injection and the expense if you have severe osteoporosis.

Treatment is restricted to a period of no more than two years. That's because there's been no evaluation of the safety or effectiveness of teriparatide for more than two years. Also, you cannot use it if you have high levels of calcium in your blood (hypercalcemia), or if you've had previous x-ray therapy. Side effects include leg cramps, dizziness, nausea, headache, and sore throat.

Non-hormonal Medication Options

Now, if you either cannot take estrogen or prefer not to take estrogen, there are alternative therapies which don't involve hormones. The wonderful thing about these products is that they have the same ability as estrogen to protect bone against osteoporosis. They are the SERMs, a special category of which are the Bisphosphonates.

Selective Estrogen Receptor Modulators (SERMs)

We addressed the Selective Estrogen Receptor Modulators earlier. They are especially beneficial in the context of osteoporosis. Basically, their name means that these agents behave like estrogen in some ways, but not in other ways. They act by binding with estrogen receptors, but selectively modify the effect that estrogen has on only certain parts of the body. Thus, they don't increase the amount of estrogen in your body.[14]

Tamoxifen (Nolvadex)

The oldest SERM is a medication by the name of tamoxifen.[14] It's a drug used to treat breast cancer. It's also useful for preventing the development of breast cancer in women at high risk for that disease.[14] Tamoxifen also prevents osteoporosis and heart attacks.[14] The risks of tamoxifen include an increase in cancer of the uterus, blood clots, and disorders of the eye.[14]

The most notable side effect with tamoxifen is that it increases the thickness of the uterine lining and causes uterine cancer. If you use tamoxifen and you still have your uterus, you'll need to be diligent about having your uterus examined regularly to ensure that there's no indication of uterine cancer. The necessary tests include an ultrasound to look at the uterus, and a biopsy of the uterine lining to examine the cells. It's sort of a pain! Of course, if you don't have a uterus, it's easy (and painless) to take tamoxifen.

Raloxifene (Evista)

The most well known SERM for use in menopause is a pharmaceutical product called raloxifene. Most people recognize it by its trade name, Evista. Evista is more selective for the purpose of menopause than tamoxifen.[14] Evista prevents osteoporosis to a degree equal to that of estrogen. It prevents spinal fracture, but may not prevent hip fracture.[14] It increases bone marrow density by 2% to 3%, and decreases the risk of spine fracture by 35% to 50%. Unfortunately, it has the same risk of causing blood clots that estrogen has. For this reason, you can't take both estrogen and Evista. The two fall into the either/or category.

The good thing about Evista is that it has no effect on your breasts. Thus, it's an ideal choice if you've had, or are concerned about, breast cancer. Evista also has no effect on your uterus, so it's a good choice if you're concerned with uterine cancer. Another benefit of Evista is that it helps prevent heart attack.[14] It decreases lousy LDL, and increases healthy HDL, both of which are desirable in preventing heart attack.[14] It may or may not alleviate the symptoms of menopause to the same degree that estrogen does, and it has the side effect of actually *causing* hot flashes. The standard dose of Evista is 60 mg daily.

Bisphosphonates

A special category of SERMs is the bisphosphonates. Three of the pharmaceutical preparations in this family of drugs are alendronate (Fosamax), risedronate (Actonel), and ibandronate sodium (Boniva). None of these agents has an effect on anything other than bone. Thus, they don't ameliorate any of the symptoms of menopause; nor do they have an effect on the heart, uterus, breast, or blood vessels (blood clotting). They're great if you want to target bone only, but have no desire to address any other aspect of menopause.

Because they don't have any negative effects on the heart, uterus, breast, or blood vessels, it's perfectly safe to combine any of these with estrogen or with calcium, or with both estrogen and calcium. But you can't combine them with parathyroid hormone medications like teriparatide. Like hormone replacement, bisphosphonates are only beneficial *while* you're taking them. Once you discontinue them, your increased risk of osteoporosis will return. However, they do hang around for a short time. If you've taken them for two to three years, your DEXA scan will not change significantly for one year after discontinuing them.

Alendronate (Fosamax)

Alendronate (Fosamax) is most effective for women who have actual osteoporosis (T score < -2.5) or a previous fracture of the spine.[2] It works better on the *spine* than at any other location in preventing or treating bone fracture. The dose for prevention (T score > -2.5) is 5 mg daily, while the dose for treatment (T score < -2.5 or previous fracture) is 10 mg daily. It's also available in a 70 mg tablet that you only have to take once a week, and in a raspberry flavored liquid.

The most common side effect of alendronate (Fosamax) is inflammation of the esophagus. To prevent this, it's necessary to sit or stand upright for at least 30 minutes after taking the medication. You also have to take it on an empty stomach with at least eight ounces of water.

Risedronate (Actonel)

Risedronate (Actonel) has a significant positive effect on fractures in *any* location. The dose is 5 mg daily for both prevention and treatment. It doesn't have the severe effect on the esophagus that's characteristic of alendronate (Fosamax). Its side effects include headache, nausea, joint pain, abdominal pain, diarrhea, ringing in the ears, and inflammation of the sinuses.[2]

Ibandronate Sodium (Boniva)

Ibandronate sodium (Boniva) is a bisphosphonate that comes in a once a month dose of 150 mg. It significantly reduces fractures of the spine by 52%. It is similar to the other bisphosphonates in its tendency to cause irritation of the esophagus, so you still have to take it in the morning on an empty stomach and sit upright for 60 minutes instead of just 30 minutes. It isn't safe to take if you have kidney disease.

Which SERM to Choose?

Comparing raloxifene (Evista) to the bisphosphonates (Fosamax, Actonel, and Boniva), it may be important to note that both categories of agents decrease fractures in the spine. But only the bisphosphonates decrease fractures in both the hip and the spine.[13] So, if you're at high risk for bone fracture, a bisphosphonate is a good choice. In this context, you're "high risk" if you're elderly, you're frail, or you've had previous spine fractures.[13] Bisphosphonates have a higher chance of causing or aggravating stomach ulcers.[13] So, if you have ulcers, Evista is a better choice.[13] Some women are candidates for both a bisphosphonate and Evista together. If you have severe osteoporosis, you may need to take both of these agents. [13]

Once again, let me reiterate that it's important to take calcium (1500 mg per day) and vitamin D (400 – 1200 IU per day). Remember, however, that these serve the purpose of *strengthening* your bone. They don't prevent bone *loss*, and they aren't a substitute for any of the therapeutic options I've mentioned in the sections on hormonal or non-hormonal medications. They're intended for use *in addition* to the agents listed above.

CHAPTER 30: BREAST CANCER

Statistics

Here's another topic of great concern. Let's start with the statistical information. Breast cancer is the most common cancer among women. It is not, however, the most common cause of death from cancer in women. Lung cancer has that distinction. One out of every seven women suffers from breast cancer at some time in her life. I know that sounds like a high incidence, but this statistic only pertains to women who live beyond the age of 81. In reality, your risk of breast cancer increases with age. In other words, one out of seven women at every age does not have breast cancer. But one out of every seven women from ages 81 – 90 does. To have a risk as high as one out of seven, you have to live until you're in your 80s. Until you reach that age, your risk is much lower than that. If you broke it down into risk at various ages, it would look like this:

From age 30 – 40, 1 out of every 252 women gets breast cancer.
From age 41 – 50, 1 out of every 68 women gets breast cancer.
From age 51 – 60, 1 out of every 35 women gets breast cancer.
From age 61 – 70, 1 out of every 27 women gets breast cancer.
From age 71 – 80, 1 out of every 25 women gets breast cancer.
From age 81 – 90, 1 out of every 7 women gets breast cancer.[1]

Risk Factors

The causes of breast cancer are many. All of the following are factors which contribute to the high incidence of breast cancer:

1. **Personal history of breast cancer**
   A previous breast cancer increases your risk of a *subsequent* breast cancer.
2. **Family history**
   (maternal first degree relatives only)
   If your biologic *mother, sister, or daughter* has had breast cancer, you have a much higher risk of having it also. This may be due to a genetic mutation called BRCA-1 or BRCA-2.
3. **Age**
   The *older* you get, the greater your likelihood of getting breast cancer.
4. **Age at the time of your first full term pregnancy**
   The later the pregnancy, the higher your subsequent risk of breast cancer. A first pregnancy *after the age of 30* carries an increased risk of breast cancer.
5. **Number of pregnancies**
   Fewer pregnancies increases your risk of breast cancer.
6. **Age when your first period occurred**
   Younger age is associated with increased risk. If you were *younger than 12*, your risk is increased.
7. **Age when *post*-menopause occurs**
   The later menopause occurs, the greater your risk. Menopause *after age 55* carries higher risk. Early menopause and surgical menopause decrease the risk of breast cancer.

Note: *Thus far in the list of risk factors, notice that there is a relationship in the number of menstrual cycles you've had and your risk of breast cancer (indicated by items 4 – 7). The more cycles you've had, the greater your risk.* (We'll discuss this shortly.)

8. **Tobacco use**
   Smoking increases your risk of breast cancer.
9. **Activity level**
   The *less active* you are, the greater your risk of breast cancer.
10. **Body weight**
    The *heavier* you are, the higher your risk of breast cancer.
11. **Diet**
    The *more fat* there is in your diet, the higher your risk of breast cancer.

12. **Benign breast disease**
    This actually makes it more difficult to *diagnose* breast cancer early.
13. **Regular alcohol consumption**
    The *more alcohol* you consume, the higher your risk of breast cancer.
14. **Exposure to intense radiation**
    Radiation therapy for other cancers can cause breast cancer.
15. **Dense breasts**
    The density of your breasts is related to how much time you've spent *pregnant* or *breastfeeding*.

If you have any of these risk factors, you're at increased risk of breast cancer. Breast cancer is an extremely important part of any discussion about menopause. That's because menopause is all about estrogen, and many of these factors have to do with the presence, quantity, or duration of estrogen in your body. Overall, the more menstrual cycles you've had, the higher your risk of breast cancer. That's why starting your periods early and/or reaching menopause late increases your risk. And notice that it's only the *cyclic* fluctuations in estrogen that count. High levels of estrogen, as in pregnancy, actually protect you against breast cancer. That's why later and/or fewer pregnancies increase your risk.

You may wonder why *cycles*, rather than absolute levels of estrogen or progesterone, increase your risk of breast cancer. Here's why: With each cycle you have, your breast tissue proliferates (multiplies) before your period, and resolves afterwards. Proliferating cells are programmed to stop proliferating once your period starts. A *cancer cell* is a proliferating cell that has lost control. So, it doesn't stop proliferating. Instead, it goes wild and proliferates rapidly and continually. Each cycle you have increases the opportunity for a normal proliferating cell to lose control and become a cancer cell.[2]

Because the number of cycles you've had is so important, we have a formula for calculating the number of cycles you've had during your lifetime. We call this your "*menstrual life*." Here are the calculation and the parameters for your risk category.

MENOPAUSE

(Age at menopause – Age at first period) X 13
- Months of breastfeeding
- Months of pregnancy
ANSWER

a.) Answer < 350 cycles / lifetime = low risk
b.) Answer between 350 - 450 cycles / lifetime = high risk
c.) Answer > 450 cycles / lifetime = very high risk

The magic number is 350. Your risk of breast cancer increases once you've had 350 menstrual cycles.

One of the dilemmas that arises in managing menopause is whether or not to take some form of estrogen to replace the estrogen that's lost in the process of menopause (estrogen replacement therapy). Some studies have suggested or questioned the possibility that estrogen replacement therapy *may be* associated with a higher risk of breast cancer. To date, we have no consensus on the issue. Thus, it's important to consider each of these factors in deciding whether or not to take any form of estrogen replacement therapy.

The interesting thing is that data from the last 30 to 50 years is consistent in showing that neither current nor past use of birth control pills increases the risk of breast cancer. This is true even for women with a high risk of breast cancer. It's even true for women with genetic mutations that place them at the highest risk of breast cancer. That's odd, given the fact that birth control pills contain much higher doses of both estrogen and progesterone than hormone replacement therapy for menopause.

In most instances, because we don't know absolutely whether or not estrogen replacement therapy increases the risk of breast cancer, most physicians recommend that women who have had breast cancer refrain from using estrogen. I'll give you a lot more information about that later in this section.

WORKSHEET TIMEOUT:
Answer question # 7 on your worksheet.
Circle all <u>your</u> risk factors for breast cancer.

Management Options

Focus on Risks

Despite the fact that breast cancer has a hereditary component, there are a multitude of things you can do to decrease your risk of breast cancer. Reflect back on the factors which contribute to breast cancer. The list includes a previous personal history of breast cancer, family history, age, age at first full term pregnancy, number of pregnancies, age at first period, age at menopause, benign breast diseases, and exposure to intense radiation for other cancers. You *can't change* any of these! (Okay, depending on your age, you may be able to change the number of pregnancies you have…but do you really want to go to such extremes at this extreme of your reproductive life?) The best you can do is know the facts, and use those facts to manage your menopause wisely. There are a bunch more that you *can change*, and we'll discuss those later.

One of the most important things for you to understand is how your family history affects your risk of breast cancer. Most women aren't aware of which family members are pertinent to their own risk of breast cancer. Let's clear that up. Not every family member has a bearing on your risk. You might just be surprised, even relieved, to discover which ones have an influence on your risk, and how much of an influence they have.

If *your mother* has had breast cancer, your risk increases from 1 in 7 to 1 in 4. If *your sister* has had breast cancer, it increases from 1 in 7 to 1 in 6. If your *maternal grandmother* had breast cancer, your risk remains at 1 in 7 (no increased risk). If *your mother and your mother's sister* have had breast cancer, your risk increases from 1 in 7 to 1 in 4. (Notice that your aunt's breast cancer did not change your risk at all!) If *your mother and your sister* have had breast cancer, your risk increases from 1 in 7 to 1 in 2. Breast cancer in a *grandmother or aunt* involves a second degree relative, making the increase in risk for you negligible or irrelevant. Focus on your *first degree relatives*. They include your mother, sisters, and daughters.

MENOPAUSE

If your ___ had breast cancer, your risk increases from ____ to _____.

mother	1 in 7	1 in 4
sister	1 in 7	1 in 6
mother and mother's sister	1 in 7	1 in 4
mother and your sister	1 in 7	1 in 2
grandmother OR aunt (second degree relatives)	No change	

The medical profession doesn't know whether or not estrogen *causes* breast cancer. However, because so many of the risk factors for breast cancer have to do with estrogen production in the body, it's a safe assumption that there is *some relationship* between the two. For instance, the relationship of age at first full term pregnancy has to do with the fact that pregnancy arrests the cyclic process of estrogen production. While there are very high levels of estrogen in the body during pregnancy, they are not *fluctuating* levels. This absence of fluctuating estrogen appears to have a protective effect on the breast. So, the younger you were when you had your first pregnancy, the lower your risk of breast cancer.

Likewise, the number of pregnancies you've had is important in calculating your risk of breast cancer. That's because the more instances in which your body has had a break from the cyclic production of estrogen, the more your breast is protected against breast cancer. So, the more pregnancies you've had, the lower your risk of breast cancer. By the way, twins count as a single pregnancy, as do triplets, etc. And, we're not talking about pregnancies that end in the first trimester. Remember, the critical factor is the break from cyclic activity. A first trimester loss doesn't involve a significant long term break from having cycles.

The relationship of breast cancer risk to age at first period and age at menopause are based on the same logic. Both early onset of periods and late menopause create a longer period of time that the breast is exposed to fluctuating levels of estrogen.

Now, if you're beyond childbearing age, it's not possible to adjust either the age of your first full term pregnancy or the total number of pregnancies you've had. So, take these statistics into consideration in weighing your concerns for breast cancer and then move on.

Age is pertinent simply because of the fact that the older you get, the more time you have to develop breast cancer. This isn't so bad, mind you. Such is the case with a vast number of diseases when you think about it. Live long, but decrease your risk of breast cancer by adopting good health habits.

The risk factors over which you have total control are the ones on which you should focus. I have often pondered about the extent to which women agonize over the factors they *can't* change, while failing to concentrate on the factors over which they have complete control. Many of these factors have to do with lifestyle and habits. Like many other things, they include diet, exercise, weight control, tobacco use, and alcohol use.

Diet and Lifestyle Options

No Smoking

I can't emphasize enough how much you help yourself by discontinuing smoking. Breast cancer is only one of many cancers related to smoking. In fact, I have difficulty thinking of any cancer that isn't related in some way to smoking. I urge you to do whatever it takes to discontinue smoking. Seek help from your physician if necessary. Try hypnosis or acupuncture if you wish. Avoiding tobacco is one of the best things you can do for yourself.

At the age of menopause, a heavy smoker has *four times greater risk* of breast cancer than a non-smoker. "Heavy smoking" isn't clearly defined for purposes of its effect on breast cancer. So let's arbitrarily define it as smoking ten or more cigarettes daily. While this may not match your definition of heavy smoking, use it for purposes of assessing your risk of breast cancer. In this case, it's better to err on the side of being too careful than too careless. That four-fold increased risk with heavy smoking is associated with the presence of an enzyme abnormality in many smokers. So, in essence, smoking increases your risk of breast cancer regardless of whether or not it's heavy smoking.

Exercise

Exercise has been the topic of many studies on breast cancer. Inevitably, all studies agree that exercise decreases the risk of breast cancer. In one study, the risk of breast cancer in post-menopausal women who exercised moderately for only a few hours a week decreased by 18% compared with inactive women.[3] The risk decreased even more for women who engaged in moderate exercise for more than a few hours per week.[3] Women who exercise for one hour, four times weekly, decrease their risk of breast cancer by 30%. In general, higher levels of physical activity provide modest protection against breast cancer.[3]

Studies that evaluate the effect of previous strenuous exercise *before* the onset of menopause also reveal significant benefits of exercise.[3] Thus, exercise has a lasting effect in decreasing your risk of breast cancer, but is most effective when it's ongoing. The greatest benefit of exercise occurs in women who are close to ideal body weight. The benefit decreases with greater degrees of obesity. That's because obesity, in and of itself, is a risk factor for breast cancer.

The mechanism by which exercise has an effect on breast cancer is complex. Basically, though, regular exercise normalizes insulin levels and blood sugar levels. This results in decreasing excess body fat. So, as you can see, a little exercise goes a long way in protecting your breasts against breast cancer.

Weight Control

Obesity is an independent risk factor for breast cancer. That's because fat cells produce estrogen. The risk of breast cancer is directly proportional to the extent of obesity. So, the more overweight you are, the higher your risk. Losing even 10% of your body weight can make a significant difference in reducing your risk of breast cancer.

Obesity contributes to breast cancer in another way, also. Not only does it increase the chance of developing breast cancer; it also decreases the likelihood that you will *discover* it early. Why? Because breast tissue is primarily composed of fat. And when you're overweight, your breasts will be larger due to excess fat. This excess fat obscures your ability to feel small masses in your breasts that constitute early breast cancer. The probability of finding the cancer at a much *later* stage, with a much *worse* survival rate, skyrockets. So does the probability of failing to find it at all.

Diet

The dietary factor of greatest consideration with regard to breast cancer is fat consumption. There's substantial research showing a strong relationship between a high fat diet and breast cancer. A low fat, high fiber diet results in the excretion of excess estrogen, thus decreasing the likelihood of stimulating your breast tissue.

Now, I know you wish it were that simple, but, of course, it isn't. Breast cancer is also associated with sugar and refined carbohydrates. Both of these substances cause insulin to rise. These high insulin levels suppress Sex Hormone Binding Globulin (SHBG), which normally binds and inactivates estrogen. In essence, sugar and refined carbohydrates result in higher estrogen levels, which stimulate breast tissue.

So, the best dietary principles for breast health include the following:

1. Eat five servings each of fruits and vegetables every day.
2. Make soy products a regular part of your diet.
3. Eat 1 tsp – 1 tbsp of crushed flaxseed (which provides lignans) daily.
4. Limit sugar and refined carbohydrates.
5. Include omega 3 fats in your diet (salmon, swordfish, flaxseeds, or DHA [docosahexanoic acid] 100 – 400 mg daily).
6. Take a coenzyme Q10 supplement (10 – 100 mg daily for most women; 70 – 100 mg daily for high risk women and women taking cholesterol-lowering drugs).

Limit Alcohol Intake

The risk of breast cancer increases with the amount of alcohol you consume. This relationship has been demonstrated in a large number of studies. In fact, the risk of breast cancer is *60% higher* in women who consume *one or more alcoholic beverages daily* than in women who do not drink alcohol. This is due to the fact that alcohol has an effect on the liver, which interferes with its ability to metabolize estrogen.

Think back about the effect of alcohol on your risks of heart attack and osteoporosis. One alcoholic drink a day is *good* for your heart, *borderline* for your bones, and *bad* for your breasts. These differences in the effects of alcohol on your heart, bones, and breast are a perfect example of the importance of focusing on *your own risks* for various diseases. Your friend may have a high risk of breast cancer, and decide that she needs to limit or eliminate alcohol from her diet. You, on the other hand, may have a high risk of heart attack, and decide that a glass of wine a day is a good thing for you. With every option, you must balance the benefits of the option against the risks of the option. Put together a plan that, on balance, is best for **you**.

Hormonal Medication Options

Estrogen

Does Estrogen Cause Breast Cancer?

Research and Facts

Earlier, I stated that the medical profession *doesn't know* whether or not estrogen causes breast cancer. Now, you may have balked at that comment. Or you may have thought it was a mistake. Most likely, you probably responded with, "Please elaborate." If you had any of those reactions, this section is precisely for you.

First, let's clarify some definitions. The word "*cause*" is a very powerful word. It means that there is a cause – effect relationship, rather than simply an association, or a link, or any relationship other than a cause – effect relationship.

When we ask the question, "Does estrogen *cause* breast cancer?" we're asking if the presence of estrogen *induces* normal breast cells to become cancer cells. We're asking if estrogen serves to *begin* the process of transforming normal cells into cancer cells.

When we ask the question, "Does estrogen *cause* breast cancer?" we're *not* asking if estrogen and breast cancer are simply related in some manner. There are many ways in which estrogen may be related to breast cancer, but not actually cause it. I think we've already established that the cyclic activity of estrogen (along with progesterone) increases your risk of breast cancer. Now, we're going to address whether or not estrogen actually sets the stage and initiates the process of cancer formation.

In order to answer such a question about the cause of cancer, we look at many factors. These are the factors that are common to other agents that clearly cause cancers. In other words, for a substance to qualify as a causative agent for a cancer, it must pass certain tests. Let's see how the data on estrogen stands up to these tests.

Consistency

In any area of medical research, there are many studies devoted to a single topic. The topic here seeks to answer the question as to whether or not there is a cause – effect relationship between estrogen therapy and breast cancer. To have confidence in the relationship between the two, it's necessary for the relationship to be *consistent* in the research studies and published articles. That means all the studies must come to the same conclusion.[3] Sometimes, it's acceptable if a majority of the studies come to the same conclusion. Such is *not* the case with regard to research studies or published articles on breast cancer and estrogen.[3] In essence, for every study claiming that estrogen causes breast cancer, there are many more claiming the opposite. *There is no consistency between studies on the relationship between estrogen and breast cancer.* So, estrogen fails this first test as the cause of breast cancer.

Dose Relationships

If breast cancer is indeed initiated by estrogen, you'd expect the effect to be dose related.[3] This means that it would be logical for higher doses of estrogen to be associated with higher rates of breast cancer. Alternatively, it would be logical for higher doses of estrogen to be associated with more severe or more aggressive forms of breast cancer. However, the studies don't show a consistent dose response effect.[3] *Higher doses of estrogen are not associated with higher rates of breast cancer or worse forms of breast cancer.* So, estrogen fails this second test as the cause of breast cancer.

Estrogen Alone Versus Estrogen Plus Progesterone

If estrogen causes breast cancer, there should be a difference in the incidence of breast cancer in women who take estrogen alone versus those who take estrogen plus progesterone. Overall, 82% of studies on estrogen alone show no significant difference in the incidence of breast cancer in women taking estrogen for menopause than in those who don't.[3] Additionally, 80% of studies on estrogen plus progesterone show no significant difference in the incidence of breast cancer.[3] Both categories (estrogen alone and estrogen plus progesterone) compare the incidence of breast cancer to women who took no hormones. Only 13% of studies demonstrate a significant increase in breast cancer with the use of estrogen alone, while 10% demonstrate a significant increase in breast cancer with estrogen plus progesterone.[3] Believe it or not, some studies even show a *reduction* in the incidence of breast cancer with hormone use. This is true for 2% of the studies with estrogen alone, and for 10% of the studies with estrogen plus progesterone.[3] *Overall, though, the medical literature does not support any difference between estrogen alone and estrogen plus progesterone in their effects on breast cancer.*[1] So, estrogen fails this third test as the cause of breast cancer.

Persistence

If there is a cause – effect relationship between estrogen and breast cancer, any increased risk should persist even after discontinuation of estrogen therapy.[3] If the risk doesn't persist for some time after discontinuing therapy, then the relationship is usually just a reflection of the increased probability of detection during therapy.[3] Virtually all studies that demonstrate an increase in breast cancer in women using estrogen reveal that only *current* users, but not past users, have an increased risk.[3] Additionally, there's a rapid *disappearance* in the increased risk after discontinuation of estrogen therapy.[3] *The bottom line is that the increased risk of breast cancer disappears once estrogen is stopped.* So, estrogen fails this fourth test as the cause of breast cancer.

Think about this for a minute. Remember our discussion of why cycles are to blame for an increased risk of breast cancer? I explained that a cancer cell is a normal cell that goes wild and transforms into a rapidly growing cancer cell. Once it's a cancer cell, it's not going to transform back into a normal cell. The point is that a cancer cell *loses control.* It's not going to decide to stop growing. That's why cancer doesn't disappear once the causative agent is withdrawn. Anything that *causes* cancer will get the process started, and the cancer will continue to grow regardless of whether or not there is continued exposure to the causative agent. This "persistence test" is a critical one.

Type of Breast Cancer

Another interesting observation is the fact that when a woman receives a breast cancer diagnosis *while* she's receiving estrogen therapy, the *kind* of breast cancer is different than that of a woman not receiving estrogen.[3] *Breast cancer diagnoses during estrogen therapy are consistently less aggressive, more responsive to treatment, and less fatal.*[3] In essence, they aren't as serious as breast cancers in women who aren't taking estrogen. This would suggest that, if estrogen does cause breast cancer, that it causes a milder form of cancer than other possible causative agents. So, estrogen fails this fifth test as the cause of breast cancer.

Now it could be that women who are taking estrogen are more likely to see a physician regularly, more likely to have regular mammograms, and more likely to have follow up than women who aren't taking estrogen.[3] If so, this may account for the fact that breast cancers discovered in the presence of estrogen tend to be less serious. However, those factors can't explain the less aggressive nature of those cancers. Aggressiveness of a cancer depends on the type of cell that grows into a cancer, which has nothing to do with how much a woman sees her physician.

Growth Rate

Breast cancer takes many years to grow from a single cell to a tumor that is large enough to diagnose.[3] In fact, it takes a breast cancer **seven years** (yes, I said seven years) to grow from a single cell to the size of a small grape. This confuses the *timing* of estrogen's effect on breast cancer. Did the estrogen cause the first cancerous cell to appear? Or, was that first cancerous cell there already? If it was there already, did the estrogen accelerate its growth? Or could the estrogen possibly have slowed its growth or made the cancer less aggressive? These are all questions that are very difficult to answer. And, the answers may vary from one woman to another. Most likely, the appearance of breast cancer within three or four years of starting estrogen therapy is too soon to be a result of that therapy.[3] *Because breast cancer grows so slowly, it's difficult to determine if and when estrogen might have had an effect on it.* So, estrogen fails this last test as the cause of breast cancer.

So the final answer to the question, "Does estrogen cause breast cancer?" is, **"We don't know!"**

I know that you probably don't like it that there is no answer for such an important question. Currently, however, that's just the way it is. Research is ongoing to discover the answer to this question, and, hopefully, we'll know the final word on this soon. For now, you just have to accept the fact that we don't know everything. Work with the knowledge you have, and do the best you can.

Caution

In general, the medical profession has taken the approach of withholding estrogen from any woman who has had breast cancer *herself.* Because progesterone and testosterone are closely related to estrogen in their chemical structure, most physicians also withhold them from women who have had breast cancer. As you've already discovered, these two hormones have the ability to transform into estrogen under certain circumstances. Until we have more concrete answers, most physicians probably won't give *any* hormones to women who have had breast cancer.

However, physicians don't typically refrain from giving estrogen to a woman who has a *family member* with a history of breast cancer. You are free to take hormones if a family member had breast cancer, even if she was a maternal first degree relative. Despite this practice, you need to assess your own comfort level with the idea of taking estrogen given the unknown relationship between estrogen and breast cancer. We tend to fear the unknown, so if you prefer to avoid estrogen because of this uncertainty, that's okay. There are other options available to you. Realize, though, that estrogen is not taboo for women who have not had breast cancer themselves.

To summarize:

- The studies on breast cancer and estrogen are inconclusive and inconsistent.
- There is no dose related effect between estrogen and breast cancer.
- There's no overall difference in breast cancer rates between women taking estrogen alone versus those taking estrogen plus progesterone.
- The increased risk of breast cancer disappears when estrogen is discontinued.
- The kind of breast cancer in women taking estrogen is less serious than in women not taking estrogen.
- Breast cancer takes a long time to grow to a detectable size, and may begin long before estrogen therapy starts.

I've given you a great deal of information here. My goal is for you to have the facts. I seek neither to persuade you to take estrogen nor to make you fearful of doing so. My goal is to simply give you all the available information in as simple a manner as I can. You have your own threshold for comfort with the available information. Your comfort level may differ from that of other women. You may place much more weight on this information than your friend does. That's the purpose of an unbiased presentation. You know yourself better than anyone else does. Take all that I've given you and apply it to your own situation.

Progesterone

There may be a difference in synthetic progesterone and bioidentical progesterone on breast tissue. While evidence suggests that synthetic progesterone doesn't protect against breast cancer, the same may not be true for bioidentical progesterone, such as ProGest cream or Prometrium pills. The medical profession simply doesn't have the answer on this issue. It's possible that bioidentical progesterone could have a protective effect on your breasts by protecting your breasts from overstimulation by estrogen. For now, this is still an unknown.

Breast cancer is usually classified as *estrogen receptor positive* or *estrogen receptor negative*. All estrogen receptor positive cancers are also progesterone receptor positive. This is a good thing because positive progesterone receptors make the cancer receptive to progesterone's balancing effects. So, progesterone may be therapeutic in estrogen receptor positive breast cancers. In general, estrogen receptor positive breast cancers are slower growing, less aggressive, and more responsive to treatment.

Postmenopausal Hormone Replacement Therapy

Current use of post-menopausal hormone replacement therapy is associated with an increased risk of breast cancer.[3] This is especially true for estrogen plus progesterone. *Past* use of post-menopausal hormone replacement therapy does not increase the risk of breast cancer. The increased risk with current use is small, and this information requires careful application to your individual situation. In and of itself, this information isn't significant enough to deter all women from using estrogen plus progesterone for menopause. Estrogen vaginal creams tend to pose no additional risk of breast cancer.[3]

Non-hormonal Medication Options

Tamoxifen (Nolvadex)

Tamoxifen is most well known for its use in decreasing the risk of getting breast cancer in the first place, as well as avoiding recurrences of the disease. Many women who are at high risk of breast cancer take this drug as a preventive measure. A convenient positive side effect of tamoxifen is that it also prevents bone loss (if you're *post*-menopausal), making it a good option if you have concerns about both breast cancer and osteoporosis. Another benefit is that tamoxifen decreases lousy LDL and decreases your risk of heart attack. Tamoxifen's beneficial effects on the breast are most significant in the first five years of use. Thereafter, the benefits may subside.

The negative side effects of tamoxifen include thickening the lining of your uterus (increasing your risk of uterine cancer), hot flashes, memory loss, blood clots, visual disturbances, and depression. Once again, remember that you have to monitor your uterus (if you have one) with regular ultrasounds and biopsies if you use tamoxifen.

Aromatase Inhibitors

Aromatase is the set of enzymes which convert androgens (male hormones) into estrogens (female hormones). Converting androgens to estrogens is a normal process. In most cases, it's desirable, too. But in the case of breast cancer, it's not desirable if the breast cancer is fed by estrogen. There are three drugs, known as the aromatase inhibitors, which are available only to *post*-menopausal women for treating breast cancer. They block the conversion of androgens to estrogens. They are as follows:

1. Anastrozole (Arimidex)
2. Letrozole (Femara)
3. Exemestane (Aromasin)

These three drugs decrease the recurrence and the spread of breast cancer more effectively than tamoxifen. Unlike tamoxifen, they *do not* prevent osteoporosis or heart attacks. In fact, the most significant problem with them is that they *cause* bone loss that leads to fractures. Side effects include hot flashes, joint pain, muscle aches, and decreased sex drive. Compared to tamoxifen, they cause less thickening of the uterine lining, fewer blood clots, and fewer hot flashes.

Self Breast Examination

This section on self breast examination and mammograms focuses on early *detection* of breast cancer. Face it: when it comes to breast cancer, timing is everything. Breast cancer is a very treatable disease… **IF** you detect it early. So, do everything you can to prevent it, and *also* do everything you can to detect it early if you happen to get it. This section will help you save your own life.

There are two basic features that we use to detect breast cancers early. We either attempt to feel them on breast examination or we try to see them on a mammogram. Not all breast cancers behave in the same manner. Some show up on a mammogram before you can feel them. With others, you can feel them long before they show up on a mammogram. My goal in presenting this material is to ensure that you understand the importance of both self breast examination *and* mammograms in finding breast cancer early. They do not fall into the "either/or" category. You need to understand them both, and you need to utilize them both.

Checking your own breasts is one of those things that is quick, free, and without adverse effects. It simply makes *no sense* to forgo the opportunity to perform a self breast exam when it can serve to help you discover breast problems much earlier than you would otherwise.

The real purpose of self breast exam is for you to become so familiar with what's **normal** for your own breasts, that you know them better than anyone else does. Think of it this way: If *you* check *your* breasts on a monthly basis, and you check no breasts other than *your own*, and your physician checks *many* breasts every day, and only checks yours once a year, who's more likely to recognize a subtle change in *your* breasts the earliest? **You are!** The goal of self breast exam is for *you* to become the world's greatest expert on *your own* breasts. It's simply a matter of knowing your own body, which isn't difficult.

In order to perform breast exam adequately, you must know three things:

(1) How to check your breasts;
(2) When to check your breasts; and
(3) What to feel for when you check your breasts.

We'll cover each of these in turn.

How to Check Your Breasts

Positions

Self breast check takes place in two positions:

(1) Lying down, which is the feeling position; and
(2) Sitting or standing in front of a mirror, which is the looking position.

Lying Down

First, **lie down** on your back on a flat surface. This allows your breast tissue to spread out flat over your chest. Place one hand behind your head and use the other hand to check the opposite breast. Extend the first two fingers on your breast-checking hand. Imagine that your breast is the face of a clock. Place the two breast-checking fingers at twelve o'clock just above and at the edge of your nipple. Press down to your rib, feeling through the entire depth of your breast tissue. Lift your fingers, and place them at one o'clock, pressing down to your rib again. You must press deeply enough to feel your ribs with each step.

Move in a circular, clockwise motion, until you have done this all the way around your breast. Depending on the size of your breast, you may have to go around more than once. *Almost all* breasts are large enough to require more than one circle. Start close to the nipple and work your way outward with each new circle. Once you've covered all the breast tissue around the nipple, push down on the nipple itself.

Now there's another part of the breast of which you might be completely unaware. You see, *your breast isn't round*! It's actually shaped like a bird's wing. In other words, in addition to the round mound of breast tissue that you can see, there's also a "tail" of tissue that extends up into your arm pit.

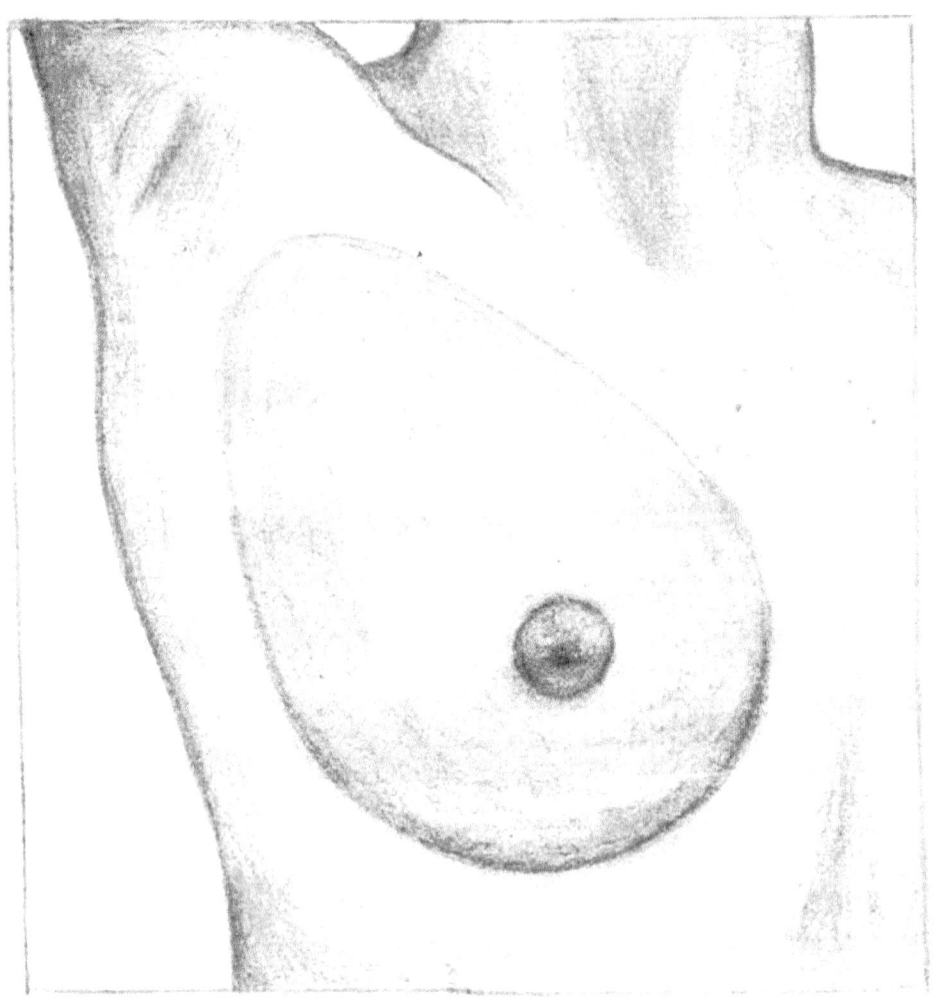

Figure 16: Breast, with tail of tissue extending into the arm pit

So, after you check your breasts in the circular clock face fashion I've described, you need to reach up into your arm pit and press down to your rib there, also. Press into the arm pit in the same way you did over your chest. Be sure to press deeply enough to feel your ribs. Check the entire area. Take your time and make sure you cover the entire breast. Even if this takes fifteen minutes, that's not a lot of time to devote to the opportunity to find something while it's very small and curable.

BREAST CANCER

Sitting or Standing in Front of a Mirror

Next, **sit or stand in front of a mirror.** Look at your breasts from the front and the sides. Notice the skin, the nipples, and the overall shape of your breasts. Specifically, make sure the nipples aren't pulled inward (unless they have always been that way), make sure the skin doesn't have large pores like an orange peel, and make sure there's no puckering of the skin.

Look for any asymmetry that's unusual for you. By the way, most breasts are *not* perfectly symmetrical. One may be larger than the other, hang lower than the other, or have a shape that differs from the other. All of these things are okay if that's the way your breasts have always been. If not, and you discover an asymmetry that's new, it warrants an evaluation by your physician.

First, make all of these observations with your arms relaxed at your sides. Second, make the same observations with your hands on your hips, pushing inward to tense your chest muscles. Third, make these observations with your hands raised over your head.

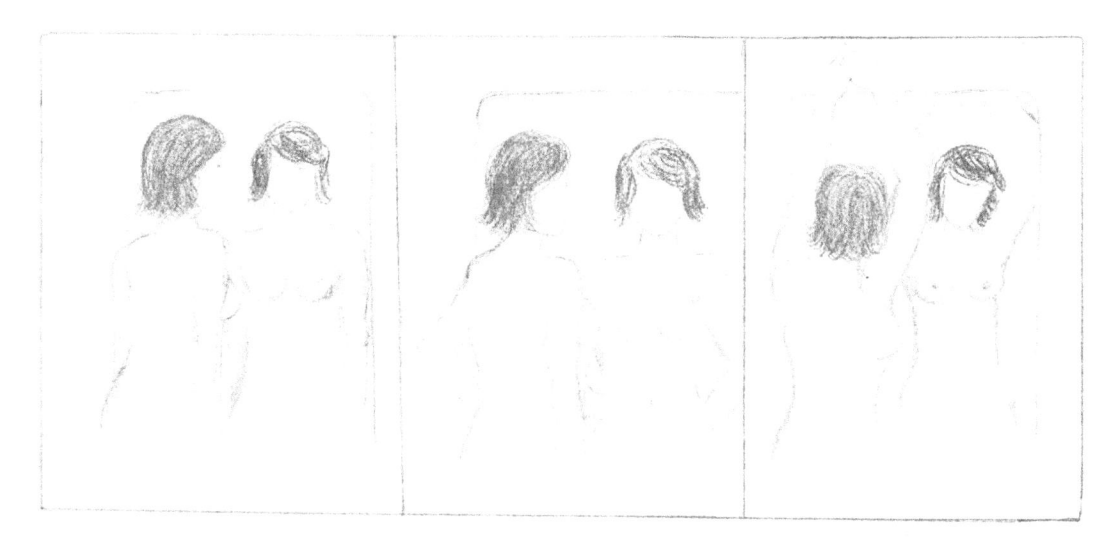

Figure 17: Look at you breasts sitting or standing in front of a mirror:
    (1) First, with your hands resting at your sides;
    (2) Second, with your hands pressing in on your hips;
    (3) Third, with your hands raised above your head.

Exclusions

Notice that I have *not* included the shower as one of the places where you should perform your breast exam. That's because you can't lie down and get your breasts to spread out flat over your chest when you're in the shower. If you're like most people, you *stand* in the shower, and you can't feel all your breast tissue when you're standing. You also can't press all the way down to your rib when you're standing. Finally, you don't have access to an adequate mirror in the shower. If you like the idea of having slippery fingers for your breast check, then feel free to apply lotion, Vaseline, or water to your fingers when you do your breast check lying down. I find those shower-breast-check-reminders quite disturbing. They imply that the shower is the place for breast checking, although it isn't. So, the next time you see one of those breast check reminders hanging in a shower, just make a note to do your breast check in the appropriate place and at the appropriate time, as indicated below. Don't let it induce you to do your breast check in the shower!

You might ask, "What about the bathtub?" At which point I will ask, "Are you able to lie flat in your bathtub and do a diligent breast check without drowning?" Remember, breast checking requires you to lie on a *flat* surface. Your breasts have to spread out like a pancake. So, no bathtub checks!

When to Check Your Breasts

For purposes of timing your breast checks, you fall into one of two categories. You are either still having cycles (making you a "cycler"), or you aren't (making you a "non-cycler"). We'll discuss the timing guidelines for each category.

Cyclers

If you're still having periods or cycles, either spontaneously or as a result of hormone therapy, there's only one specific time in your cycle to check your breasts. There are *no* exceptions. Check your breasts *just after your period ceases* each month. Remember, you count the days of your cycle by designating the day you begin your period as day one. So, if your period lasts five days, check on day six of every cycle.

The purpose behind breast checking is for *you* to become so familiar with your breasts that you can find an abnormality when it is very tiny. That means **your breasts must be the same each time you check them**. If you're still having cycles, your breast tissue is changing throughout each cycle. By adhering to the exact same time of each cycle, your breasts should be identical every time you check them.

The worst thing you can do is to check at different times during your cycle. That's because your breasts differ throughout your monthly cycle. And, if your breasts are different every time you check them, you'll never know what "normal" is.

Another huge mistake is to think that more is better. In other words, if you check more often than once a cycle, you'll lose your ability to know what normal is because your breasts will be *different* every time you check them, plus you'll lose your ability to discover an abnormality when it's tiny. *The "more is better" mentality defeats the whole purpose.* It's probably the most common mistake women make. Unfortunately, it's the most costly one, also.

Think of it this way: If it takes seven years for a breast cancer to grow to the size of a small grape, and you're checking your breasts more often than once a cycle, how well do you think you'll be able to tell that something's growing? **You won't!** It's a lot like seeing a little child every day. You can't see that he/she is growing because you see that child so often. However, when you haven't seen that little child in a long time, your first comment is that he/she has gotten so big. You notice how much he/she has grown because there's been enough time between visits for you to easily notice the difference. Breast checking is the same. If you check too often, you sabotage your ability to notice changes early on. It's actually detrimental in the sense that it *increases* the chance that you'll *miss* something.

Remember that forgetfulness is part of menopause. Even if forgetfulness isn't one of the symptoms you have, I highly recommend that you provide yourself with a reminder for breast checking. The important thing about this reminder is that you must make sure you see it ***only*** when it's time for your breast check. If you see it more frequently than that, you'll train yourself to ignore it.

If you're taking birth control pills or patches, or using cyclic hormone replacement therapy (HRT), you can put a reminder on the new, unopened package. Since your period will end just before you begin a new pack, seeing the reminder on the day you open the package is perfect.

Alternatively, if you use light pads or mini-tampons at the end of your period, you can put a reminder on the box of pads or tampons. Be sure it's not on the box of hygiene products you use for your entire period. You'll be sure to forget to do your breast check if you've seen the reminder day after day throughout your period.

Whatever you do, *do not* put your reminder in the shower.

Non-Cyclers

If you no longer have periods or cycles, your breast tissue is *not* changing from day to day. It isn't responding to hormones, so it'll feel the same from one day to the next. If that's the case, just pick a day of the month to check your breasts, and check them on the **same day each month.** For example, you could check on the first day of each month, or on the day of the month you were born each month.

Under *no* circumstance should you check your breasts more often than once a month. That's because checking too frequently can actually make it more difficult for you to detect small changes in your breasts, thus delaying your ability to find changes early. Remember, the majority of breast cancers grow slowly, so slowly that it takes seven years for a breast cancer to grow to the size of a small grape. If you're checking too frequently, you'll be unable to notice changes in the size of a breast mass. The analogy I used above about being unable to see growth in a small child that you see every day applies to non-cyclers, also. If you didn't read the section for the cyclers, do so.

As with the cyclers, you'll need to remind yourself when it's time for your breast check. Since you're not having cycles, and all of the cycler's reminders are linked to the end of their period, I think the best way to remind yourself if you're a non-cycler is to mark the day for breast checking on your calendar. If you have a pocket PC with a calendar, you can put it on that calendar and even program it to sound an alarm to remind you.

Whatever you do, *do not* put your reminder in the shower.

Exclusions

I've emphasized caution against placing your reminder in the shower and against doing your breast exam in the shower. There's a good reason for that.

First, how often do you get in the shower? How often should you check your breasts? Get it? The purpose of your reminder is for you to see it **only** when it's time for your breast check. So, unless you shower only once a month, and it's at the time your breast check is due, a reminder in the shower serves no purpose at all.

Notice also that the shower is not the place to check your breasts. Why? Because you shower standing up, which prevents you from feeling all of your breast tissue during the feeling portion of your breast check. And even if you have a mirror in your shower, it won't be adequate for you to visually examine your breasts during the looking portion of your breast check. Your breast exam should be a separate activity dedicated solely to breast checking.

Okay, what about having your partner do your breast check for you? Are you kidding me? Your partner doesn't want to check your breasts in the clinical sense. Your sexual partner touches your breasts in the sexual sense! Breast checking is something you have to *do* yourself *for* yourself. You can't count on anyone else to do it for you. Besides, your partner probably wants to touch your breasts much more often than once a month!

What to Feel for When You Check Your Breasts

Ban on the Word "Lump"

I have a problem with the word "lump." That's because it's a vague word with different meanings for different people. Additionally, **normal** breast tissue is lumpy. So, if I tell you to feel for "lumps" in tissue that is, by its very nature, "lumpy", there's a pretty good guarantee that it will only serve to confuse you. To avoid the confusion, I'll refrain from using the word "lump," to describe what to feel for when you check your breasts. Instead, I'll use it to describe the *normal* tissue in your breasts. I hope you do the same.

Normal breast tissue contains soft, poorly defined areas that are *not* smooth. These "lumps" are ill-defined. That means there are no well-defined borders around them. They are bumpy, but they mesh with the surrounding tissue. The bumpiness isn't discrete.

Let's do an experiment. Lie down in the manner I described for doing a breast exam, and feel your breast. Do you notice that lumpy tissue I've referred to? Now, draw what you're feeling on a piece of paper. Are you having a bit of difficulty drawing it? If you are, I'm not surprised. The point is that the normal lumpy tissue in your breasts isn't discrete enough for you to draw it on paper. It's vague and irregular. The name of this lumpy tissue is "fibrocystic tissue." It's the normal stuff of which the breasts are made. It's *not* a disease. There's no such thing as "fibrocystic disease."

Rocks or Pebbles

When you check your breasts, you aren't feeling for that lumpy, poorly defined stuff. You're feeling for *"rocks" or "pebbles"*. That's right! The abnrmalities that you're checking for feel just like a rock or a pebble in your breast. They're firm, well-defined, masses. They may not be as hard as rocks or pebbles, but they're definitely harder than that normal lumpy stuff. They are so distinct from the surrounding tissue that you can feel the borders of the rock or pebble. You can describe the shape and size, and you could even draw them on paper if you needed to.

So, think about rocks and pebbles when you check your breasts. And if you feel a rock or pebble, it warrants an evaluation by your physician. It doesn't mean that it's cancer. It just needs closer examination. In fact, most rocks and pebbles are benign.

Now don't worry about any of the *details* of the rock or pebble. Every rock and pebble gets evaluated, no matter what else you may notice about it. It may be painful or painless. It may move or it may be stationary. It may have smooth edges or rough edges. It may be isolated or multiple in number. It may be behind the nipple, in the surrounding breast tissue, or in the arm pit. None of these things change the need to evaluate it. Please don't assume that any of these features or any others that you may notice free you of the need to see your physician. And remember, don't assume it's cancer, either.

It's common for women to arbitrarily assume that some aspect of a rock or pebble makes it unnecessary to have it evaluated by a physician. I've heard all kinds of incorrect assumptions. The fact that a rock moves does not mean that it doesn't require evaluation. A rock in your arm pit requires evaluation just as much as one behind your nipple. Sadly, many of those myths have resulted in fatal breast cancers that were curable had the woman simply responded to the mere *presence* of the rock or pebble rather than assuming that some characteristic of the rock or pebble made it unnecessary to evaluate it.

Likewise, never let a physician tell you that a rock or pebble is nothing to worry about, without having some diagnostic tests to prove it. The "feel" of a rock or pebble is not enough to make it worry-free. Be sure that all rocks and pebbles undergo surveillance by ultrasound, mammography, MRI, biopsy, aspiration, or whatever else gives you a final answer.

It's always surprising to hear a woman say that the reason she refrains from checking her breasts is because she's afraid she just *might find* something. Believe it or not, such a comment is quite common. But it makes no sense, because you should be more afraid of *not* finding something. By finding something when it's small, you greatly increase the chance that it will be curable. Breast cancer is a very treatable disease, but only if you discover it early. So, don't fear self breast examination. It's your friend. It empowers you to feel secure, not only in your ability to know what's normal for your own breasts, but also to find things early so that they're amenable to treatment and cure.

Time Investment

No matter how large your breasts, the maximum amount of time you'll invest in breast checking is **30 minutes per month!** Let's see, you probably spend more time than that drinking coffee or tea, watching television, maybe even watching commercials on television every day. Doesn't 30 minutes a month seem like a worthwhile investment in yourself? Isn't finding breast cancer early enough to cure it a good return on those 30 minutes? I think so! For 30 minutes per month, you could save your own life by finding breast cancer when it's early and curable.

Mammograms

Guidelines

The guidelines for mammograms are as follows:

For women with average risk of breast cancer (1 in 7):

1. Baseline mammogram at age 35
2. Mammogram every one or two years beginning at age 40
3. Mammogram, and/or ultrasound, and/or MRI, and/or aspiration, and/or biopsy any time there is breast pain, a breast rock or pebble, or other symptoms indicative of possible breast rock or pebble

For women with higher than average risk of breast cancer (> 1 in 7):

1. Baseline mammogram at age 30 to 35
2. Mammogram once a year beginning at age 35
3. Mammogram and/or ultrasound, and/or MRI, and/or aspiration, and/or biopsy any time there is breast pain, a breast rock or pebble, or other symptoms indicative of possible breast rock or pebble

Sometimes, an ultrasound can clarify or further define the mammogram findings. Even MRI (magnetic resonance imaging) of the breast is helpful at times. And sometimes, a biopsy (tissue sample) or aspiration (fluid analysis) is necessary to adequately evaluate a breast rock or pebble or findings on a mammogram.

In the realm of breast concerns, I believe that peace of mind is your greatest ally. You owe it to yourself to do whatever it takes to attain peace of mind any time you have a breast concern. Many women at high risk of breast cancer establish a relationship with a breast specialist, whom they visit annually for breast exams, and consult any time they have a concern regarding their breasts.

It sometimes happens that a woman consults a physician over a breast issue, and the physician advises her to "just watch it." I completely disagree with that approach. Never allow a healthcare practitioner to convince you to "watch" anything that gives you cause for concern in your breasts. What are you going to watch it for? Are you going to watch it become a larger rock, pebble, or mammogram finding that's more difficult to treat if it is a cancer? Are you going to watch it grow large enough to obscure something else? Are you going to watch it while you worry yourself silly? The only situation in which I believe it's reasonable to "watch it," is if you're a cycler, and you re-evaluate it at a different time in your cycle. That's because your normal breast lumpiness (fibrocystic tissue) changes throughout your cycle. That would entail waiting only six weeks to re-evaluate it. Otherwise, if your healthcare provider recommends "watching it," consult another. Be persistent in gaining peace of mind on your own terms. You deserve it.

Limitations

Now, a bit about the limitations of mammograms. In order to help you understand the limitations of mammograms, please reflect on the fact that your breasts change in various ways as you age. When it comes to mammograms, the pertinent change that affects mammograms is the consistency of your breast tissue.

When you're *young*, before you've had pregnancies and breastfed your babies, your breasts are very *dense*. That means that they're firm, shapely, and more "lumpy." This "lumpy" tissue is called "**fibrocystic tissue**." It's the *normal* tissue of which your breasts are composed. It is *not* a disease. So, it seems like an oxymoron to refer to this normal fibrocystic breast tissue as "fibrocystic disease."

Menopause

This dense, firm consistency of your young fibrocystic breasts is what allows you to win the wet t-shirt contest in your adolescent or young adult years. But, it's also the tissue that makes it very difficult to read a mammogram. On mammogram, dense breast tissue is thick, producing a cloudy appearance, and obliterating detail. It's like trying to look through a glass of milk. The difficulty in reading the mammograms of young women is what sets the stage for recommending baseline mammograms beginning at age 35 rather than earlier. That's also the reason that ultrasounds are used in conjunction with or instead of mammograms in young women.

© Copyright Photo researchers, Inc.

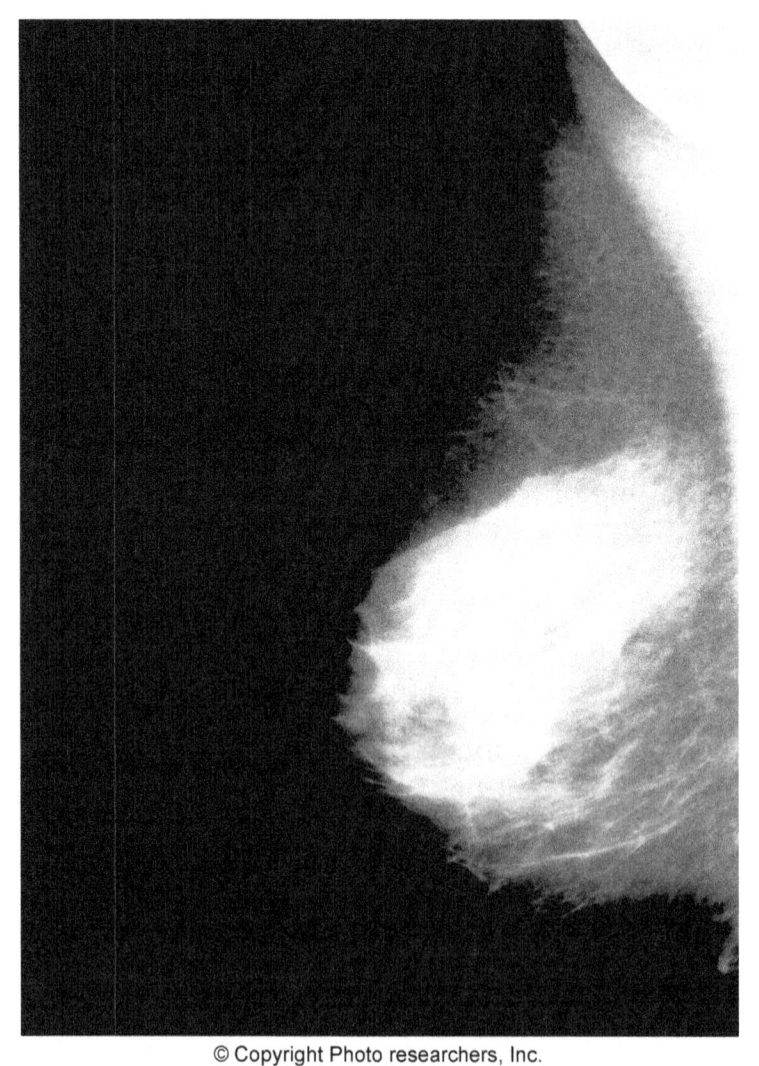

Figure 18: Mammogram of dense breast

BREAST CANCER

Now, as you get *older*, have pregnancies, and breastfeed, your breasts lose that firm, dense consistency. They become softer; they sag more; they attain a consistency that's more gelatinous. That's because the fibrocystic tissue is **replaced with fat** as you age. While they're much less attractive, and any hope of winning the wet t-shirt contest is lost, they're much more conducive to mammograms. The mammogram film of the older breast is clear and easy to read. It's like looking through a glass of water. This is the time when mammograms are most beneficial.

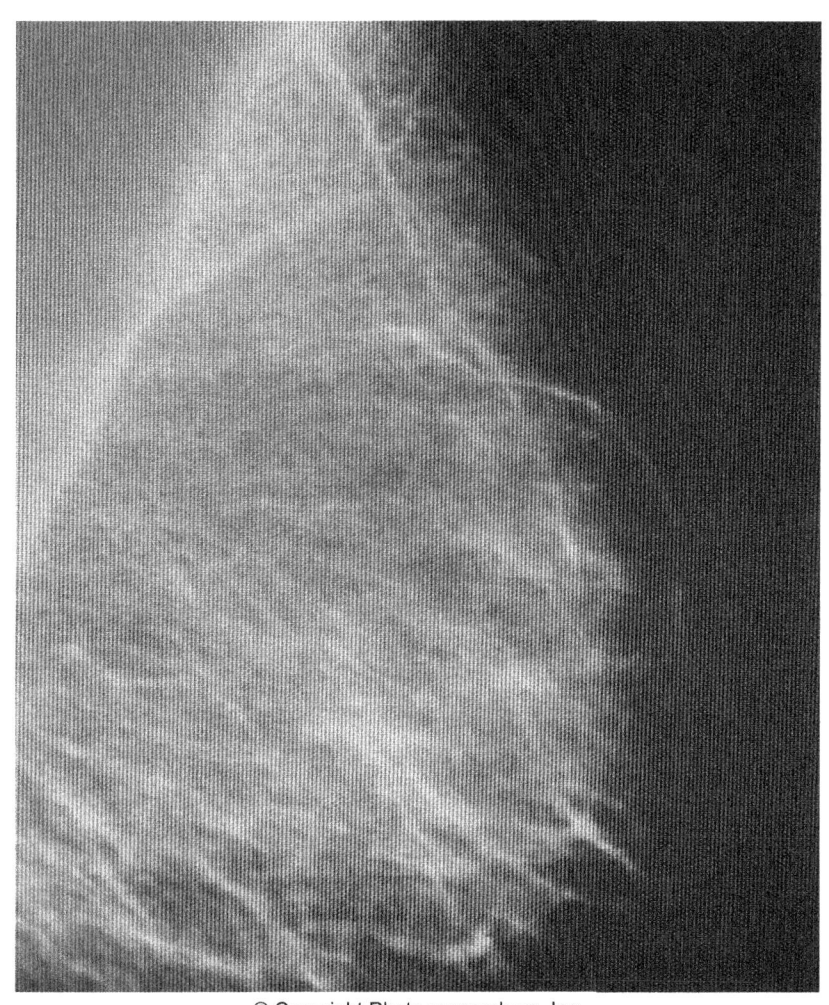

© Copyright Photo researchers, Inc.

Figure 19: Mammogram of fatty breast

So, here's the bottom line:

Younger Breasts	**Older Breasts**
Firm	Soft
Perky	Saggy
More dense	Less dense
More lumpy	Less lumpy
Fibrocystic tissue	Fatty tissue
Cloudy mammogram	Clear mammogram

My message to you is this:

If you: (1) are young; (2) haven't ever been pregnant; (3) haven't ever breastfed; or (4) have naturally dense or lumpy breasts, be prepared for mammograms that are "inconclusive." If the radiologist tells you that further studies are necessary to evaluate your "routine or annual" mammogram, don't immediately start worrying about breast cancer. Realize that the most likely reason for further studies is that it's just difficult to interpret the mammogram because of your normal, dense, fibrocystic tissue. If you find out that everything's okay, enter a wet t-shirt contest. You'll probably win!

On the other hand, don't be cavalier and dismiss the recommendation for additional testing. Women with extremely dense breasts *do* have a higher risk of breast cancer than those without dense breasts. In fact, the risk is four to six times higher. You may have to undergo ultrasound, biopsy, aspiration, or MRI of your breasts to get a final answer. Do whatever it takes. It's worth it.

What it boils down to is this: The more time your body has spent reproducing (pregnancy, breastfeeding), the less dense your breasts will be, and the lower your risk of breast cancer. On the contrary, the less time you've spent reproducing, the more dense your breasts, and the higher your risk of breast cancer.

Chapter 31: Uterine Cancer

Incidence

You may be inclined to skip this section if you don't have your uterus any longer. Remember, you don't have your uterus if you've had either a "Total Hysterectomy," meaning removal of your uterus and your cervix, or a "Subtotal or Partial Hysterectomy," meaning removal of your uterus without removal of your cervix. Without your uterus, you may think that you don't really need this chapter. Well, think again. Actually, you may learn quite a bit that helps you manage your menopause, even without your uterus.

Uterine cancer doesn't cause as much of a stir as breast cancer. That's odd, because uterine cancer is the most common female gynecologic cancer in the United States. It's intimately related to the aging process. Thus, 70% of all uterine cancers occur in women between the ages of 45 and 75. Only 8% of uterine cancers occur in women younger than age 45.

Anatomy

Any discussion of uterine cancer begins with a definition and description of the tissue that lines the inside of the uterus. The tissue that lines the inside of the uterus is called the **endometrium**. Sometimes, we refer to it as the endometrial lining. It's the tissue that you shed with each menstrual period. During your reproductive years, when you're having menstrual periods, estrogen causes this lining to thicken. Then progesterone ultimately causes this lining to shed. This principle is very important in understanding many aspects of menopause and hormone therapy. *The critical thing to remember is this:* **Progesterone** *is the magic hormone that prevents thickening of your uterine lining, and thus prevents uterine cancer.*

The Effect of Estrogen on the Uterus

When menopause occurs, the ovaries stop producing estrogen to thicken the lining of your uterus. The ovaries also stop producing progesterone to stabilize that thickened lining and subsequently cause it to shed. So, shedding of your endometrial lining ceases. This makes sense, right? So far, we've just reviewed the basics.

Now, what if you were to continue getting estrogen from a source *other than your ovaries?* Go back to the section on Categories of Hormones and Their Sources, and notice how many sources there are of estrogen. The "other source" could be a food, an herb, or a hormonal medication. And what if you weren't getting any progesterone along with that estrogen? What do you think would happen in such as situation?

Well, let's see...the estrogen you received from another source (foods, herbs, hormonal medications) would cause the lining of your uterus to thicken. And since there wouldn't be any progesterone to stabilize that lining and limit how thick it gets, it would become *extremely thick.* And that's not all.

Since shedding of your uterine lining requires a *drop* in progesterone, and there's no progesterone in the first place, you wouldn't shed the lining at all. This means that your thickened uterine lining would become progressively thicker and thicker. It would spiral out of control.

When there's no control over proliferating cells in the human body, those cells become *cancer* cells. They grow and replicate uncontrollably. And that's exactly what would happen in this case. You'd end up with uterine cancer.

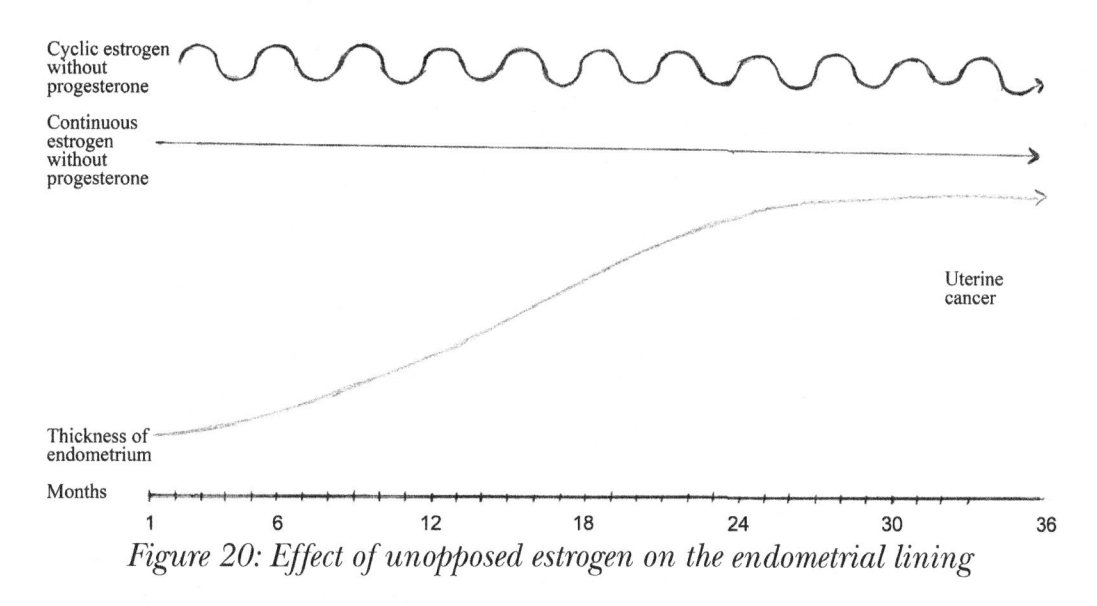

Uterine Cancer

Figure 20: Effect of unopposed estrogen on the endometrial lining

The key word is "excess." It's not that any estrogen will thicken the lining of your uterus; it's just that excess estrogen will. You've had estrogen production from your ovaries throughout your reproductive life. It's a normal substance. Estrogen, in and of itself, isn't harmful. The important thing is that you've had progesterone to control the estrogen. It's the *balance* between the two that's critical. Excess estrogen *without progesterone* is dangerous.

Another term for estrogen alone or estrogen without progesterone is "**unopposed estrogen**." Think of it this way: Estrogen and progesterone oppose one another. Estrogen thickens your uterine lining while progesterone causes it to shed. Without progesterone to oppose it, estrogen alone is not kind to your uterus.

If you don't have a uterus, none of this pertains to you. You can take estrogen without progesterone and have no concerns about uterine cancer. In that regard, you're lucky.

One of the most common sources of estrogen is *fat* cells. You already knew that, didn't you! Fat produces estrogen. The significance of this is that women who are overweight produce more estrogen than those who aren't overweight. So, if you're overweight, you're at highest risk of developing uterine cancer because of the estrogen produced by your fat cells. Therefore, in making management decisions for menopause, you must keep this in mind.

Because estrogen thickens the uterine lining, use of estrogen without progesterone can be harmful during menopause. With regard to uterine cancer, use of progesterone *in addition to* estrogen (estrogen plus progesterone) is important to protect against uterine cancer. Of course, if you've had your uterus removed (hysterectomy), use of estrogen alone is safe.

Okay, it's one of those instances in which I need to give you the simplistic version. Here's how I would simplify all that complicated stuff I just told you about your uterus:

Your uterus has a very basic view of the world. To your uterus, estrogen *causes* cancer, and *progesterone* prevents cancer. That's it! It's not the way other parts of your body see the world, but to your uterus, it's that simple.

Irregular Vaginal Bleeding

It would be incomplete to omit some comments about unexpected vaginal bleeding during menopause. If you experience unexpected vaginal bleeding during peri-menopause or post-menopause, it warrants an investigation. "Unexpected" means bleeding more often than once a month whether or not you're using hormones. Never assume that bleeding more frequently than once a month is normal. It could indicate any number of things, including inadequate hormone dosages, pregnancy, a thickened uterine lining that isn't cancerous, or uterine cancer. So don't conclude that all irregular or unexpected vaginal bleeding indicates cancer. In most cases it doesn't. It's just that you really need to have it evaluated.

An evaluation of irregular bleeding can involve a variety of tests, including: (1) a blood test for pregnancy; (2) an ultrasound to view the uterus and the thickness of its lining; and (3) a biopsy to examine the cells lining the uterus. It isn't always necessary to do all three. Your physician will tailor your evaluation to your personal situation. Your job is to call the bleeding to your physician's attention.

Risk Factors

Unlike some of the other disease entities pertinent to menopause, uterine cancer does not have a long list of risk factors. There are only a few, and almost every case of uterine cancer is associated with at least two of them. They are as follows:

1. **Age**
   Uterine cancer is a disease of middle-aged and elderly women. It's quite rare to find uterine cancer in a woman under the age of 45. Only 8% of uterine cancers occur in women under the age of 45. It increases in frequency with age, also.
2. **Obesity**
   Obesity is almost always present in spontaneous cases of uterine cancer. By "spontaneous," I'm referring to the cases that are not a result of hormonal influence from external sources of estrogen, like medications. Obesity is commonly associated with uterine cancer because uterine cancer is a result of excess estrogen, and fat cells produce excess estrogen. Simply put, the more fat cells you have, the more estrogen there is in your body, and the higher your risk of uterine cancer.
3. **Excess estrogen**
   If you refer back to the section entitled "The Effect of Estrogen on the Uterus," you'll recall my emphasis on the key word "excess." This means that estrogen that isn't *balanced by progesterone* causes uterine cancer. As long as you take both estrogen *and progesterone* in balanced proportions to one another, you don't have to worry.

Let me define the word "balance" for purposes of preventing uterine cancer. As you learned earlier in this book, estrogen and progesterone work together in producing your menstrual cycles. Estrogen builds up the uterine lining. Progesterone stabilizes the lining and then causes it to shed. All of that happens automatically when your own body is producing these two hormones in balanced proportions.

But now you're peri- or post-menopausal, and *you* have to balance estrogen and progesterone. *"Balance" means that you have to have enough progesterone to protect your uterus from uterine cancer.* If you take cyclic hormone replacement therapy, you have to have enough progesterone to make your uterine lining *shed* periodically. If you take continuous hormone replacement therapy, you have to have enough progesterone to *prevent build-up* of your uterine lining in the first place. If you take botanicals or herbs which contain estrogen, you need to take some kind of progesterone, also. If you eat mass quantities of soy products, you need to counteract the estrogen with some progesterone.

Now that you understand this, it seems fairly straight-forward. But you'd be surprised at the number of women with a uterus who take estrogen *without* progesterone.

WORKSHEET TIMEOUT:
Answer question # 8 on your worksheet.
Circle all *your* risk factors for uterine cancer.

Management Options

This section pertains to you only if you still have your uterus at the time of peri-menopause or post-menopause. If you've had your uterus removed surgically (hysterectomy), you have an advantage with regard to this section. You don't have to worry about any of the risk factors for uterine cancer. You may pursue any option you wish without having to balance that option with regard to its effect on the uterus. You still have to balance all the other issues that pertain to you, but you can ignore this one.

If you do still have your uterus, then you'll take into account the benefits and risks of the various options with regard to your uterus as well as everything else you're balancing. It's not that much more complicated, and you'll do just great.

Diet and Lifestyle Options

Weight Control

The most important and most beneficial thing you can do to prevent uterine cancer is watch your weight. Watch to make sure that it's not excessive. Try to maintain ideal weight because fat cells are the culprit in producing excessive estrogen that causes uterine cancer. By keeping your weight in the normal range for your height, you decrease the amount of estrogen available to thicken the lining of your uterus, and thus decrease your chances of developing uterine cancer. Menopause just seems to give you a whole new list of reasons to get your weight under control, doesn't it?

Diet

Throughout this book, I've mentioned a lot about how healthy a diet rich in soy can be. And it's true that soy products in your diet are very good for you because of the phytoestrogens they contain. So, I don't want to contradict anything I've said about the benefits of soy.

The key is to realize that estrogen from *any* source has an effect on your uterus. And that includes the estrogen in soy foods. The principle to remember and practice is that of balancing your estrogen intake with some form of progesterone. You want to avoid an excess of estrogen and a deficiency of progesterone. Eat plenty of soy in your diet, and also include some form of progesterone. It can be an herb, a cream, a gel, or a pharmaceutical product. Take your pick.

Botanical and Herbal Options

Chasteberry (Vitex agnus-castus)

Chasteberry is a convenient way to prevent an excess of estrogen and its thickening effect on the lining of your uterus. That's because it increases the production of progesterone in the body. The only challenge will be in knowing exactly how much to take in order to do the trick. You may need to test your hormone levels or use an ultrasound to examine the thickness of your uterus. The good thing is that progesterone is pretty safe. The whole herb and the powdered drug are available as capsules, drops, film tablets, and compound preparations.

Dosages are as follows:

> Capsules: 40 – 100 mg
> Liquid extract: 1:1 aqueous – alcoholic extract, 30 – 40 mg
> Dried extract: 100 gm containing 0.2 gm dried extract in a ratio of 1:5 in either ethanol or water

Wild Yam (Dioscorea villosa)

It would be great if you could just eat soy and wild yams together in a balanced combination to achieve the right estrogen to progesterone ratio. But it's not that simple. While the quantities of estrogen in soy foods are significant enough to have an effect on your uterine lining as well as on your symptoms of menopause, the quantities of progesterone in wild yams aren't. You'd have to consume mass quantities of wild yams to get enough progesterone to accomplish your goal.

You're better off using Wild Yam in the form of a cream or gel. Progesterone creams and gels are available in health food stores. You can rub them on your abdomen, buttocks, or thighs. Once again, it may take extra effort to get the balance of estrogen and progesterone just right.

The *root* of the Wild Yam plant is a precursor for manufacturing both progesterone and estrogen. Because of this, Wild Yam may have an additive estrogenic effect when combined with estrogen. In other words, depending on how your body metabolizes Wild Yam, you could get a double dose of estrogen rather than a balance between estrogen and progesterone. Wild, isn't it! What that means is that you could be getting more estrogen than you intended, and no progesterone at all. That's why you've got to tell your healthcare provider if you're using this stuff. Just be careful if you choose Wild Yam as your progesterone source.

Dosages are as follows:

> Capsules: 200 mg, 400 mg, 505 mg, 535 mg
> Liquid: 1:1 or 1:2 of 250 mg/ml

Hormonal Medication Options

Beware of Estrogen Alone

Earlier, I alluded to the fact that there's a direct cause – effect relationship between the use of estrogen and an increased risk of uterine cancer. To review, I stated that estrogen is the hormone that builds up the inner lining of the uterus. When there are no menstrual periods to shed this lining, it remains thick and develops into uterine cancer.

The causative hormone with regard to uterine cancer is **estrogen alone**. Combinations of estrogen plus progesterone do not count in this section. In fact, uterine cancer develops specifically *because* there is no progesterone to counteract the estrogen. So, don't make the mistake of including progesterone in your understanding of the causes of uterine cancer. I'm referring to ERT (estrogen replacement therapy) as the culprit, not HRT (hormone replacement therapy). When I refer to estrogen alone, I'm referring to all forms of estrogen, including phytoestrogens, herbs, plant-based products, and pharmaceutical preparations. You don't avoid this problem by taking a "natural" or herbal preparation. So, beware; balance your estrogen and progesterone, regardless of the source of estrogen.

Evidence that estrogen alone causes uterine cancer is everywhere. This isn't one of those gray areas or relationships that we're unsure about. There's no clear cause – effect relationship between estrogen and breast cancer. But there is an undeniable, blatant cause – effect relationship between estrogen and uterine cancer. Remember the cause – effect tests we discussed for estrogen and breast cancer? There, estrogen failed all of the tests for a causative agent. That's not the case with uterine cancer. It passes every one of them.

First, there is consistency in all studies examining the relationship between estrogen alone (or unopposed estrogen) and uterine cancer. They all conclude that estrogen causes uterine cancer. Second, there is a dose response relationship between estrogen alone and the development of uterine cancer.[1] This means that *the higher the dose* of estrogen alone, the greater the risk of developing uterine cancer.[1]

Third, there is a completely different result in women who take estrogen alone versus those who take estrogen plus progesterone. Estrogen and progesterone together *prevent* uterine cancer. Fourth, the risk of developing uterine cancer *persists* for at least five years after you discontinue taking estrogen alone.[1] This is typical for a cancer-causing agent. Another factor that further confirms the cause – effect relationship between estrogen alone and uterine cancer is that the risk of uterine cancer increases substantially the *longer* you take estrogen alone.[1]

Now, the hero hormone in the case of uterine cancer is progesterone. Progesterone is the hormone that either causes shedding of the thickened uterine lining or prevents thickening in the first place. So, the key to protecting the uterus is to combine estrogen with progesterone. It's that simple. Estrogen alone isn't allowed if you have a uterus. You'll gain all the benefits of estrogen without creating the risk of uterine cancer by combining the two. We'll refer to this option as <u>estrogen plus progesterone</u>.

Cyclic Versus Continuous Estrogen Plus Progesterone

Going back to the beginning of this book, I explained that menopause is a process. It takes months or years to complete the process and reach the stage of post-menopause. Post-menopause is defined as the time when you've had no menstrual periods for 12 consecutive months. I'm repeating all this because it dictates the way in which you may need to take estrogen plus progesterone.

There are two groups of uterus-bearing women experiencing the phenomenon of menopause. The first is the group who is having symptoms of menopause but *has not yet discontinued* menstrual cycles for 12 consecutive months. The second is the group who is having symptoms of menopause and also *has discontinued* menstrual cycles for 12 consecutive months or longer. Because there are two different groups, and because progesterone (the hero hormone of the uterus) has the job of getting rid of that thick uterine lining, there are two different ways to take progesterone.

Let me explain what I'm getting at here. Just imagine yourself as a post-menopausal woman who hasn't had a period for three years. Hallelujah! Now, if you decided to take estrogen plus progesterone, and I gave you a combination of the two that caused you to have monthly vaginal bleeding, you'd probably find a way to hurt me. So, we have a regimen for you if you've completed your periods, and we have a different regimen for you if you haven't. This allows us to work in harmony with Mother Nature even though you're taking hormones.

Because of all this, there are two different regimens for estrogen plus progesterone. The first is the "cyclic regimen" of estrogen plus progesterone. The word "cyclic" refers to the presence of cycles, menstrual cycles, that is. The second is the "continuous regimen" of estrogen plus progesterone. "Continuous" means that you don't have cycles of your own and the hormone replacement therapy doesn't create cycles for you. So, let's elaborate on these two regimens.

Cyclic Regimen of Estrogen Plus Progesterone

The first regimen is called a "cyclic regimen." This term derives from the fact that the hormones are designed to mimic the menstrual cycle that you're already having. As such, this involves taking estrogen during the first half of your cycle, and adding progesterone to the estrogen during the last half of your cycle. For most women, this results in a shedding of the uterine lining just as if it were a real menstrual period. The bleeding is usually very light. This regimen is ideal for you if you're still having menstrual periods, but need hormones to control the symptoms of menopause. There are two ways to accomplish the cyclic regimen of estrogen plus progesterone. They include: (1) low dose birth control pills or skin patches; and (2) cyclic hormone replacement therapy (cyclic HRT). They differ with regard to the dosages of hormones they contain.

Low Dose Birth Control Pills or Skin Patches

One option for accomplishing the cyclic regimen of estrogen plus progesterone is to take low dose birth control pills. The dosages of estrogen and progesterone in low dose birth control pills are much higher than they are in cyclic hormone replacement therapy. That's because the younger you are, the more estrogen you need. So, the higher dosages of hormones in low dose birth control pills are sometimes the perfect answer for the early years of peri-menopause.

With the primary focus being on the uterus for now, you'll be glad to know that low dose birth control pills result in an overall decrease in your risk of uterine cancer by up to 70% if you use them for at least 12 years. Of course, if you start using them for peri-menopause, you may not use them that long. But your uterus will still benefit greatly from them even if you only take them for a few years. Even if you use them for as little as one year, you'll reduce your risk of uterine cancer by 40%. That protection will last for 20 years after discontinuing birth control pills. The longer you take birth control pills, the lower your risk of developing uterine cancer, at least until age 65.

Typically, early peri-menopause is a very confusing time. You still have periods, but they may be unpredictable, both in timing and in character. It's more difficult to know when you're likely to get pregnant, and you feel strange in a multitude of ways. So, low dose birth control pills kill two birds with one stone. They provide hormone replacement for menopause in cyclic fashion, and they prevent pregnancy. This is a good option, because the hormones designed specifically for menopause (called "hormone replacement therapy" or HRT) are very low dose, too low to prevent pregnancy. Mind you, pregnancies can, and do, occur during peri-menopause. It is always a great surprise when this happens.

You're probably already familiar with birth control pill packs, and the low dose ones are no different. They come in a 28 day supply to represent a single cycle. The days of the week are indicated on the pack, and you just punch out a pill each day. It's best to take your pill at the same time every day, because they're so low dose that a delay may increase your chances of getting pregnant.

Low dose birth control pills will mask all the symptoms of peri-menopause. You won't even know it's happening. It's like sleeping through adolescence and never experiencing the slightest hint of that hormonal rollercoaster. There are some additional, long-term advantages to birth control pills, also. You'll protect your bones against osteoporosis, decrease your risk of ovarian cancer by 50%, increase healthy HDL, and decrease lousy LDL.

Beware: Birth control pills are prohibited for smokers over the age of 35. So, do yourself a favor and avoid smoking completely. Even if you smoke only an occasional cigarette, cigar, pipe, or marijuana, you increase your risk of heart attack and stroke too much to take low dose birth control pills. I emphasize this deal breaker because it's always heartbreaking for a woman who plans on using low dose birth control pills as a segue from pre-menopause to post-menopause to discover that she's not eligible because she's a smoker.

Conditions that make physicians refuse to give you low dose birth control pills are listed below. The risks are just too high.

1. Personal history of blood clots
2. Heart attack in the past
3. Previous stroke
4. Breast cancer
5. Pregnancy
6. Smoking

If you don't like the idea of taking a pill, but you do like the idea of the higher doses of hormones for peri-menopause, you have the option of using a skin patch that delivers the same hormones as a pill. The difference with a patch is that the hormones pass into your body after absorption through your skin. You may not have to change the patch very often, depending on the formulation you use, and the patch allows the hormones to bypass your liver. Both of these are advantages over the pills.

Cyclic Hormone Replacement Therapy (Cyclic HRT)

Cyclic HRT involves using the medications that are specifically designed for menopause. They replace your estrogen and progesterone at minimal doses, prevent the symptoms of menopause, and also mimic your cycle.

The dosages of estrogen and progesterone in cyclic HRT are only a fraction of the dosages in low dose birth control pills. As a result, you can forget about pregnancy protection with these. You still have to use some method of birth control if you don't want a surprise pregnancy.

With cyclic HRT, you take estrogen alone during the first half of your cycle and then you take estrogen plus progesterone during the second hlaf of your cycle. The addition of progesterone limits the build-up of your uterine lining, and causes you to shed that lining in the form of a period. All in all, you mask the symptoms of menopause and you protect your uterus against uterine cancer.

These formulations are available in a variety of dosages. The goal is to find the one that relieves all your symptoms of menopause, prevents osteoporosis, and balances the amount of estrogen and progesterone. While there are "standard" dosages that suffice for the majority of women, be true to yourself and take the dose that works best for you, personally. You may discover that you can manage on a lower dose than the majority of women. Then again, you may realize that you're experiencing every symptom of menopause with the standard dose, indicating that you need more.

You can take advantage of cyclic HRT in either of two ways. If you like the concept of cycle packs, you can use the formulations that are prepackaged. These packs look just like birth control pill packs. There are 28 pills per pack. The first 14 contain estrogen alone. The second 14 contain both estrogen and progesterone in balanced proportions in a single pill. All you have to do is punch out the pills in sequence each day.

Alternatively, if you wish to take a dosage combination of estrogen and progesterone that's different from the standard, or you wish to adjust the number of days that you add progesterone to the estrogen, you can take the pills separately. As such, you would take only an estrogen pill for the designated number of days during the first part of your cycle, and then you would take both an estrogen and a progesterone pill for the remaining days. Some women even have some pill-free days, in which they take no hormones at all.

As you can see, there are a variety of ways to take cyclic HRT. This allows you to tailor the regimen to your unique needs. Be sure that you don't manipulate things on your own, though. Consult your healthcare provider. There have been many women who caused themselves harm by experimenting without guidance. You could end up with a pregnancy, osteoporosis, or uterine cancer if you aren't careful.

Continuous Regimen of Estrogen Plus Progesterone (Continuous HRT)

The second regimen is called a "continuous regimen." The word "continuous" refers to the fact that the progesterone is taken continuously with the estrogen, resulting in an absence of cycles. Of course, you have to have attained the status of post-menopause by having *no periods for 12 consecutive months* to be a candidate for this regimen.

In the cyclic regimen, it's the use of estrogen alone for the first half of the cycle that builds up the lining in the uterus. Since this continuous regimen doesn't have any days in which you take estrogen alone, there is no opportunity for your uterine lining to thicken in the first place. Instead of allowing the uterine lining to thicken, in which case it then must shed, this regimen prevents thickening of the uterine lining altogether. As such, there is no shedding of the uterine lining at all.

This regimen comes in those dial packs with the days of the week designated, also. All the pills are the same, though, and the dosages are standard. The dial pack serves more as a reminder for you to take the pill than it does to make sure you balance your hormones. Alternatively, you can get separate prescriptions for estrogen and progesterone, and take a pill of each daily. Doing so allows you to tailor the dosages of each to your personal needs.

I know that you wish you could use this regimen from the start of peri-menopause and just forget all about periods once and for all. But you can't overcome the forces of nature and turn off your normal bodily functions just because you want to. Unfortunately, it's not possible to use this regimen if your body isn't yet ready to stop having menstrual periods, even if they're only occasional. *Any* bleeding on the continuous HRT regimen requires an evaluation, including ultrasound and biopsy of your uterus.

Progressive Estrogen Plus Progesterone Regimens

You may find it easiest to progress from one form of hormone therapy to another over time. This allows you to graduate from one regimen to another smoothly, without having to experience any symptoms of menopause at all. For example: You may begin low dose birth control pills in your early 40s (if you're a non-smoker), and continue them until your late 40s or early 50s. At that time, you may switch to the cyclic regimen of estrogen plus progesterone for the transitional perimenopausal years. Finally, when you are past the age of 53 or so, you may switch to the continuous regimen of estrogen plus progesterone. All during this time, when asked about symptoms of menopause, you'll probably answer with something like: "Menopause? What's menopause? I've never had a single hint of it?"

CHAPTER 32: OVARIAN CANCER

Incidence and Risk Factors

In general, ovarian cancer is a very rare disease. It occurs in one out of every 70 women.

It's difficult to say exactly what causes ovarian cancer. The most significant causes are **genetic**. Some families carry genes with abnormalities called "*mutations*" which place them at much higher risk of ovarian cancer. Usually, there is a family history of breast, ovarian, and colon cancer in first degree (mother, sister, daughter) and second degree (aunt, grandmother) relatives. The risk is higher if the person with ovarian cancer had it at a young age. About 10% of ovarian cancers are a result of an inherited tendency to develop the disease. To put this in perspective, the lifetime risk of ovarian cancer for women without these genetic mutations is 1.8%. But it is 20% to 60% for women with these genetic mutations. The good thing is that only 0.15% of the general population carries these mutations. It's most common in people of Icelandic, Swedish, Dutch, and Ashkenazi Jewish ancestry. Women with no family history have a 1.8% lifetime risk of ovarian cancer, while women with one first degree relative with ovarian cancer have a 4% to 5% lifetime risk.

Other factors that increase your risk are listed below:

1. **A personal history of breast cancer**
   If you've had breast cancer, you have a higher risk of ovarian cancer, also. Both of these cancers share some of the same risk factors, and they both have a lot to do with your reproductive

and hormonal history. BRCA-1 and BRCA-2 genetic mutations increase the risk of both breast cancer and ovarian cancer.

2. **Age**
The most common time for ovarian cancer to develop is *post-menopause*. In fact, half of the cases of ovarian cancer occur in women over the age of 63.

3. **Obesity**
The *heavier* you are, the greater your risk of ovarian cancer. In very obese women, the risk is 50% greater than in non-obese women.

4. **Number of menstrual cycles**
Things that increase the number of menstrual periods you've had in your lifetime increase your risk of ovarian cancer. Having your *first period before age 12*, having had *no children*, having your *first child after the age of 30*, and becoming *post-menopausal after age 51* are all contributors to a higher risk of ovarian cancer. *(Notice that the actual ages at which your risk increases with regard to these factors differ for ovarian cancer and breast cancer.)*

5. **Infertility**
Because infertility is associated with *more menstrual periods*, it increases your risk of ovarian cancer.

6. **Infertility drugs**
Prolonged use of infertility drugs may increase your risk of ovarian cancer.[3] This is especially true if you failed to achieve pregnancy with the drugs. The association has to do with the way these drugs increase ovulation and raise the levels of sex hormones. And, of course, use of infertility drugs is related to having fewer or no pregnancies, also.

7. **Hormone replacement therapy for menopause**
This one is questionable. Some studies suggest that hormone use for menopause increases the risk of ovarian cancer, while others show no effect of postmenopausal hormone therapy on ovarian cancer risk. Of the studies that demonstrate a relationship between hormones and ovarian cancer, some show a relationship only between estrogen alone and ovarian cancer, while others reveal a relationship between both estrogen and progesterone and ovarian cancer. Clearly, this is an area where we really don't have the answer.

The confusion is very similar to what you learned about breast cancer and hormone therapy.[2] In the case of ovarian cancer, the uncertainty stems in large part from the small number of cases of ovarian cancer.[2] The incidence of ovarian cancer is so low, that the length of time and the number of patients necessary to clarify the relationship between estrogen and ovarian cancer is difficult to attain.[2] Currently, the theory is that estrogen alone may slightly increase the risk of ovarian cancer, while estrogen plus progesterone may not.[2] Notice that I used the word "may" for both scenarios. We really don't have good information on this stuff. There is little data on the effect of estrogen vaginal cream on ovarian cancer.[2]

8. **Talcum powder in your genital area**
   If you apply talcum powder to your genital area, sprinkle it in your underwear, or put it on a sanitary napkin, it may increase your risk of ovarian cancer. This association may stem from contamination of talcum powder with asbestos, which was common years ago. Fortunately, it's not common any more, although talc is similar to asbestos in structure.[3] And there's no evidence that powders made from cornstarch have any relationship to ovarian cancer. However, it doesn't seem safe or necessary to have any kind of powder in your underwear creeping up your reproductive tract and *spilling out into your pelvis.*

9. **A high fat diet or a low fiber diet**
   Here we go again. As you can see, your diet really does matter. A high fat diet makes you fat, and being fat increases your risk of ovarian cancer. Likewise, a low fiber diet does the same thing.

WORKSHEET TIMEOUT:
Answer question # 9 on your worksheet.
Circle all your risk factors for ovarian cancer.

Symptoms

The most worrisome aspect of ovarian cancer is that it doesn't have typical early warning signs that make early diagnosis possible. Most commonly, ovarian cancer is pretty advanced at the time of diagnosis.

More than 70% of women with ovarian cancer have advanced disease, with spread beyond the ovary, at the time of diagnosis.[1] That's unfortunate, because cure rates are high (90%) if ovarian cancer is discovered early, when it's confined to the ovary.[1]

The inability to diagnose ovarian cancer early is what makes it a devastating and highly fatal disease. In fact, it's the deadliest of all the female cancers. Many women with ovarian cancer will have sudden bloating, enlargement of the abdomen, and the urge to urinate as the first signs.[2] But the cancer is fairly extensive once these symptoms occur.

Diagnosis

The other thing that makes ovarian cancer so complicated is that there isn't an accurate screening test for ovarian cancer. We don't have anything that serves the purpose of screening all women for signs of the disease. Unfortunately, there's a lot of misunderstanding about this. It's one of those areas in which many women think they have the facts, when they actually don't.

Many women think that CA-125 is a screening test for ovarian cancer. Unfortunately, it isn't. CA-125 is a common blood test that may be elevated in the presence of ovarian cancer, but the test is *not specific* for that purpose. This means that an abnormal result can indicate many things other than ovarian cancer. An elevated CA-125 can be the result of an infection, benign tumors, endometriosis, or ovarian cancer. An elevated CA-125 can even be the result of inflammation in parts of the body distant from the reproductive tract, like the pancreas or colon. So, it isn't very useful in diagnosing ovarian cancer early. To make it even less useful, only 50% of women *with* early ovarian cancer will have an elevated CA 125.[1]

CA-125 *is* useful for following the progression of ovarian cancer if someone has full-blown disease. But that's not the same thing as screening for early disease. The distinction is that CA-125 is a *monitoring* device for advanced ovarian cancer. It isn't a screening test for detecting the disease early.

Ovarian Cancer

Even the "normal range" for CA-125 is variable. A normal CA-125 for post-menopause is less than 30 – 35 U/ml, depending on the laboratory. But, for pre-menopause, it's less than 200 U/ml. Interpreting the CA-125 can be quite confusing.

It's possible to use ultrasound to look at the ovaries, but ultrasound only gives us information on the *size* of the ovaries. Not only are there many things that can enlarge the ovaries (some of which are normal), but ovarian cancer doesn't always begin with enlarged ovaries. The bottom line is that the diagnosis of ovarian cancer is one of the more difficult diagnoses to make.

There were plans to introduce a commercial screening test in 2004, but that didn't happen because the FDA (Food and Drug Administration) was worried about the reliability of the test. It didn't define whether or not ovarian cancer was present in a consistent manner. So, it would have created a lot of confusion and concern, but no valid information. What it boils down to is the unfortunate fact that the only way to diagnose ovarian cancer before it's extensive is with surgery.

Oddly enough, the most common situation involving an early diagnosis of ovarian cancer is accidental discovery. It happens like this: A woman decides to have a hysterectomy for a reason totally unrelated to any concern about ovarian cancer. She has heavy bleeding, or fibroids (benign tumors in her uterus), or something else that adversely affects her quality of life. Let's say she's 45 or older. Her physician gives her the option of having her ovaries removed or leaving them in place. She opts for removal of her ovaries since she knows she'll be going through menopause soon and won't need them after that. On the day of surgery, the physician performs a Total Hysterectomy (removes her uterus), performs a Bilateral Salpingo-oophorectomy (removes her fallopian tubes and ovaries), and sends all these specimens to the pathology lab (where the pathologist examines all tissues that are removed from all bodies). To the surgeon's naked eye, the ovaries appeared to be completely normal. However, in a couple of days, the pathologist calls the surgeon and informs him/her that there was an ovarian cancer confined to the ovary. He states that it was a good thing he/she removed the ovaries because the woman had ovarian cancer that she didn't know about. This is not an uncommon scenario. It illustrates the fact that ovarian cancer doesn't identify itself early.

Management Options

Diet and Lifestyle Options

Diet

It seems that high saturated fat has a role in increasing your risk of ovarian cancer, so the easiest thing you can do is to **limit the saturated fat** in your diet. Since we've discussed this as a beneficial lifestyle change a number of times now, it isn't new to you. We all have different thresholds for changing our behavior, and we respond to different incentives for doing so. If none of the other reasons for limiting saturated fat in your diet has fazed you, maybe decreasing your risk of ovarian cancer will.

The other important dietary measure for preventing ovarian cancer is **increasing the fiber** in your diet. Fiber is really good for you, and there are so many sources of it all around you. Popcorn, oatmeal, grainy breads, fruit, and vegetables are perfect.

Weight Control

Obesity is associated with ovarian cancer because fat cells produce undesirable changes in your hormones. Maintaining ideal body weight is the key. You've heard it before. This is one more reason to just do it.

Avoidance of Talc

Some women use talcum powder or other talc-containing powders in their underwear or panty hose in an effort to stay dry. It's similar to an antiperspirant for the underarms. The problem is that it can get into the vagina, ascend into the uterus and fallopian tubes, spill out the ends of the fallopian tubes, and into the belly and pelvis.

Now that may not seem like a big deal at first, but the problem is that talc is similar to asbestos in structure.[3] As such, it has the potential for increasing your risk of ovarian cancer if it creeps up into your pelvis.

It's not possible for talc to enter your pelvis if you've had a hysterectomy or had your tubes tied. And, as you might expect, women who've had either of those procedures have lower risks of ovarian cancer.[3]

It appears that there's a greater risk of ovarian cancer with more frequent and longer duration of talc exposure.[3] So, if you use talc, stop it now.

Hormonal Medication Options

Birth Control Pills

Good news! Birth control pills significantly decrease your risk of ovarian cancer. In fact, they're one of the things recommended for prevention of the disease. There's a 10% decrease in risk every year for five to seven years of using birth control pills.[3] The protection lasts for over 20 years after you no longer take birth control pills.[3]

Preventive Surgery

It's not uncommon for a woman who's witnessed ovarian cancer in family members, or who's had breast cancer, to be so concerned about her risk that she requests removal of her ovaries to avoid being an ovarian cancer victim herself. While it may seem like a drastic measure, it can make sense. Removing the ovaries in a preventive fashion to avoid ovarian cancer does significantly reduce the risk, but it doesn't completely erase it. If you have the gene mutation for ovarian cancer (BRCA), removal of your ovaries decreases your risk of ovarian cancer by more than 90% and your risk of breast cancer by more than 50%.[3]

Most doctors think that preventive surgery is only appropriate for women who have gene mutations or a strong family history of ovarian cancer. Again, that's because the benefits of the surgery should outweigh the risks of the surgery, and all surgery carries some risk.

Chapter 33: Alzheimer's Disease

Description

Alzheimer's disease is a brain disorder in which memory, reasoning, and independent thinking become impaired. There is limited understanding about the cause of this disease, but a genetic component is readily apparent. Alzheimer's disease is important in menopause because there seems to be a link between Alzheimer's disease and estrogen. And the association appears to be a favorable one for estrogen. This is one area where females may have an advantage over males, at least until the age of menopause.

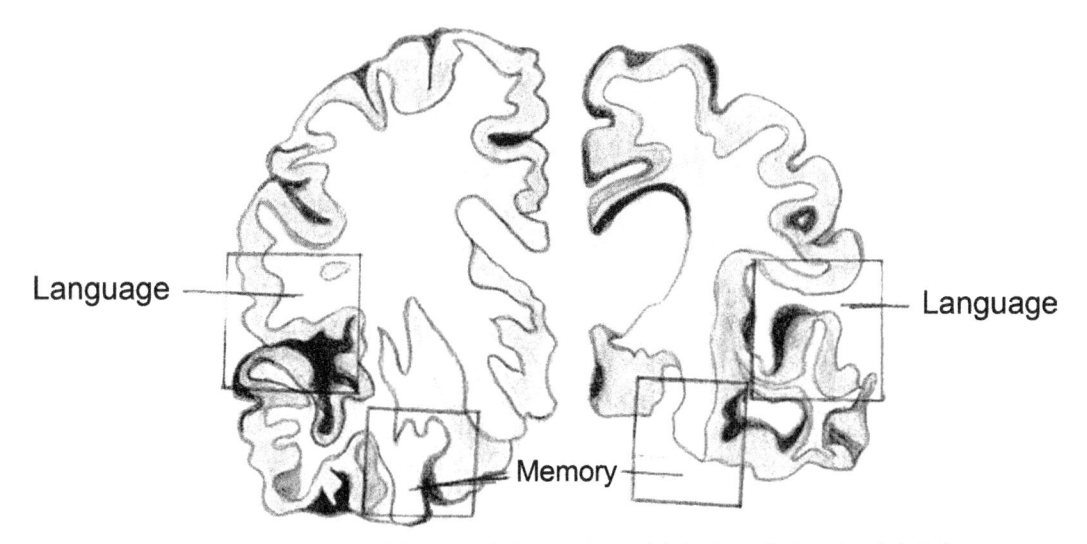

Figure 21: Normal brain (left) versus Alzheimer's brain (right)

Alzheimer's and Estrogen

Estrogen increases blood flow to the brain. Specifically, it enhances blood flow to the areas involved with memory, increases the activity of the hormones which regulate brain function, and stimulates growth of brain cells that communicate with one another.

Preliminary studies suggest that your body's natural estrogen decreases the risk, and delays the onset, of Alzheimer's disease. It seems that there may even be a relationship between the quantity of estrogen and the risk of Alzheimer's, because women with the highest levels of estrogen have the lowest incidence of Alzheimer's.[1] The length of time that estrogen is present in the body may also be a factor. Early menopause and surgical menopause are associated with higher rates of Alzheimer's disease than late or natural menopause.[2] Alzheimer's disease is rare before menopause.

Most studies on Alzheimer's disease have addressed three key areas, which include: (1) The relationship between natural estrogen levels and declining brain function; (2) Development of brain deterioration in women already taking hormone replacement; and (3) The role of estrogen or other hormone replacement in treating dementia or other forms of decreased brain function.[3] The brain is one of the many organs that has estrogen receptors. Because of this, changes in estrogen levels can modify the symptoms of Alzheimer's disease or influence its occurrence.

Risk Factors

There are risk factors for Alzheimer's disease. They are as follows:

1. **<u>Age</u>**
   Age is the most important and most consistent risk factor for Alzheimer's. Your *risk increases with age*. The number of people with Alzheimer's doubles every five to ten years beyond the age of 65.
2. **<u>Gender</u>**
   Gender is the second most significant risk factor. Being *female* is a risk all by itself. This may be partially due to the fact that

females have longer life spans than males. The female to male ratio for Alzheimer's disease is 2:1.

3. **Genetics**
Genetics plays a part in Alzheimer's, also. There are familial forms of Alzheimer's disease, and family history is a very consistent risk factor. *A positive family history of Alzheimer's* makes your risk four times higher at any age. In addition, a positive family history is associated with a younger age of onset of the disease.

4. **Previous traumatic head injury**
Perhaps brain damage can manifest later in life in the form of Alzheimer's.

5. **Lower educational level**
Educational level has to do with how much you exercise your brain. The *less* you use your brain, the higher your risk of Alzheimer's.

6. **Possibly, risk factors for heart attack and stroke**
These include *high blood pressure, high cholesterol*, and *low levels of folate*.

WORKSHEET TIMEOUT:
Answer question # 10 on your worksheet.
Circle all your risk factors for Alzheimer's disease.

Management Options

Diet and Lifestyle Options

Diet

The most basic dietary recommendation to prevent Alzheimer's disease is to avoid processed, refined foods. Fresh foods, whole grains, wheat germ, and lecithin are beneficial in feeding your brain an anti-Alzheimer's diet.

Exercise

Exercise increases the blood flow to your brain, and increased activity levels are associated with increases in brain function. Apparently, a good workout helps you think more clearly in the short term as well as in the long term.

Trying *new* exercises is the best thing for your brain. Have you ever noticed that when you're learning a new physical activity, like dancing or step aerobics, that you feel mentally exhausted afterwards? That's because you actually work your brain as well as your body when you learn a new physical activity. Those balancing exercises I discussed in the section on osteoporosis constitute another physical activity that's also mental.

Play Mind Games

Do you remember when you were a kid, and you played board games, cards, and memory games. Do you remember building puzzles? When was that last time you did any of those things? Did you stop playing mind games at some point in your adult life? If so, why? The point is this: Playing mind games is absolutely wonderful for keeping your mind sharp. You actually grow new connections between brain cells when you exercise your mind in this manner. If you've put all your games away, pull them out again, and start playing them. You'll have fun and you'll decrease your risk of Alzheimer's disease at the same time.

Going to school, learning a language, learning to play an instrument, or doing anything that challenges you mentally is vital for your brain health. You're never too old to learn something new. Go take a class in some subject you never imagined you'd pursue. Expand your horizons...and your brain.

Vitamin and Mineral Options

Vitamin B1

Vitamin B1 (thiamine) is good for many things. It has particular utility in brain function. Thiamine is especially important for women who drink alcohol. The recommended dose is 100 mg daily. Most multivitamins contain vitamin B1. Check to make sure the dose is adequate.

Vitamin B3

Vitamin B3 (niacin) is essential in the prevention of senility. Likewise, it's beneficial in preventing Alzheimer's. Pure niacin is available in slow release capsules of 250 mg each. The dose is 3 - 4 capsules three times daily with meals.

Nicotinic acid is a less active, but more tolerable form of the vitamin. The dose is 500 mg daily for three days. Increase by 500 mg daily, maintaining the dose for three days with each higher dose. The minimum effective dose is 3000 mg (or 3 gm).

Vitamin C

Vitamin C in a dose of 3 gm daily is useful in preventing Alzheimer's disease. That's a lot of vitamin C. You'll probably need more than what you find in most multivitamins. It's not harmful to take high doses of vitamin C, so add to your multivitamin if necessary.

Vitamin B6, Magnesium, and Zinc

This combination is invaluable in maintaining mental stability. It's available in a single tablet or capsule. The desired dose is 3 - 6 pills daily.

Vitamin E

Vitamin E, in a dose of 1000 – 1500 mg daily, assists in clearing arteries of fatty deposits. That includes the arteries in your brain. This is a higher dose of vitamin E than present in most multivitamins, and it's higher than generally recommended. But, it's the dose needed to prevent Alzheimer's.

Lecithin

Lecithin helps to clear your arteries of plaque, and improves the blood supply to your brain. The necessary dose is 2 tbsp daily or two 1200 mg capsules daily.

Botanical and Herbal Options

Ginkgo (Ginkgo biloba)

This is the same great herb that helps with the forgetfulness typical of menopause. It has beneficial effects on memory and brain function in both the short term and the long term. In the short term, it helps with reducing forgetfulness. In the long term, it helps with reducing Alzheimer's.

Hormonal Medication Options

Estrogen

Estrogen can enhance brain function through a variety of mechanisms.[2] It can enhance growth of neurons, protect your brain cells from injury, and increase blood flow to your brain.[2] While this is definitely true of your natural estrogen, and it is true at the beginning of post-menopause, later use of estrogen is more questionable. Whether you begin estrogen replacement immediately at the time of post-menopause or some later time may affect its impact on your brain. Overall, use of estrogen replacement is associated with a lower risk of Alzheimer's disease.

The results of early studies supported the fact that estrogen users developed Alzheimer's disease later than nonusers. Additionally, use of estrogen for more than one year was associated with a greater reduction in risk of Alzheimer's disease.[3] Some later studies have shown no benefit in estrogen therapy in preventing or treating Alzheimer's disease.[4]

The differences in conclusions as to whether or not estrogen prevents Alzheimer's disease result from timing. If you begin estrogen replacement early, before Alzheimer's begins, your risk will be reduced by 2.5 times in ten years.[5] However, if you begin estrogen therapy after Alzheimer's disease has already begun, there's no benefit. Estrogen doesn't have the ability to slow or reverse Alzheimer's disease.[5] That's because by the time there are symptoms of Alzheimer's disease or dementia, 40% of brain cells are already dead. The brain has an amazing capacity to compensate until that time, and then it begins to decay. After that, it's too late to intervene.[5]

The length of time that you use estrogen also has an effect on decreasing your risk of Alzheimer's disease. Long-term use is much more protective than short-term use. It's most beneficial before the age of 65. So, think of estrogen as a preventive measure for brain deterioration. If you start estrogen early in your peri- or post-menopausal years, it's effective for reducing your risk of Alzheimer's disease. If you wait until you're 65 to start estrogen, it won't help you avoid Alzheimer's.

Dehydroepiandrosterone (DHEA)

DHEA is an effective hormonal option for you if you have fears or risks for which you choose to avoid estrogen. It produces the benefit of protecting the brain, without the side effects of estrogen.[1] It's an androgen that may have some masculinizing side effects, like acne or growth of hair on your chin and chest.

Summary

If you've read all the forgoing information, you've probably noticed some recurring themes. The most common recommendations to improve your quality of life have been a healthy diet, exercise, maintaining ideal body weight, and not smoking. Of all the means for attaining and maintaining health and a high quality life, diet and exercise are more important than anything else. They provide the greatest benefit over the long term, while having significant short-term benefits as well.

I hope you can see why no two women are alike. Even if they have risks for the same diseases, they may have different degrees of risk. They may have totally different lifestyles and body types. Their comfort levels and preferences for traditional versus alternative and complementary medicine may vary. Each must honor her preferences and do what is right for her.

You may have risks for more than one disease. In that case, some of the benefits for one may be risks for the other. You have to balance those things. (I've actually created a slide chart covering all the options for all the combinations of all these diseases, but it's too large to fit in the book, and it's three dimensional. You can purchase one on Amazon.com.)

Remember to revisit this book and your worksheet from time to time. As you evolve, your needs may change. As new information becomes available, your desires may change. That brings us to the next section.

Section IV:

Research Studies and For the Guys

Chapter 34: "What About the Research Studies?"

Introduction

Doesn't it seem as though, just when you get comfortable on a medical therapy of some sort, you hear a media release warning you of some hazard associated with your medication? What's with that? Doesn't anyone test this stuff beforehand? Actually, they do. Here's what's happening.

Types of Research Studies

Research studies come in many flavors. There are studies which follow groups of people over time while imposing no control over them, studies which match subjects and then give one person a drug and give their match a placebo, studies which conceal who's getting what from the researchers or the subjects (single blind) or both (double blind), and studies which just review the other studies. Some studies are prospective, moving forward in time as the events occur. Others are retrospective, looking at things after the fact. Some studies are huge, examining multiple populations of people, conducted by multiple researchers. Other studies are small, involving just a small number of subjects and a single researcher. Almost all studies have a specific objective. Sometimes, the findings and conclusions pertain to that objective. Sometimes they don't.

Significance of Research Results

Study results are defined in terms of whether or not the findings are "significant." Now, although that's a common word, it has a specific meaning in the world of statistics. Not only does it pertain to the population as a whole rather than to you as an individual, but what's significant to a statistician may or may not be significant to you. For instance, a study may conclude that a risk is "insignificant." And it may well indeed be insignificant in terms of a large population of people. The risk may only be 1 per 10,000 people. But, if you're the one, it's pretty significant, don't you think? On the other hand, a risk of 1 per 10,000 may actually strike you as being so unlikely that you feel more secure about the likelihood that you won't be the one. And, of course, the odds are in your favor that you won't be the one. Regardless of the nature of a study, there is one thing that no study takes into account… *you*.

There are thousands of studies taking place at any one time. Usually, multiple studies examining the same matter reveal different results. Some will conclude that a drug is harmful in a certain way, while others will conclude that it isn't. The reasons for the differences are many. They range from flaws in the design of the study, to differences in populations, to variability in the effects of the study drug.

In many cases, we're left with an indefinite answer. Recall the explanation that I gave you earlier on the issue of whether or not estrogen causes breast cancer. If we're lucky, the vast majority of the studies will agree with one another, and we'll have new knowledge of which we feel certain…that is, until another study comes along to make us think otherwise.

Every so often, the media presents the results of a study. I'm sure you can think of one or two right off the top of your head. Did you think that those were the only studies out there and that the media is able to present them all? Or are you aware of the fact that the media picks and chooses which studies to present? If you guessed that they pick and choose, you're right. And they're pretty choosy.

What About the Research Studies?

It's also important to realize that there's usually an emphasis on certain aspects of the study, and a glossing over of others. The most dramatic, startling, attention-getting findings get center stage. There may be other findings that are significant, or that diminish the importance of the startling ones, but oftentimes, they're overlooked.

The media is in the business of journalism and entertainment. It's their job to present things that are interesting, to do so in a way that will get your attention, and to use dramatic ways to accomplish that goal if necessary, even if they have to scare you in the process.

Now, I have nothing against the media. I actually appreciate and respect what they do. They provide us with valuable information, and they do so in a way that focuses on the main issues. My message to you is that you need to use that information wisely. Don't use it as your only source of medical information. Don't let it scare you. Don't let it induce you to change your medical regimen without guidance from your healthcare provider. Always remember, no study has studied you as an individual. Some of those study findings may have nothing to do with you. You're unique. Take note of the results, discuss them with your healthcare provider, plug yourself into the information, and use it to determine whether or not you need to change anything at all.

Other factors play into the world of research, also. Sometimes, drug companies sponsor or fund the research. Sometimes the researcher is determined to prove something in particular, and designs the study in a manner that makes it likely that the desired results will manifest themselves.

All in all, research is good. Without it, we'd have very little progress in medicine. Likewise, the media is good. So are drug companies and researchers. You just need to be aware of these nuances as you evaluate research studies. First, know that for every study you hear about, there are hundreds that you don't hear about. Know that the results differ among the studies on a single topic, and that the medical community supports what the majority of them reveal. Don't let a single study, in and of itself, sway you or make you think that it's the final answer. Add it to the mix, weigh its merits, and consider it along with all the others. Don't forget that studies pertain to populations of people. They're like averages. The results don't translate into personal statistics. Finally, apply the information to *yourself* as a unique individual.

Factors Which Affect Research Studies

Let's list the factors which affect a research study. These are the things to which you need to pay attention as you assess the merit of any study on you as an individual:

1. Study design
2. Size of the study population
3. Characteristics of the study population
4. How much you resemble the study population
5. Criteria for excluding subjects
6. Duration of the study
7. Study objectives (purpose)
8. How well the conclusions pertain to the objectives
9. Actual conclusions
10. Sponsorship for the study
11. Market forces
12. Economics
13. Competition
14. Media reporting, drama, sensationalism

With that as your foundation, let's review the chronologic development of the studies and reactions that have been pivotal in the realm of hormones for menopause. This will help you understand why the information and recommendations seem to change from time to time. Remember, these are just the most notorious and publicized items. There are a multitude of others that didn't have as great an impact.

Postmenopausal Hormone History

In this section, we'll review the history and chronological development of postmenopausal hormones. In so doing, you'll identify the various forces that brought us to where we are today. You'll see how the media, drug companies, public reaction, drama, scientific data,

What About the Research Studies?

and market forces have interacted to create the current practices and demands for post-menopausal hormones.

As you read through each historical event, refer to the list above. Consider which items in that list are pertinent. The idea is not for you to know everything about postmenopausal hormone history! It's for you to see how the listed items have played a part in the evolution of postmenopausal hormone history. I want you to practice scrutinizing the research with these items so that you can do the same when you hear about new research studies. So, here we go.

The desire to slow, arrest, or reverse the aging process isn't new. It's been around since the late 1800s.[1] Back then, scientists tried to preserve youth, health, sex, and vitality with injections of hormones, drugs, potions, and animal parts. In Europe, gonads from pigs, dogs, and other animals were the sources of these substances.[1]

In 1928, a German scientist synthesized the first estrogen, called estrone. Not much else happened for the next ten years, until a British scientist synthesized another estrogen by the name of diethylstilbesterol. You may recognize it by the name DES. It was used to prevent pregnancy loss rather than for menopause, but it set the stage for the synthesis of hormones for various purposes. (Let the *competition* begin!)

In 1942, a pharmaceutical company by the name of Ayerst patented an estrogen called Premarin. It was a mixture of estrogens extracted from the urine of pregnant mares (Pre = pregnant, Mar = mare, In = urine). It was approved by the FDA (Food and Drug Administration) for menopausal hormone replacement. Thereafter, estrogen replacement for menopause became commonplace, largely because of the heavy marketing of Premarin to gynecologists. That also led to the production of many other estrogen products for menopause.[1] (This is an example of market forces, economics, and competition, items **11**, **12**, & **13**.)

In 1952, a study assessing the effect of estrogen on the brain showed that it enhanced verbal memory in elderly women. This began our understanding of how estrogen relates to Alzheimer's disease.[1] (Consider items 2, 3, 4, 5, 6, 7, **8**, 9, & 10.)

In 1959, two doctors wrote a paper in which they described *"menopausal syndrome."* They defined it as a combination of symptoms, including hot flashes, insomnia, fatigue, moodiness, and undesirable changes in lipids (elevated lousy LDL, lower healthy HDL). They asserted that women could avoid this syndrome by taking estrogen for menopause.[1] (Do you think calling menopause a "syndrome" makes it sound like a disease that requires treatment? Let's apply items 3, 6, 7, 8, 9, 10, 11, 12, 13, & **14**.)

In the same year, an article in *JAMA (Journal of the American Medical Association)* touted the benefits of long term estrogen therapy for protecting bones and relieving the symptoms of menopause. It also said that "Fear that breast and cervical cancer may result from this therapy appears unfounded."[1] (Could it be that the researchers or those funding the study needed to persuade people to have a positive opinion about estrogen? Items **1**, 2, 3, **4**, 5, 6, 7, **8**, 9, **10**, 11, 12, 13, &14.)

In 1962, a gynecologist by the name of Robert Wilson published an article in *JAMA* describing his treatment of 304 women between the ages of 40 and 70 with estrogen and progesterone. He had expected that 18 of them would develop some kind of cancer during treatment. None did, so he concluded that estrogen and progesterone *prevented* breast and gynecologic cancers.[1] (Do you see how surprising results brought about conclusions that hadn't really been tested? There's a huge difference between absence of a disease and prevention of a disease. Just because the hormones didn't *cause* cancer doesn't mean that they *prevented* it. This is an example of conclusions that don't pertain to the objectives.) (Think about items 1, 3, 5, 6, 7, **8**, & **9**.)

In 1966, instead of presenting his research findings to just the medical community in a medical journal, Dr. Wilson wrote a book called *Feminine Forever*, in which he recommended hormone replacement therapy as the "cure" for "*the tragedy of menopause.*" He stated that "women who use the drugs will be much more pleasant to live with and will not become dull and unattractive." He also repeated his belief that estrogen prevented breast and uterine cancer. There was suspicion that Wilson's studies were sponsored by drug companies, but it was never proven. Eventually, the FDA (Food and Drug Administration) concluded that

What About the Research Studies?

his recommendation went beyond approved uses for hormones, and would no longer accept his data. But the public response to his book was very positive. By 1973, sales of estrogen quadrupled.[1] (How would you respond to the "tragedy" of menopause if there were a book called *"Feminine Forever"* to save you from such a "tragedy?" This is an example of items 10, 11, 13, & **14**.)

In 1969, *Everything You Always Wanted to Know About Sex*, by David Rueben promoted estrogen as a menopausal cure-all. In it, he said, "As the estrogen is shut off, *a woman comes as close as she can to being a man*.... Increased facial hair, deepened voice, obesity, and decline of the breasts and female genitalia all contribute to a masculine appearance. To many women, the menopause marks the end of their useful life."[1] (Somewhat dramatic...and attention-getting, wouldn't you say? How about items 10, 11, 13, & **14**.)

In 1973, an article in *Harper's Bazaar* asserted: "There doesn't seem to be a sexy thing estrogen can't and won't do to keep you *flirtatiously feminine* for the rest of your days...a real package deal that *spruces up your vagina*. Prevalent medical opinion is that the safety and benefits of ERT (estrogen replacement therapy) have been convincingly demonstrated."[1] (I don't know about you, but if someone offered me something that would "spruce up my vagina," and keep me "flirtatiously feminine," I'd give it a try. This illustrates items 10, 11, 12, 13, & **14**.)

At the same time, a study in which *men* took Premarin to prevent heart attacks and strokes was discontinued because they were having more heart attacks and blood clots.[1] (Do you remember the chapter on Heart Attack? How much do men resemble women with regard to heart attacks? This a good place to apply items 1, 2, 3, **4**, 5, 6, 7, 8, 9, 10, & 11. How much you resemble the study population is especially important.)

In 1975, the *NEJM* (*New England Journal of Medicine*) published two studies showing that women who took estrogen for menopause had a four fold increased risk of developing uterine cancer over those who didn't. The longer they took it, the greater the risk. At the same time, other clinical trials were ongoing in which progesterone was administered with the estrogen. The idea was to mimic the natural menstrual cycle. By that time, over 30 million prescriptions for estrogen were written every year. Half of all menopausal women were using it for an average of five years.[1] (Do you think some of the women taking estrogen suddenly stopped it? If so, do you think they applied the information to themselves and their own situation, or do you think they just responded to this information with fear? Consider items 1, 2, 3, **4**, 5, 6, 7, 8, 9, & 10.)

In 1976, scientist Robert Hoover presented the first study showing a link between estrogen for menopause and breast cancer in the *NEJM* (*New England Journal of Medicine*). He studied women in just one private practice, involving only 1800 women. It made estrogen sales plummet. By 1979, estrogen was approved *only* for treating hot flashes and vaginal dryness.[1] (Remember when we analyzed the data on whether estrogen causes breast cancer? A "link" between estrogen and breast cancer isn't the same thing as a cause – effect relationship between estrogen and breast cancer. This small study created a large response! Apply items 1, 2, 3, 4, 5, 6, 7, **8**, 9, **10**, **11**, & **13**.)

In 1980, an article by R. Ben Gambrell in *Obstetrics and Gynecology* reported that adding progesterone to estrogen actually resulted in a decline in uterine cancer. And in 1982, he published an article in *Fertility and Sterility* stating that the estrogen plus progesterone combination may help osteoporosis and have "protective effects against cardiovascular disease." At the same time, several experts in *Cancer Research* said that hormones for menopause were a major factor in causing cancer.[1] (This is an example of conflicting data. Who's correct? What should you believe? How should you react to this conflicting information? What if you knew how much you resemble each of the study populations? Would that enable you to decipher the information more easily? Think about items 1, 2, 3, 4, 5, 6, 7, **8**, 9, 10, & 14.)

In 1985, there was a campaign to create public awareness of osteoporosis. In the same year, the Framingham Heart Study showed that 1,234 women using estrogen had more heart attacks than women who didn't use it. Their risk was 50% higher for heart attacks, strokes, and blood clots. The women in that study were older, at greater risk in the first place, and some had received higher dosages of estrogen than that in menopausal formulations. On the other hand, the Nurses

What About the Research Studies?

Health Study sent questionnaires to 121,964 female nurses between 30 and 55 years of age showing that, among those who took estrogen, the risk of heart attack actually decreased. They concluded that among the 32,300 post-menopausal women, hormone users had half the rate of heart attack as those who had never taken hormones for menopause.[1] (Let's see...one study with 1,234 subjects, and another study with 121,964 subjects. Which one is more valid? It might depend on study design, or characteristics of the study population, or how much you resemble the study population. Consider items 1, **2, 3**, 4, 5, 6, 7, 8, 9, 10, 11, & 14.)

Before long, researchers were coming out with all kinds of studies showing the beneficial effects of hormones for menopause. They asserted that hormones prevented heart attack, hardening of the arteries (atherosclerosis), and bone loss, while having no increase in the rates of cancer, stroke, or blood clots. They even showed that hormones reduced death from all causes, including accidents and homicides! As is typical with research subjects and patients who visit doctors regularly, the women who were taking estrogen were more educated, wealthier, and more compliant, which adds up to research bias. Also, all the while, the *PDR* (*Physician's Desk Reference*) stated that estrogen should not be prescribed to women with heart disease, high blood pressure, or diabetes. So, women with heart problems were not receiving these hormones. It was no surprise that the ones who were had fewer heart attacks.[1] (My! There sure was a lot going on! It sounds like someone is trying to find a panacea for everything that ails you. Notice the confounding of data which results with the exclusion of women with heart disease, while also asserting that estrogen prevents heart attacks. Refer to items 1, 2, 3, 4, 5, 6, 7, **8**, 9, 10, &14.)

In 1987, a clinical trial called the Postmenopausal Estrogen/ Progesterone Intervention Trial (PEPI) began. It studied the effects of hormones on key risk factors for heart disease, such as lipids, blood clotting, and weight gain. It lasted three years and showed that, while hormone replacement therapy reduced some risk factors (lousy LDL), it increased others (triglycerides).[1] (Oh, so it's possible for a hormone to have some beneficial effects *and* some detrimental effects? Go figure! This is reality. That's why you have to apply the information to your unique circumstance. Think about items 1, 2, 3, 4, 5, 6, 7, **8**, 9, 10, & 13.)

In 1989, a Swedish study appeared in the *NEJM* (*New England Journal of Medicine*). It involved 23,244 women who had used either estrogen alone or estrogen plus progesterone, and showed a slight increase in breast cancer among those who took estrogen alone. When they then switched to estrogen plus progesterone, their risk for breast cancer more than doubled. The study received wide media coverage. It was the first evidence that progesterone for protection of the *uterus* might increase the risk of *breast* cancer.[1] (As you've learned, a hormone can be beneficial for one aspect of your menopause management, and detrimental for another. Note that the findings in this study are inconsistent with the findings of other studies on the same topic. Refer to items 1, 2, 3, 4, 5, 6, 7, **8**, 9, & 13.)

In 1990, the NIH (National Institutes of Health) launched a very large, multi-site clinical trial on women's health. It covered heart attacks, breast cancer, colon cancer, osteoporosis and bone fractures in relationship to the roles of hormone therapy, diet, vitamins, and calcium in preventing these diseases. They called it the "Women's Health Initiative" (WHI). (Wow! Is it even possible to study so many things at once? What was the actual objective of the study? How can a researcher pay attention to so many variables at once? Consider items 1, 2, 3, 4, 5, 6, **7**, 8, 9, & 10.)

At the same time, the pharmaceutical company Wyeth (formerly Ayerst) was allowed to list protection against heart attacks on its label for Premarin.[1] (Sounds like market forces and competition to me. Could this be an example of putting the cart before the horse? Refer to items **11**, 12, & **13**.)

From 1990 to 1995, Premarin was the most frequently prescribed prescription drug in America. Several other small drug companies offered generic estrogens, but Wyeth attempted to get them off the market by alleging that they released estrogen into the blood stream too quickly. Despite these allegations, a new estrogen by the name of Cenestin did make it into the marketplace. Within the same time frame, Wyeth began marketing Prempro, which provided both estrogen and

What About the Research Studies?

progesterone in a single pill.[1] (Ready, set, go! Who will win the race to sell more product and make more money? Don't get me wrong; all these products make management of your menopause easier. You have many options from which to choose. Some are more popular than others. But, it's not a popularity contest. Apply items 11, 12, **13**, & **14**.)

In 1992, two books hit the market. The first was *The Silent Passage* by Gail Sheehy. It focused on the losses entailed with the process of menopause. The second was *The Change* by Germaine Greer. It stated that it was fine for women to give up sex and embrace the "crone" years.[1] (I'm not sure what she meant by "crone" years. I certainly don't think of menopause as a time to shrivel up and stop enjoying life. I also find it a little interesting that previous books, written by men, promised flirtatiousness and a spruced-up vagina, while these women are throwing in the towel. Don't you think you deserve the facts and the opportunity to manage your menopause your way?)

In 1996, the Heart and Estrogen/Progestin Replacement Study (HERS) began. It was the first major placebo controlled trial of hormone replacement therapy showing that hormones did not help women who had already had a heart attack. In fact, it caused a 50% increase in heart attacks and strokes. By the end of the second year, it was clear that there was no hope of showing any benefit to the heart from hormones. In 1998, the HERS investigators reported their findings, and shocked the medical community, which had firmly believed the opposite. (Well of course they believed the opposite. Premarin listed protection against heart attacks on its label!) That study subsequently came to a halt.[1] (In other words, they discontinued the study before completion. How does that affect the data? Does it provide an actual answer to the questions the study attempted to answer? Or does it render the findings incomplete? Could it be that the results might have changed over time (short-term versus long-term results)? Who discontinued the study? Was it the financial sponsors, the medical community, or the researchers? Did a pharmaceutical company have a stake in the matter? Be inquisitive! Consider items 1, **2**, 3, 4, **5**, 6, 7, 8, 9, & 14.)

In 2002, after 5.2 years of follow-up, the Women's Health Initiative, discontinued one arm of the study (the estrogen plus progesterone arm). It was designed to focus on *prevention* of heart attack, breast cancer, colon cancer, and osteoporosis in healthy post-menopausal women. Discontinuation was due to "risks that *outweighed* the benefits." A year and a half later, the other arm of the study (the estrogen alone arm) was discontinued because the "benefits of estrogen *did not exceed* the risks."[1] The media covered discontinuation of the study heavily and sent both patients and their physicians into a frenzy. (This is an example of items 1, 2, 3, 4, 5, 6, 7, **8**, **9**, & 14.)

Since this is the latest of the really big events in the history of hormonal therapy, we'll analyze it thoroughly to illustrate how the data were interpreted. It's probably the one you've heard about. You may have questions about it, so I don't want to gloss over it. The fact is, we're just getting over all the panic this study created.

Women's Health Initiative (WHI)

Purpose (Objective)

The Women's Health Initiative was a national, large-scale study sponsored by the National Institutes of Health (NIH). Its planned duration was 8.5 years. Its primary purpose was to examine how well hormone therapy during menopause *prevented heart attack*. Its secondary purpose was to examine how well hormone therapy during menopause also prevented *breast cancer, colon cancer,* and *osteoporosis.* So, it was assessing how well hormone therapy could be used in a manner to do something other than manage menopause. It was designed to assess how well hormones prevented medical problems, especially heart attack. ***It didn't assess the effect of hormones on menopause at all!*** It was a ***preventive*** trial rather than a therapeutic trial.

The fact that it was a "preventive trial" is significant for a variety of reasons. It means that it assessed whether or not hormones could *prevent* diseases, rather than whether or not they could *treat* diseases or the symptoms of menopause. It also means that very low thresholds were set for any negative outcomes.[2] In essence, as a preventive trial, its threshold for failure was quite low. Finally, it's important to realize that proving that hormones don't *prevent* a disease is not the same thing as proving that they *cause* a disease.

Two Arms of the Study

Estrogen Plus Progesterone Arm

There were two groups (arms) in the study. The first group was the "Estrogen Plus Progesterone Group." It consisted of 50 to 70 year old women, each of whom still had her uterus.[3] They received either estrogen plus progesterone, or a placebo (fake pill). This group "demonstrated risks which outweighed benefits."[3] Therefore, this portion of the study was discontinued after 5.2 years.[3]

Estrogen Alone Arm

The second group was the "Estrogen Alone Group." It consisted of 50 to 70 year old women, each of whom had no uterus.[3] They received either estrogen alone, or a placebo (fake pill).[3] This group did not demonstrate risks which outweighed benefits.[3] It did show a decrease in the risk of hip fracture, a possible reduction in the risk of breast cancer, no effect on the risk of heart attack, as well as an increased risk of stroke. Nevertheless, this portion of the study was discontinued after 6.8 years simply because "continuation of the study would not have changed the results."[3]

Soon after the media reported the results of the WHI study to the public, 40% of postmenopausal women who were using *any* type of estrogen and/or progesterone to **manage menopause** discontinued their hormones. They did so because of the reports indicating the possibility of increased risks for some diseases.

Analysis of the Estrogen Plus Progesterone Arm

Now, let's look closely at the data and the conclusions. You may have already heard about this study, but I have a feeling that you'll be surprised when you hear the results from a source other than the media.

The primary goal of this arm of the study was to answer the question: "Does postmenopausal hormone therapy (estrogen plus progesterone) *prevent heart attack* and, if it does, what are the risks of *using it for this purpose?*" The overall answer based on the findings from this arm of the WHI was: "Estrogen plus progesterone is unlikely to prevent heart attack. That's because the risks of heart attack and cancer outweigh the benefits. The increases in risks of various diseases were too high a price to pay for any possible preventive benefits."[4]

The results of the study were reported to the general public without clearly distinguishing between use of estrogen plus progesterone for symptoms of menopause versus use of estrogen plus progesterone for purposes of preventing heart attack. What you heard was the following:

Estrogen plus progesterone causes:

- A 100% increase in blood clots

- A 41% increase in strokes

- A 29% increase in heart attacks

- A 26% increase in breast cancers

- A 22% increase in all heart diseases, including heart attacks

In essence, these results were generalized to *all* uses of estrogen plus progesterone. Frankly, I know of no one who actually uses estrogen plus progesterone for the primary purpose of preventing heart attack. If indeed this combination does prevent heart attack, it would be an ancillary benefit rather than the primary reason for using hormone replacement therapy.

Even though there were some positive results, they weren't publicized to the same extent, or at all. Just so you know, here are the beneficial findings of estrogen plus progesterone from the WHI study:

What About the Research Studies?

Estrogen plus progesterone causes:

- A 37% decrease in colon cancers

- A 33% decrease in hip fractures

- A 24% decrease in all types of fractures

- No difference in deaths from all causes

Risks

Now, let's translate those percentages that you heard in media reports to the general public into actual numbers. First, we'll look at all the risks due to estrogen plus progesterone that this study revealed. Specifically, the breakdown of diseases would be as follows in a group of **10,000 women per year:**

- 8 more blood clots

- 8 more strokes

- 7 more heart attacks

- 8 more breast cancers

These actual numbers are much less alarming than the percentages that the media reported to the public, aren't they?

Benefits

You never heard about the benefits of estrogen plus progesterone that this study revealed. Overall, the combination of estrogen plus progesterone prevents the occurrence of diseases in some women, so that, **for every 10,000 women**, fewer would suffer from certain diseases **each year**.[3] Specifically, the breakdown would be as follows:

- 6 fewer colon cancers

- 5 fewer hip fractures due to osteoporosis

Overall, the combination of estrogen plus progesterone might account for 20 more health problems *per 10,000 women per year.* (You arrive at this number by subtracting the number of benefits per 10,000 women per year from the number of risks per 10,000 women per year, which is 31 − 11 = 20.)

	Media Report	**Translation**
Blood clots	100% increase	8 more/10,000 women/year
Strokes	41% increase	8 more/10,000 women/year
Heart attacks	29% increase	7 more/10,000 women/year
Breast cancers	26% increase	8 more/10,000 women/year
Colon cancers	37% decrease	6 fewer/10,000 women/year
Hip fractures	33% decrease	5 fewer/10,000 women/year
All fractures	24% decrease	4 fewer/10,000 women/year

The question I have for you is this: When you heard the media report, did you think that a "100% increase in blood clots" pertained to you personally, and that you had a 100% chance of having a blood clot? Or did you know that it pertained to a population of 10,000 women per year? Furthermore, did you know that the "100% increase" actually meant that only eight more women out of 10,000 would suffer a blood clot each year? In other words, did you realize that instead of eight women having blood clots, there would be 16 having blood clots each year in a population of 10,000 women? Do you think that the public reaction to this study would have been as drastic if the media had reported the actual numbers rather than the percentages? And what about *you*? Would *you* have reacted differently? After all, what you really care about is how the study findings affect *you*, not how they affect a population of 10,000 other women.

The WHI study did *not* address the short-term benefits of hormone replacement therapy (estrogen plus progesterone) for the purpose of treating the symptoms of menopause. That's unfortunate because *nine out of every ten* women who begin estrogen plus progesterone do so for the specific purpose of controlling the symptoms of menopause. Many of them intend to take hormones for only a few years. Any benefit in terms of *improved quality of life* was not taken into consideration in assessing the risk to benefit ratio. And for them, the benefits may outweigh the risks, even if only temporarily.

Reflect back on the section entitled "The Balancing Act." It referred to considering all the factors, placing them on a scale, with the benefits on one side and the risks on the other, to see which side weighs more. This study didn't do that. It noted some alarming things, and forgot to take note of the other factors that may hold significant weight for some women.

As you assess your own options for managing menopause, don't let a single study, a single risk, or a single benefit hold all the weight for you. Go ahead and take the time to put *all* the factors on the scale. Unlike any study, only *you* can add yourself to the scale and consider those things that matter to *you* the most. Don't forfeit your chance to do just that.

Analysis of the Estrogen Alone Arm

Now, let's dissect the estrogen alone arm, just as we did the estrogen plus progesterone arm.

The primary goal of this arm of the study was to answer the question: "Does postmenopausal hormone therapy (estrogen alone) *prevent* heart attack and, if it does, what are the risks of *using it for this purpose?*" The overall answer based on the findings from this arm of the WHI was as follows: "Estrogen alone may or may not prevent heart attack. We can't answer that question because we discontinued the study before its completion." Of course, that's not the answer that was presented to the general public. Instead, they were told that the study was discontinued because "continuing it would not have changed the results." Might economic concerns have been the real reason?

<u>The Bottom Line of the Estrogen Alone Arm</u>

Let's put the findings into perspective so that you are more able to apply them to your personal situation. We'll analyze this arm according to age groups since the age at which you use hormones for menopause is the crucial variable.

In the youngest age group of women (aged 50 to 59), the risk of heart attack was decreased by almost half. This is the age group most representative of the majority of women who begin estrogen therapy for menopause.[5]

The risk of stroke in the youngest age group (aged 50 to 59) was increased only slightly.[5]

The risk of blood clots was increased in all age groups. The degree of risk increased with age.[5] This is consistent with what happens in the real world.

The risk of breast cancer was decreased in all age groups.[5]

The risk of colon cancer was decreased in the women who were 50 to 69 years of age. It was increased in women aged 70 and older.[5]

There was an overall reduction in the risk of bone fracture. However, there were an unusually high number of fractures in the youngest women (aged 50 to 59).[5] This is confusing, as studies like this often are. Maybe they were very athletic and injured themselves.

During the study, the death rates were lowest for the youngest women (aged 50 to 59) on estrogen compared to those on placebo. They were the same for the middle age range (aged 60 to 69) on estrogen and placebo. They were higher for the estrogen users in the oldest age range (aged 70 to 79).[5] Isn't that true as women age anyway?

Limitations of the WHI Study

In order to make sense of the study results, you have to know some of the limitations of the study. If you take them at face value, they're deceiving, primarily because the results pertain to a large group of women. The women who were tested in the study may or may not be representative of you as an individual. I'm sure you want to use the information for your own personal reasons, and you can't do that if you don't delineate some of the factors that sway, limit, invalidate, or validate the information *for you.*

What About the Research Studies?

The word "limitation" is not positive or negative in terms of your personal use of the information. Sometimes a limitation of a study makes it invalid for you personally. Other times, it makes it more specific to you, and therefore more useful. It's important to be aware of the limitations of any study before you jump to conclusions.

The WHI evaluated women ranging in age from 50 to 70 at the start of the study. This means that the average age of women in the study was 63.6 years. All the women initiated use of hormones at the start of the study, at various ages. This isn't typical of how most women use hormones.[5] Most commonly, they begin hormones at age 50 to 52 to control the symptoms of menopause. The older a woman is, the greater her risk for certain health problems by virtue of her age alone (breast cancer, osteoporosis, heart attack, and stroke). Because this trial examined the ability of hormones to *prevent* these diseases, the results may have been different if the women had started hormones at younger ages. Maybe some of these diseases had already begun to develop *before* the study began.

Another important point is that, although the study was designed as a trial of "healthy" postmenopausal women, at least 50% of them had been smokers, 33% were overweight, 4% had diabetes, 33% had high blood pressure, and 15% had a family history of breast cancer.[5] You might consider this a flaw in the study. Or you might think that it represents the "average" older American woman at 63 years of age.

Although the WHI was designed to use hormones as a form of preventive therapy, many of the women in the study already had some of the health problems of concern.

One of the limitations of the WHI study is that it only tested a single dose of only one brand of oral estrogen (0.625 mg of conjugated equine estrogen, which is better known as Premarin), and one dose combination of only one brand of estrogen plus progesterone (0.625 mg of conjugated equine estrogen and 2.5 mg of medroxyprogesterone acetate, which is better known as Prempro).[5] Since you have the option of a variety of dosages and many different brands of estrogen and progesterone, testing other types and dosages of estrogen and progesterone may have produced different results.

Also note that WHI evaluated only a continuous estrogen plus progesterone regimen.[5] While that's common for women once they reach post-menopause, what about all those women who use some form of cyclic estrogen plus progesterone? And don't forget that the majority of women who take hormone replacement therapy do so when they're *peri-* or early *post-menopausal*, and may not have the option of using a continuous regimen.

Since the WHI study, further research has revealed that non-oral forms of estrogen have fewer risks than oral forms of estrogen.[5] The differences are significant. It appears that non-oral forms of estrogen decrease triglycerides, and have no tendency to increase blood clots. So, it may be a lot less risky to use an estrogen patch or vaginal ring than it is to take an estrogen pill. Just be aware of the fact that all forms of estrogen are not created equal.[6]

Women who were more than 20 years post-menopausal were at the greatest risk of heart attack after beginning hormone therapy. In contrast, women less than ten years post-menopausal had no marked increased risk of heart attack.[5] This makes sense because women who are within ten years of being post-menopausal are fairly young and have a naturally lower risk for heart attack anyway. Women who are 20 or more years beyond menopause have a higher risk for a heart attack based on their age alone.[2]

In general, the results of the WHI study don't apply to young women who become menopausal prematurely, either from natural causes or as a result of surgery, x-ray therapy, or chemotherapy. These women benefit from hormone therapy, and the benefits outweigh the risks for them.

Likewise, do not apply the results to your personal situation if you're peri-menopausal or very recently post-menopausal, with severe symptoms. Such women were not included in the WHI trial.[2]

The WHI eliminated women who had significant menopausal symptoms, even though that's the group of women who is most likely to opt for use of hormones in the first place.

What About the Research Studies?

Interpretation of Results

In analyzing these results for your own decision-making process, realize that all these results are expressed in terms of increased risk or benefit per 10,000 women per year. None of these results refer to you personally.[3] As you can see, the absolute risk for any individual woman remains small.[3]

Unfortunately, the results of this study caused overreaction by both physicians and patients with regard to use of hormones for menopause. The appropriate response would have been for each patient to re-examine her options in view of the new data and with the guidance of her physician. Few women would have discovered a need to change their management choices for menopause. Instead of this rational approach, most patients and physicians discontinued all post-menopausal hormone therapy. This decreased the quality of life for many women and robbed them of the opportunity to consider other options that would have provided benefits without the risks. Many physicians became reluctant to prescribe post-menopausal hormones to any patients, for fear of litigation.

Lesson

Here's the lesson in presenting all of this to you: Whenever you hear about the results of a study, don't panic. Don't let just a single study rob you of your options. Remember that there are hundreds of other studies that you didn't hear about. Sit down with your doctor, and apply the information in the study to your personal situation. If you realize that none of the concerns apply to you, don't change a thing. If you realize that adjusting your regimen is warranted by changing your dosage or length of treatment, do so. If you realize that the new information has significant disadvantages for you, then consider other alternatives. There are many hormone formulations from which to choose, and they aren't all created equal. And, there are many non-hormonal medications, botanicals, herbs, vitamins, and minerals that may take the place of hormones. Of course, your lifestyle matters a great deal, also. Always remember, you want to maximize the benefits and minimize the risks.

The underlying purpose of the WHI study was to determine if hormones for menopause were beneficial for the primary purpose of *preventing* heart attack. The bottom line is that they aren't. So, if you're a thin, athletic, health nut, with no family history of heart attacks, and you have no increased risk for breast cancer, but miserable symptoms of menopause, you may decide that it improves your quality of life to take hormones. You already do all kinds of other things to prevent a heart attack, and the benefits of taking hormones may outweigh your risks. Alternatively, if you're an obese, sedentary, junk food lover, with a strong family history of heart attacks, a high risk of breast cancer, and few symptoms of menopause, you may decide that it does nothing to improve your quality of life to take hormones for any reason. You can mix up any of the descriptive factors that I listed here, and you can weigh them any way you want.

New Recommendations

As you learned from the section on the history of hormones, research studies and the public reaction to research studies create new recommendations for how to use medications. The results of the WHI sent panic waves throughout the world of gynecologists and patients alike. Unfortunately, few people took the time to really assess the information and apply it to their own situation. Now that some time has passed, various organizations have restructured their guidelines as to the recommendations for hormone use. So, here are the new recommendations. Remember, they're for "women in general." They may or may not apply to you personally.

Do not use estrogen plus progesterone specifically for the purpose of preventing heart attack. Instead, adopt lifestyle changes in diet, exercise, and cessation of tobacco for this purpose.[3]

Weigh the benefits against the risks of using estrogen plus progesterone to prevent osteoporosis. Don't use it specifically for this purpose if you don't have actual osteoporosis already.[3] Consider some of the alternatives and use hormone replacement therapy as a second-line alternative. Consider it a good choice if your risk of fracture from

What About the Research Studies?

osteoporosis greatly exceeds your risk of heart attack, stroke, and blood clots.[7]

Assume that use of estrogen alone for more than five years may increase your risk of breast cancer.[8]

Regular self breast examinations and mammograms are a must.[3]

The primary reason to use estrogen alone or estrogen plus progesterone is treatment of moderate to severe symptoms of menopause, especially hot flashes.[9]

Local estrogen in the form of a cream or ring is best if the sole purpose is to treat vaginal dryness or urinary symptoms.

Hormone replacement therapy is appropriate as a first line therapy only if you become post-menopausal before the age of 45.[7]

Although specific brands and types of hormones may produce different benefits and risks, it's reasonable to generalize the information to all similar products unless there is evidence to the contrary.

The primary purpose of progesterone is to prevent uterine cancer if you have your uterus.

Do not start using estrogen plus progesterone after age 65 for the primary purpose of preventing dementia or treating Alzheimer's disease.[8]

I would imagine that these new guidelines make sense to you now. Pay particular attention to the ones which hold the most weight for you. If I had to summarize all of these findings from the WHI study, and give you my simplistic version, I'd sum it up like this: For women who begin hormone therapy (estrogen and progesterone/HRT or estrogen alone/ERT) for menopause in peri- or early post-menopause, the benefits outweigh the risks early on for the vast majority. With time, the risks may outweigh the benefits for some women, mostly due to the aging process.

Hopefully, you now have a greater understanding of all the factors that intertwine to bring about media reports of research studies. Like everything else in medicine and in life, it's all a balancing act. Take the time to weigh all the factors and apply them to your unique situation. It will give you peace of mind and good quality of life…now and later.

WORKSHEET TIMEOUT:
Answer question # 11 on your worksheet.
Circle all the terms which describe your body type and fill in the blanks.

Answer question # 12.
Circle all the terms which describe your diet.

Answer question # 13.
Fill in the blanks and circle the terms which describe your lifestyle.

AND FINALLY,
Re-answer questions # 14 and # 15.
How do your current choices compare with the ones you chose before?

YOUR BALANCING ACT:

On the last page of your worksheet, use the answers from all the previous worksheet questions to weigh and balance all your positives and negatives. List all the factors that you view as an advantage under the positive column, and all the factors that you view as a disadvantage under the negative column. Some of your positives and negatives may be universal to all women. Some of them may be personal to you.

For example: A personal history of breast cancer may be a negative for any woman, whereas absence of a uterus may be viewed as a positive by some and a negative by others.

WHAT ABOUT THE RESEARCH STUDIES?

Use your worksheet to consider options and weigh them according to your personal needs and preferences. You now have the knowledge to do this, and knowledge is power. Remember, your menopause is all about you, and you know yourself better than anyone else does.

All right! Now it's time for you to hand this book to your partner. I've included a chapter for him, too. See, isn't this great? You've probably been telling him for years that it's all about you. Well, now I'm going to tell him for you!

Chapter 35: For the Guys

This final chapter has three parts, serving three purposes. First, it summarizes the fundamental biologic process of menopause, giving you guys just enough to understand what's really going on during menopause, and also serving as a review for the women ("Menopause in a Flash"). Secondly, it explains the ways in which the male manifests the effects of aging ("Male Menopause"). Lastly, it guides you guys in how to be supportive for the menopausal women in your life, whether they be your wife, your girlfriend, your mother, your sister, or your friend ("Men in Support of Menopause"). Hopefully, it'll be just what you guys have been looking for.

Menopause in a Flash

Anatomy

I could have called this section "Menopause in a Nutshell," but since hot flashes are the most recognizable aspect of menopause to most people, "Menopause in a Flash" makes more sense. Let's start with the scientific stuff. This will give you a basic understanding of menopause so that you can put it all in perspective. The parts of the female reproductive system that are involved with menopause are the *ovaries*. That's where a woman's eggs are stored throughout her lifetime. Until menopause begins, the eggs are released from the ovaries, one at a time, on a monthly basis. That's what produces a woman's cycles, as evidenced by her monthly periods.

Estrogen

Estrogen is the hormone that fuels a woman's cycles. Without it, the process of egg release stops. And that's exactly what happens during menopause. Now, it might be more efficient for the cycles to stop suddenly, as if a switch were turned off, but that's not how Mother Nature designed things. Instead, menopause is a *process*. That means that it takes place over time, slowly and gradually, unless it results from removal of the ovaries during surgery, or damage to the ovaries from radiation therapy or chemotherapy.

Just as it takes years to complete puberty and adolescence, the same is true for menopause. Think about your own puberty. Was it fun? Was it instantaneous? Was it easy? For most individuals, the answer to all three questions is a resounding, "No," regardless of whether you're male or female. Well, menopause is, in essence, puberty in reverse. For females, puberty marks the beginning of their reproductive years, and menopause marks the end of their reproductive years. So, it makes sense that they'd resemble one another.

Phases of Menopause

There are three phases of menopause. They represent the time frames before (pre-menopause), during (peri-menopause), and after (post-menopause) the transition into menopause. *Pre*-menopause is the time before any of this transition begins. Periods are still monthly and everything seems routine. *Peri*-menopause is the time during the transition when all of these changes occur. It can last months or years. It's the phase that resembles puberty and adolescence, with physical and emotional changes that are blatantly obvious. *Post*-menopause is when the transition is complete. Things settle down. Some of the changes that took place during the transition are here to stay. Others have resolved spontaneously.

When you think about it, Mother Nature is responsible for many things in life, some of which are magnificent. However, there are things about Mother Nature's design that you may find a little flawed. Nonetheless, they're normal and natural. So, don't try to fix them!

For the Guys

Accept them as they are, and deal with them in the most positive way possible. Menopause is one of those things.

Signs and Symptoms of Menopause

Reflecting back on puberty and adolescence in both males and females, the ultimate purpose of the entire process was simply to convert the non-reproductive body into one that has the potential for reproduction. So, why all the acne, mood swings, irritability, feelings of confusion, and behavioral issues that accompany the process? Aren't the physical changes enough?

Applying the same analysis to menopause, not only does the female body stop producing eggs and estrogen, it also endures a multitude of other new features. The list seems endless and includes the following:

1. Periods that become farther apart, rather than monthly
2. Hot flashes
3. Night sweats
4. Insomnia
5. Fatigue
6. Forgetfulness
7. Mood swings
8. Irritability
9. Depression
10. Cravings for sweets, carbohydrates, alcohol
11. Breast pain
12. Joint stiffness and joint pain
13. Dry skin
14. Hair loss on the scalp
15. Hair growth in undesirable locations
16. Dryness of the vagina
17. Urinary problems, like infections and leaking urine
18. Weight gain
19. Decreased sex drive or increased sex drive
20. Acne
21. Headaches

Menopause

Now, as you look at that list, there are some items which are similar to puberty and adolescence:

1. Mood swings
2. Irritability
3. Depression
4. Cravings for sweets and carbohydrates
5. Weight gain
6. Acne
7. Increased sex drive
8. Headaches

Some resemble pregnancy:

1. Hot flashes
2. Night sweats
3. Insomnia
4. Fatigue
5. Mood swings
6. Irritability
7. Cravings for various foods
8. Breast pain
9. Urinary leakage
10. Weight gain

Some resemble aging:

1. Less frequent periods
2. Insomnia
3. Fatigue
4. Forgetfulness
5. Joint stiffness and joint pain
6. Dry skin
7. Hair loss on the scalp
8. Hair growth in undesirable locations
9. Dryness of the vagina
10. Urinary infections and leakage
11. Weight gain
12. Decreased sex drive

And, alas! It appears that all the symptoms of menopause are accounted for when you examine them in the context of adolescence, pregnancy, and aging.

So, you might say that menopause represents a time when there's a combination of hormonal and aging processes. That's a lot to handle all at once! Wouldn't you agree? That's why menopause seems so drastic. The more severe the symptoms of menopause, and the longer the transition drags on, the more difficult it can be for everyone. That includes the woman herself, her partner, family members, friends, and co-workers.

Male Menopause

Male Reproduction

Males have neither the pleasure nor the pain of a menopausal experience similar to that of females. That makes sense, because males don't perform the reproductive process of pregnancy and childbearing. Additionally, the reproductive phase of a man's life is indefinite. A male can father children at any age. He continues to produce sperm his entire adult life. There's no need to reverse the process of puberty in the male.

The Male Aging Process

Nonetheless, males do age. You do so gradually, over many decades, rather than over a few months or years.[1] You become forgetful with age; you experience stiffness and joint pain; your skin becomes dry and wrinkled; you have thinning of your hair throughout your adult life; you notice hair growth in undesirable locations, such as your ears and nose; you develop urinary problems, such as dribbling and frequent urination; you gain weight; and your sex drive decreases.

In the male, these changes are so gradual that they aren't as noticeable as the more sudden changes that occur during menopause in a female. I can't say that it's better or worse that way. It's just the way it is. You can't change it or fix it. There are management options for these changes in the male, though. And it probably isn't surprising that many of the management choices I present for female menopause are beneficial for males, also. This may induce you to read the chapters that precede this one. You'll be glad you did.

Testosterone

Men lose testosterone, just as women lose estrogen. The difference is that estrogen loss is more sudden, and therefore more noticeable, while testosterone loss is slow and gradual. The male peaks sexually at age 18, and it's downhill from there. By the time a man reaches middle age, he thinks about sex much less often than he did as a teen. The thoughts are much less overwhelming and vivid, and much easier to control. The erection of a middle-aged man is smaller, softer, and less instantaneous than it was in his teenage years. His ejaculation is also less forceful.

Emotional and Psychological Issues

Many men manifest the male version of menopause by attempting to prove to themselves and others that they're still virile. You've probably seen this behavior in someone you know, or maybe even someone you've seen in the mirror. He's a guy in his 40s or 50s, who divorces his middle-aged wife, marries a woman half his age, buys a sports car, and has a second family. That's a lot of transitioning to fix something he can't change. Please realize that virility is not the measure of your worthiness. Also realize that there are so many things that are more important than virility. However, maintenance of virility is a huge priority for many aging men. That's why drugs like Viagra, Cialis, and Levitra are so popular.

Male Mid-life Crisis

Most men experience a male form of menopause that focuses mostly on the realization that they're entering the second half of their lives. Many of the hopes and dreams they entertained in their youth may be unattainable.[1] We sometimes call this a mid-life crisis. It implies that a man reflects on the course his life has taken and evaluates the things that he has and hasn't accomplished. Some men have difficulty coming to terms with their failures. For some men, this is a time to make changes which accommodate those feelings of failure. So, job changes, new cars, sabbaticals, and new hobbies are common undertakings.

Men In Support of Menopause

Flashback

If you've had a female partner during your adult life, you've already played the role of a support system for the hormonal ups and downs of womanhood. You may have dealt with the emotional episodes inherent to PMS (premenstrual syndrome) in the days preceding your partner's monthly period. That's a time when your partner's personality seemed to change. She became short-tempered, irritable, and emotional. You may have endured many months of pregnancy, during which your partner experienced obvious physical changes in her body, as well as emotional frailties that you found odd or difficult to understand. Your sex life probably took a nose dive during and/or after the pregnancy. If you have children, maybe you're familiar with the adolescent years and all the surprises they bring, many of which are quite challenging. Maybe you remember your own adolescence. Did you give your parents a hard time? Were you unreasonable some of the time?

Menopause is just another step on this ladder of hormonal changes. It isn't worse than any of the others. Although it doesn't result in a cute little bundle of joy (as with pregnancy), and it doesn't bring you to the point of sending your prodigy off into adulthood (as with adolescence), it does bring you much closer to your partner. That is, if you choose to be loving and supportive.

Whose Role is More Difficult?

Sometimes, when a man accompanies a woman through the menopausal experience, *he* may actually find it more difficult than *she* does. During the time I was writing this book, my husband George and I went to Sunday brunch with another couple. I was meeting them for the first time. In the process of getting acquainted with one another, I told them that I was writing a book on menopause. Their reactions were very interesting. The woman was nonchalant, and said her menopause had been no big deal. Her husband, on the other hand, rolled his eyes, gestured with his hands, and slumped over as he described it as the most difficult thing he'd ever experienced. We talked about a number of things in that visit, including George's adolescent daughter, work, travel, and their new grandchildren. Our male friend did not react emotionally to these other things even remotely as much as he had to the mention of his wife's menopause. He had definitely felt more of an impact from it than she had.

Again, it's a lot like puberty and adolescence. It's sometimes harder on the parents than it is on the child. In fact, you might find it easier to deal with menopause if you just pretend that your partner is a 15 year old, confused, irritable, frustrated teenager in a grown woman's body. Treat her with the same patience, tolerance, support, and dedication, and you'll get through it all just fine.

Knowledge and Preparation

I firmly believe that there's a strong link between how much we know about something and how strongly it affects us. When it comes to our bodies and our health, our greatest fear is the unknown. If you're prepared for something, and have a basic knowledge about it, you avoid the surprises, the fear, and the angst that are present when you're clueless about it. That's why we prepare our daughters for their periods. If we didn't, they'd think they were dying at the first sight of vaginal bleeding.

Menopause deserves the same attention and preparation as periods, pregnancy, and aging. The features that are visibly obvious aren't surprising. Those that aren't cause tremendous anxiety if they come as a surprise. Menopause has plenty of both.

I'm sure you know that pregnant women have cravings for strange foods, so when your pregnant wife craved odd foods in even odder combinations, you just got them for her. Maybe you had to go out in the wee hours of the morning to buy ice cream and pickles. You probably did so with a little chuckle, even though it was a bit inconvenient. It's unfortunate that you may not be as prepared for her hot flashes. If she demands that you lower the thermostat to 60 degrees Fahrenheit, you may argue with her and tell her she's crazy rather than recognizing that this is a common sign of menopause. You may tend to disagree with her endlessly over things that you would have taken in stride during the irritable moods of pregnancy. You may see her depression as inappropriate, whereas you supported your teenagers with their depression during puberty and adolescence. But, now that you've read this chapter, you'll know better, and you'll respond more appropriately to these things. You'll be a better partner.

Most men receive very little education about female issues. In fact, most men receive little education about *male* issues. That's because women usually play the role of the health consumer in most families. The majority of men don't even maintain annual visits to a physician in their young adult years. Think about it. Most females have an annual visit to the gynecologist beginning in their early 20s. It becomes a habit, and we go to the doctor for a "well woman" exam yearly. How many men do you know who do the same thing? Most men don't visit a doctor for anything other than serious problems from their early 20s until their early 50s. If you're an exception, congratulations. If so, you probably know a lot more about the human body than most men.

Sex and Romance

While it may not make much sense to *you*, romance comes in many forms. If you're like most men, you envision menopause as a time when your sex life with your partner will either fade significantly or disappear altogether. Well, this really isn't the case. Being supportive and understanding of your partner's menopausal experience may be the most romantic thing you ever do for her. She certainly will remember your kindness, and you'll feel good about it, too. There are plenty of myths about sex being left behind as you age. Fortunately, they're just myths. For some people, sex becomes *more* frequent and *more* satisfying as they age because they're free from worry about pregnancy, privacy, and work schedules.

Show your partner that you think she's sexy. Buy her some sexy lingerie and tell her that you just know she'll look great in it. Telling her that you find her appealing is important, because menopause is a time when she may not feel very sexy. Give her reassurance that she still is. She values *your* opinion more than anyone else's.

Of course, communication with your menopausal partner goes a long way, but some people (especially men) aren't great communicators. It's really important to let your partner know that you want to support her. If you make her aware of your desire to understand what she's experiencing, she'll be much more likely to open up and share her feelings with you. She doesn't expect you to fix anything. Just listen and be supportive. I'm sure you had practice with this if you've endured a pregnancy or adolescence with anyone. In any case, the last thing she needs is for you to create a situation in which she has to deal with relationship issues in addition to menopause issues. Just be selfless for the time being and bend a little. I'm not saying that your partner should blame everything on her hormones (or lack thereof). But, as you can see, menopause isn't a walk in the park.

No Two Women Are Alike

I know you probably think all women are alike. At least that's how a lot of men perceive the opposite sex. And, I might add that many women think all men are alike, too. As surprising as it may seem to you, though, no two women are alike, especially when it comes to menopause. It's relatively easy for some, and incredibly difficult for others. This is no time to compare your partner's menopause to someone else's. Know the basics of what menopause is, and be familiar with the possible signs and symptoms that I enumerated above. Beyond that, be a good listener so that you know how the process of menopause is for your own partner. *Her* experience is the only one that matters.

Options Galore

The good news is that, unlike puberty, adolescence, and pregnancy, there are many options available to manage the unwelcome aspects of menopause. That's what this book is all about. Your menopausal partner has the choice of pursuing various options to make the process smoother. There are many categories, including dietary choices, lifestyle changes, vitamins and minerals, botanicals and herbs, hormonal medications, and non-hormonal medications.

For the Guys

While it's good for you to be aware of these options, it's not appropriate for you to impose your preferences on your partner. *Your way of managing her menopause may not be her way of managing her menopause.* I know I just told you that your opinion matters. But I was talking about your opinion of how sexy she is. I wasn't talking about her options for managing *her* menopause. When it comes to that, *her opinion is the only one that matters.* This is a time of empowerment for her. She knows herself better than anyone else does, even you. She's an adult. She has needs and preferences that she'll want to take into account in making her choices. She may have to try many different options to discover what's best for her. She may change her mind many times. As she ages, her needs may change, and she may change her management technique accordingly.

This is a time for you to support her choices. She's not trying to "fix" something. Nothing is wrong. This is Mother Nature at work, along with some modifications according to your partner's choices. Let her experiment if she wishes. She's trying to optimize things for both of you. A little understanding on your part will make all the difference.

If you remember nothing else, remember this: When it comes to menopause, *it's all about her!*

REFERENCES

Cited References by Chapter:

Chapter 1:
An Introduction to the Mystery of Menopause

1. Goldstein, I., et al. (2005). Managing the Urogenital Effects of Estrogen Deprivation: Female Health and Sexual Dysfunction. *Contemporary OB/GYN*, 1-10.
2. Northrup, C. (1997). Menopause. *Primary Care,* 24 (4), 921-948.
3. Taylor, M. (1997). Alternatives to Conventional Hormone Replacement Therapy. *Comprehensive Therapeutics,* 23 (8), 514-532.
4. ACOG Practice Bulletin, (2001). Use of Botanicals for Management of Menopausal Symptoms. *Obstetrics & Gynecology,* 28.

Chapter 2:
An Orientation to the Parts and Processes of Menopause

1. Northrup, C. (1997). Menopause. *Primary Care,* 24 (4), 921-948.

Chapter 3:
Terminology: The Language of Menopause

1. Carey, C. (Sept. 2004). Sexual Dysfunction: The Challenge of Treatment. *OBG Management,* 69-76.
2. Northrup, C. (2001) *The Wisdom of Menopause,* New York: Bantam Dell.

Chapter 4:
"How Will I Know When Menopause Comes a Knockin'?"

1. Northrup, C. (2001) *The Wisdom of Menopause*, New York: Bantam Dell.
2. Henrich, J., et al. (2006) FSH Alone Can't Diagnose Menopause. *Contemporary OB/GYN*, 17.

Chapter 5:
The Balancing Act

None

Chapter 6:
Options: Medical, Non-medical, and Everything in Between

1. ACOG Practice Bulletin, (June 2001). Use of Botanicals for Management of Menopausal Symptoms. *Obstetrics & Gynecology*, 28.
2. Taylor, M. (1997). Alternatives to Conventional Hormone Replacement Therapy. *Comprehensive Therapeutics*, 23 (8), 514-532.
3. Watt, P., et al. (2003). A Holistic Programmatic Approach to Natural Hormone Replacement. *Family Community Health*, 26 (1), 53-63.
4. Farrell, E. (2003). Medical Choices for Management of Menopause. *Best Practices: Residency in Clinical Endocrinologic Metabolism*, 17 (1), 1-16.
5. Taylor, M. (2003). Alternatives to HRT: AN Evidence-Based Review. *International Journal of Fertility in Women's Medicine*, 48 (2), 64-68.
6. Altman, A. (2007). Bioidentical Hormones: What's Fact and What's Fable? *SRM*, 5 (1), 13-16.
7. Utian, W. (2005). Bio-identical Hormones: Separating Science From Marketing. *The Female Patient*, 30, 21-22.
8. Lowes, R. (Sept. 2004). A Field Guide to Alternative Healers. *Medical Economics*, 21-25.
9. Gass, M., et al. (2001). Alternatives for Women Through Menopause. *American Journal of Obstetrics & Gynecology*, 185 (2), S47-S55.
10. Warren, M., et al. (2002). Use of Alternative Therapies in Menopause. *Best Practice & Research in Clinical Obstetrics & Gynecology*, 16 (3), 411-448.

References

11. Kass-Annese, B. (2000). Alternative Therapies for Menopause. *Clinical Obstetrics and Gynecology*, 43 (1), 162-183.
12. Israel, D., et al. (1997). Herbal Therapies for Perimenopausal and Menopausal Complaints. *Pharmacotherapy*, 17 (5), 970-984.

Chapter 7:
Categories of Hormones and Their Sources

1. Fitzpatrick, L. (2003). Alternatives to Estrogen. *The Medical Clinics of North America*, 1091 – 1113.
2. Warren, M., et al. (2002). Use of Alternative Therapies in Menopause. *Best Practice & Research in Clinical Obstetrics & Gynecology*, 16 (3), 411-448.
3. Russell, MD, Lori et al (Oct 2002) Phytoestrogens: A Viable Option? *American Journal Medical Society* 324 (4), 185-188.
4. ACOG Practice Bulletin, (June 2001). Use of Botanicals for Management of Menopausal Symptoms. *Obstetrics & Gynecology*, 28.
5. Northrup, C. (2001) *The Wisdom of Menopause*, New York: Bantam Dell.
6. Mahady, G., et al. (2002). Black Cohosh: An Alternative Therapy for Menopause? *Nutrition in Clinical Care*, 5 (6), 283-289.
7. Fedutes, B., et al. (2004). A Targeted Approach to Musculoskeletal Pain, Part 2: Management and Pharmacotherapy. *The Female Patient*, 29, 37-48.
8. Taylor, M. (1997). Alternatives to Conventional Hormone Replacement Therapy. *Comprehensive Therapeutics*, 23 (8), 514-532.
9. Watt, P., et al. (2003). A Holistic Programmatic Approach to Natural Hormone Replacement. *Family Community Health*, 26 (1), 53-63.
10. Warren, M., et al. (2004). Custom-Compounded Hormone Therapy: Is There Science to Support the Claims? *Council on Hormone Education*, 2 (4), 3-8.
11. Lewis, V. (2004). New Hormone Therapy Formulations and Routes of Delivery: Meeting the Needs of Your Patients in the Post-WHI World. *OBG Management Supplement*, 11-17.
12. Langer, R. (Nov. 2004). Strategies to Optimize the Safety of Hormone Therapy. *OBG Management*, 10-15.

13. Barbieri, R. (Sept. 2003). Latest Data on HT Side Effects: Further Reinforcement, Some Reassurance. *OBG Management,* 8- 9.
14. Archer, D. (Sept. 2004). Estradiol Gel: A New Option in Hormone Replacement Therapy. *OBG Management,* 46-66.
15. Davidson, Sonia & Davis, Susan R. (Jan/Feb 2002) Hormone Replacement Therapy: Current Controversies, *Journal of the American Pharmacologic Association* Vol 42, No 1, pp 122 - 134
16. Farrell, E. (2003). Medical Choices for Management of Menopause. *Best Practices: Residency in Clinical Endocrinologic Metabolism,* 17 (1), 1-16.
17. Hudson, T. (2001). Natural Progesterone: Clinical Indications in Women's Health. *The Female Patient,* (26), 43-48.
18. Sulak, P. (May 2004) Selecting the Option That Provides Maximum Health Benefits and Alleviates Menstrual Symptoms for the Perimenopausal Patient. *OBG Management,* 1-5.
19. Utian, W. (May 2004). Update on Menopause: An Expert's Insight on Pivotal Studies. *OBG Management,* 60-68.
20. Taylor, M. (2003). Alternatives to HRT: AN Evidence-Based Review. *International Journal of Fertility in Women's Medicine,* 48 (2), 64-68.
21. Lowes, R. (Sept. 2004). A Field Guide to Alternative Healers. *Medical Economics,* 21-25.
22. (2004). *PDR for Herbal Medicines, Third Edition* (Thompson) Montvale, NJ.
23. (2001). *PDR for Nutritional Supplements* (Thompson) Montvale, NJ.
24. (2005). *Physicians' Desk Reference, 59th Edition* (Thompson) Montvale, NJ.
25. Utian, W. (2005). Bio-identical Hormones: Separating Science From Marketing. *The Female Patient,* 30, 21-22.

Chapter 8:
Dosage Dictionary

1. Tapson, E. (2005). A Dictionary of Units. *Internet.*
2. Metric Conversion Chart. *Internet.*
3. (2005). Metric System Units. *Webdocs.*
4. (2005). Metric System. *Internet.*
5. (2005). Internet French Property Co.
6. (2005) Metric System Table. *Internet.*
7. Simetric.co.uk. *Internet.*

References

8. (2005) Infophase. *Internet.*
9. ASDOT Metric Conversion Factors. *Internet.*
10. Metric Prefixes. *Internet.*

Chapter 9:
Periods With a Personality Change

None

Chapter 10:
Hot Flashes

1. Dormire, S. (2003). What We Know About Managing Menopausal Hot Flashes: Navigating Without a Compass. *Journal of Obstetric & Gynecologic Neonatal Nursing,* 32 (4), 455-464.
2. Pradhan, A., et al. (2004). Today's Therapeutic Options for Hot Flashes. *Women's Health, Gynecology Edition,* 4 (2), 81-86
3. Kaunitz, A. (2003). Treating Hot Flashes: Options to Estrogen. *The Female Patient,* 28, 52-54.
4. Kass-Annese, B. (2000). Alternative Therapies for Menopause. *Clinical Obstetrics and Gynecology,* 43 (1), 162-183.
5. Warren, M., et al. (2002). Use of Alternative Therapies in Menopause. *Best Practice & Research in Clinical Obstetrics & Gynecology,* 16 (3), 411-448.
6. Murray, M. (2004). Black Cohosh: Nature's Best Solution for Hot Flashes. *Alive,* 48-51.
7. Taylor, M. (1997). Alternatives to Conventional Hormone Replacement Therapy. *Comprehensive Therapeutics,* 23 (8), 514-532.
8. McSweeney, J. et al., (Feb. 2005). Heart Disease in Women: Knowing the Risks, Recognizing the Symptoms. *The Female Patient,* 5-7.
9. Gass, M., et al. (2003). Amended Report From the NAMS Advisory Panel on Postmenopausal Hormone Therapy. *Menopause Management,* 12 (1), 10-18.
10. ACOG Practice Bulletin, (June 2001). Use of Botanicals for Management of Menopausal Symptoms. *Obstetrics & Gynecology,* 28.

Chapter 11:
Night Sweats

1. Gass, M., et al. (2003). Amended Report From the NAMS Advisory Panel on Postmenopausal Hormone Therapy. Menopause Management, 12 (1), 10-18.
2. McSweeney, J. et al., (Feb. 2005). Heart Disease in Women: Knowing the Risks, Recognizing the Symptoms. The Female Patient, 5-7.
3. Kaunitz, A. (2003). Treating Hot Flashes: Options to Estrogen. The Female Patient, 28, 52-54.
4. Pradhan, A., et al. (2004). Today's Therapeutic Options for Hot Flashes. Women's Health, Gynecology Edition, 4 (2), 81-86
5. Murray, M. (2004). Black Cohosh: Nature's Best Solution for Hot Flashes. Alive, 48-51.
6. Dormire, S. (2003). What We Know About Managing Menopausal Hot Flashes: Navigating Without a Compass. Journal of Obstetric & Gynecologic Neonatal Nursing, 32 (4), 455-464.
7. ACOG Practice Bulletin, (June 2001). Use of Botanicals for Management of Menopausal Symptoms. Obstetrics & Gynecology, 28.
8. Warren, M., et al. (2002). Use of Alternative Therapies in Menopause. Best Practice & Research in Clinical Obstetrics & Gynecology, 16 (3), 411-448.

Chapter 12:
Insomnia

1. Vankireddy, H. et al. (2004). Insomnia. *The Female Patient*, 29, 14-22.
2. Miller, E. (2004). Women and Insomnia. *Clinical Cornerstone*, 6, S6-S18
3. Krystal, A. (2004). Depression and Insomnia in Women. *Clinical Cornerstone*, 6, S19-28.
4. Israel, D., et al. (1997). Herbal Therapies for Perimenopausal and Menopausal Complaints. *Pharmacotherapy*, 17 (5), 970-984.

REFERENCES

Chapter 13:
Fatigue

1. Miller, E. (2004). Women and Insomnia. *Clinical Cornerstone*, 6, S6-S18
2. Israel, Pharm D, Debra & Youngkin, PhD, RNC, Ellis Quinn, (Sept/Oct 1997) Herbal Therapies for Perimenopausal and Menopausal Complaints, *Pharmacotherapy* 17 (5), 970-984
3. Vankireddy, H. et al. (2004). Insomnia. *The Female Patient*, 29, 14-22.

Chapter 14:
Forgetfulness

1. (2004). *PDR for Herbal Medicines, Third Edition* (Thompson) Montvale, NJ.
2. Healy, B. (2002, Nov. 18). The Mysteries of Menopause. *U.S. News & World Report*, 39-71.

Chapter 15:
Mood Swings, Irritability, and Depression

1. Brizendine, L. (Aug. 2004). Managing Menopause-Related Depression and Low Libido. *OBG Management*, 29-42.
2. Krystal, A. (2004). Depression and Insomnia in Women. *Clinical Cornerstone*, 6, S19-28.
3. (2001). *PDR for Nutritional Supplements* (Thompson) Montvale, NJ.
4. (2004). *PDR for Herbal Medicines, Third Edition* (Thompson) Montvale, NJ.
5. Gass, M., et al. (2001). Alternatives for Women Through Menopause. *American Journal of Obstetrics & Gynecology*, 185 (2), S47-S55.
6. ACOG Practice Bulletin, (June 2001). Use of Botanicals for Management of Menopausal Symptoms. *Obstetrics & Gynecology*, 28.
7. Hendrick, V. (2004). Effects of Hormone Supplementation on Mood in Women. *The Female Patient*, 29, 13-15.
8. Allison-Ottey, S. (2004). Depression in the Female Geriatric Patient. *The Female Patient*, 29, 19-22.

9. Taylor, M. (1997). Alternatives to Conventional Hormone Replacement Therapy. *Comprehensive Therapeutics,* 23 (8), 514-532.

Chapter 16:
Cravings for Sweets, Carbohydrates, Alcohol

None

Chapter 17:
Breast Pain

None

Chapter 18:
Joint Stiffness and Joint Pain

1. (2004). *PDR for Herbal Medicines, Third Edition* (Thompson) Montvale, NJ.
2. (2001). *PDR for Nutritional Supplements* (Thompson) Montvale, NJ.
3. Fedutes, B., et al. (2004). A Targeted Approach to Musculoskeletal Pain, Part 2: Management and Pharmacotherapy. *The Female Patient,* 29, 37-48.

Chapter 19:
Dry Skin

None

Chapter 20:
Hair Loss on the Scalp

1. Northrup, C. (2001) *The Wisdom of Menopause,* New York: Bantam Dell.

Chapter 21:
Hair Growth in Undesirable Locations

1. (2001) PDR for Nutritional Supplements (Thompson) Montvale, NJ

REFERENCES

Chapter 22:
Vaginal Dryness

1. Sand, P., et al. (1990). Nonsurgical Treatment of Detrusor Overactivity in Postmenopausal Women. *Reproductive Medicine,* 35 (8), 758-764.
2. Willhite, L., et al. (2001). Urogenital Atrophy: Prevention and Treatment. *Pharm,* 21 (4), 464-480.
3. Northrup, C. (1997). Menopause. *Primary Care,* 24 (4), 921-948.

Chapter 23:
Urinary Problems

1. Willhite, L., et al. (2001). Urogenital Atrophy: Prevention and Treatment. *Pharm,* 21 (4), 464-480.
2. Diwadkar, G., et al. (2006). Alternative Approaches to Overactive Bladder. *Contemporary OB/GYN,* 22-32.
3. Sand, P., et al. (1990). Nonsurgical Treatment of Detrusor Overactivity in Postmenopausal Women. *Reproductive Medicine,* 35 (8), 758-764.
4. Northrup, C. (2001) *The Wisdom of Menopause,* New York: Bantam Dell.

Chapter 24:
Weight Gain

None

Chapter 25:
Decreased or Increased Sex Drive

1. Wingert, P., et al. (2007, Jan.15). The New Prime Time. *Newsweek,* 38-60 (cover story).
2. Brizendine, L. (Aug. 2004). Managing Menopause-Related Depression and Low Libido. *OBG Management,* 29-42.
3. Chu, M. (May 2004). Formulations and Use of Androgens in Women. *OBG Management,* 2-5.

4. Watt, P., et al. (2003). A Holistic Programmatic Approach to Natural Hormone Replacement. *Family Community Health*, 26 (1), 53-63.
5. Northrup, C. (2001) *The Wisdom of Menopause*, New York: Bantam Dell.

Chapter 26:
Acne

1. Northrup, C. (2001) *The Wisdom of Menopause*, New York: Bantam Dell.

Chapter 27:
Headaches

1. Brandes, J. (2007) Management Strategies for Migraine in Women. *The Female Patient: Migraine Consult Collection*, 26-30.

Chapter 28:
Heart Attack

1. Mugford, J., et al. (2007). Heart Disease in Women. *The Female Patient*, 32, 39-44.
2. Kreisberg, R. (Sept/Oct 2002). HRT and Cardioprotection: Past, Present and Future. *Menopause Management*, 16-20.
3. McSweeney, J. et al., (Feb. 2005). Heart Disease in Women: Knowing the Risks, Recognizing the Symptoms. *The Female Patient*, 5-7.
4. (Jan/Feb 2003). Roundtable: Suspected CHD Risk. *Menopause Management*, 19-24.
5. Farrell, E. (2003). Medical Choices for Management of Menopause. *Best Practices: Residency in Clinical Endocrinologic Metabolism*, 17 (1), 1-16.
6. Hudson, T. (2005). Hyperlipidemia: Nutritional, Botanical, and Life-style Influences. *The Female Patient*, 30, 42-46.
7. Gass, M., et al. (2003). Amended Report From the NAMS Advisory Panel on Postmenopausal Hormone Therapy. *Menopause Management*, 12 (1), 10-18.

References

8. (2001). *PDR for Nutritional Supplements* (Thompson) Montvale, NJ.
9. Kass-Annese, B. (2000). Alternative Therapies for Menopause. *Clinical Obstetrics and Gynecology,* 43 (1), 162-183.
10. Simon, J. (2004). Assessing Risks and Benefits of Hormone Therapy for the Individual Patient: Breast Cancer, Osteoporosis, and Cognitive Decline. *OBG Management,* 7-10.
11. Speroff, L. (2007) Premenopausal Atherosclerosis. *Contemporary OB/GYN,* 84-49.
12. Rossouw, J., et al. (2007). Postmenopausal Hormone Therapy and Risk of Cardiovascular Disease by Age and Years Since Menopause. *JAMA,* 297, 1465-1477.
13. Phillips, O. (2004). WHI In Perspective – Focus on Coronary Heart Disease. *The Forum,* 2 (1), 15-18.
14. Zacur, H. et al., (July 2004). Estrogen Therapy: Is Oral Superior to Transdermal for Endothelial Function? *OBG Management,* 12-14.

Chapter 29:
Osteoporosis

1. Boyd, A. et al., (2004). Lifetime Approach to Osteoporosis. *The Female Patient,* 29, 23-29.
2. Whyte, J. (2003). Osteoporosis: Diagnosis and Treatment. *CME Resource,* 118(10), 27-46.
3. Northrup, C. (2001) *The Wisdom of Menopause,* New York: Bantam Dell.
4. Gallagher, J. (2004). Clinical Significance and Management of Accelerated Bone Loss Around the Time of the Menopause. *CME Council on Hormone Education,* 2 (2), 3-8.
5. Fitzpatrick, L. (Feb. 2004). Estrogen and Bone Health. *The Female Patient,* 4 – 9.
6. Lewiecki, E. (2004). Bone Density Testing in the Management of Postmenopausal Osteoporosis. *Women's Health,* 4 (4), 183-193.
7. Kagan, L. (June 2005). Osteoporotic Fractures and Falls: Reducing the Risk. *The Female Patient,* 7-8.
8. Audreola, N. (June 2005). Exercise: An Elixir for Osteoporosis Prevention. *The Female Patient,* 9-10.
9. Hudson, T. (2004). Nutritional Influences on Osteoporosis. *The Female Patient,* 29, 35-42.

10. Warren, M., et al. (2002). Use of Alternative Therapies in Menopause. *Best Practice & Research in Clinical Obstetrics & Gynecology,* 16 (3), 411-448.
11. Taylor, M. (1997). Alternatives to Conventional Hormone Replacement Therapy. *Comprehensive Therapeutics,* 23 (8), 514-532.
12. Kass-Annese, B. (2000). Alternative Therapies for Menopause. *Clinical Obstetrics and Gynecology,* 43 (1), 162-183.
13. Gass, M., et al. (2003). Amended Report From the NAMS Advisory Panel on Postmenopausal Hormone Therapy. *Menopause Management,* 12 (1), 10-18.
14. Phillils, O. (Nov. 2002). SERMs in Preventive Healthcare. *The Female Patient,* S1-10.

Chapter 30:
Breast Cancer

1. Fodera, S. (Sept. 2004). The Use of Endocrine Therapy in the Treatment and Prevention of Breast Cancer. *CME,* 1-27.
2. Altman, A. (2007). Bioidentical Hormones: What's Fact and What's Fable? *SRM,* 5 (1), 13-16.
3. Barbieri, R. (Sept. 2003). Latest Data on HT Side Effects: Further Reinforcement, Some Reassurance. *OBG Management,* 8-9.

Chapter 31:
Uterine Cancer

1. Thorneycroft, I. (Feb. 2004). Unopposed Estrogen and Cancer. *The Female Patient,* 19-26.

Chapter 32:
Ovarian Cancer

1. Goff, B. (2005). Screening and Early Diagnosis of Ovarian Cancer: What Primary Care Clinicians Can Do. *Women's Health,* 5, 194-206.
2. Goff, B. (2004). Ovarian Cancer: Not a Silent Disease. *Women's*

References

Health Gynecology Edition, 4 (4), 163.
3. Muto M. (Oct. 2004). Ovarian Cancer: Identifying and Managing High-risk Patients. *OBG Management,* 60-69.

Chapter 33:
Alzheimer's Disease

1. Northrup, C. (1997). Menopause. *Primary Care,* 24 (4), 921-948.
2. Jones, K. (2000). Menopause and Cognitive Function: Estrogens and Alternative Therapies. *Clinical Obstetrics and Gynecology,* 43 (1), 198-206.
3. Davidson, S., et al. (Jan/Feb 2002) Hormone Replacement Therapy: Current Controversies, *Journal of the American Pharmacologic Association* 42 (1), 122-134.
4. Henderson, V. (Jan 2005) Hormone Therapy and Alzheimer Disease: An Evidence-Based Approach to Clinical Management *The Female Patient* 30, 9-14.
5. Greene, R. (Nov. 2004). Selecting an Agent For Hormone Therapy: What to Consider. *OBG Management,* 5-9.

Chapter 34:
"What About the Research Studies?"

1. Healy, B. (2002, Nov. 18). The Mysteries of Menopause. *U.S. News & World Report,* 39-71.
2. Barbieri, R. (Dec. 2003). Hormone Therapy: For the Right Patients, Benefits Outweigh Risks. *OBG Management,* 8-13.
3. Hendrix, S. (Nov. 2002). Implications of the Women's Health Initiative. *The Female Patient,* 4-8.
4. Thacker, H. (2005). Menopausal Hormone Therapy: The Symptomatic Patient. *The Female Patient,* 30, 16-21.
5. Thorneycroft, I. (2004). WHI in Perspective: Focus on the Estrogen –Only Study. *The Forum,* 2 (2), 4-6.
6. Chervenak, J., et al. (June 2005). Hormone Therapy for the Postmenopausal Woman: Balancing Benefits Versus Risks. *The Female Patient,* 1-4.
7. Boyd, A.S. & South-Paul, J.E. (2004) Lifetime Approach to

Osteoporosis, *The Female Patient* 29 (Supp), 23-29
8. Utian, W. (2005). Postmenopausal Hormone Therapy: Clarifying the Role. *The Female Patient,* 30, 53-54.
9. (2005). The 2004 NAMS Position Statement on Hormone Therapy. *Women's Health Gynecology Edition,* 5 (1), 26-33.
10. Gass, M., et al. (2003). Amended Report From the NAMS Advisory Panel on Postmenopausal Hormone Therapy. *Menopause Management,* 12 (1), 10-18.
11. Hsia, J., et al. (2004). WHI: What Will the Estrogen Arm Show? *Women's Health Gynecology Edition,* 4, (2), 100.

Chapter 35:
For the Guys

1. Roth, D. (1999). No It's Not Hot In Here, Ant Hill Press, 146-152.

GENERAL REFERENCES

ACOG Practice Bulletin, (June 2001). Use of Botanicals for Management of Menopausal Symptoms. *Obstetrics & Gynecology*, 28.

Albertazzi, P., et al. (2002). The Nature and Utility of the Phytoestrogens: A Review of the Evidence. *Maturitas*, 25 (3), 173-185.

Allison-Ottey, S. (2004). Depression in the Female Geriatric Patient. *The Female Patient*, 29, 19-22.

Altman, A. (2007). Bioidentical Hormones: What's Fact and What's Fable? *SRM*, 5 (1), 13-16.

Amsterdam, A., et al. (2004). Managing Menopause in the Cancer Patient. *The Female Patient*, 29, 46-51.

Archer, D. (Sept. 2004). Estradiol Gel: A New Option in Hormone Replacement Therapy. *OBG Management*, 46-66.

ASDOT Metric Conversion Factors. *Internet*.

Audreola, N. (June 2005). Exercise: An Elixir for Osteoporosis Prevention. *The Female Patient*, 9-10.

Barbieri, R. (Sept. 2003). Latest Data on HT Side Effects: Further Reinforcement, Some Reassurance. *OBG Management*, 8-9.

Barbieri, R. (Dec. 2003). Hormone Therapy: For the Right Patients, Benefits Outweigh Risks. *OBG Management*, 8-13.

Basaria, S., et al. (May 2004). Safety and Adverse Effects of Androgens. *OBG Management*, 18-23.

Baxter-Jones, R. (Feb. 2003.) Preventing Colorectal Cancer: The Role of PCP's in Counseling and Screening. *Menopause Management*, 25-28.

Brandes, J. (2007). Management Strategies for Migraine in Women. *The Female Patient: Migraine Consult Collection*, 26-30.

Brizendine, L. (Aug. 2004). Managing Menopause-Related Depression and Low Libido. *OBG Management*, 29-42.

Boyd, A. et al., (2004). Lifetime Approach to Osteoporosis. *The Female Patient*, 29, 23-29.

Carey, C. (Sept. 2004). Sexual Dysfunction: The Challenge of Treatment. *OBG Management*, 69-76.

Chervenak, J., et al. (June 2005). Hormone Therapy for the Postmenopausal Woman: Balancing Benefits Versus Risks. *The Female Patient*, 1-4.

Chu, M. (May 2004). Formulations and Use of Androgens in Women. *OBG Management*, 2-5.

Davidson, S., et al. (2002). Hormone Replacement Therapy: Current Controversies. *Journal of the American Pharmacologic Association*, 42 (1), 122 – 134.

Diwadkar, G., et al. (2006). Alternative Approaches to Overactive Bladder. *Contemporary OB/GYN*, 22-32.

Dormire, S. (2003). What We Know About Managing Menopausal Hot Flashes: Navigating Without a Compass. *Journal of Obstetric & Gynecologic Neonatal Nursing*, 32 (4), 455-464.

Evans, M., et al. (2005). Management of Post-menopausal Hot Flushes With Venlafaxine Hydrochloride: A Randomized Controlled Trial. *Obstetrics and Gynecology*, 105, 161-166.

Farrell, E. (2003). Medical Choices for Management of Menopause. *Best Practices: Residency in Clinical Endocrinologic Metabolism*, 17 (1), 1-16.

Fedutes, B., et al. (2004). A Targeted Approach to Musculoskeletal Pain, Part 2: Management and Pharmacotherapy. *The Female Patient*, 29, 37-48.

Fitzpatrick, L. (2003). Alternatives to Estrogen. *The Medical Clinics of North America*, 1091 – 1113.

Fitzpatrick, L. (2003). Soy Isoflavones: Hope or Hype? *Maturitas*, 14 (44), S21-29.

Fitzpatrick, L. (Feb. 2004). Estrogen and Bone Health. *The Female Patient*, 4 – 9.

Fodera, S. (Sept. 2004). The Use of Endocrine Therapy in the Treatment and Prevention of Breast Cancer. *CME*, 1-27.

Gallagher, J. (2004). Clinical Significance and Management of Accelerated Bone Loss Around the Time of the Menopause. *CME Council on Hormone Education*, 2 (2), 3-8.

Gass, M., et al. (2001). Alternatives for Women Through Menopause.

References

American Journal of Obstetrics & Gynecology, 185 (2), S47-S55.

Gass, M., et al. (2003). Amended Report From the NAMS Advisory Panel on Postmenopausal Hormone Therapy. *Menopause Management,* 12 (1), 10-18.

Goff, B. (2004). Ovarian Cancer: Not a Silent Disease. *Women's Health Gynecology Edition,* 4 (4), 163.

Goff, B. (2005). Screening and Early Diagnosis of Ovarian Cancer: What Primary Care Clinicians Can Do. *Women's Health,* 5, 194-206.

Goldstein, I., et al. (2005). Managing the Urogenital Effects of Estrogen Deprivation: Female Health and Sexual Dysfunction. *Contemporary OB/GYN,* 1-10.

Greene, R. (Nov. 2004). Selecting an Agent For Hormone Therapy: What to Consider. *OBG Management,* 5-9.

Healy, B. (2002, Nov. 18). The Mysteries of Menopause. *U.S. News & World Report,* 39-71.

Henderson, V. (2005). Hormone Therapy and Alzheimer Disease: An Evidence-Based Approach to Clinical Management. *The Female Patient,* 30, 9-14.

Hendrick, V. (2004). Effects of Hormone Supplementation on Mood in Women. *The Female Patient,* 29, 13-15.

Hendrix, S. (Nov. 2002). Implications of the Women's Health Initiative. *The Female Patient,* 4-8.

Henrich, J., et al. (2006) FSH Alone Can't Diagnose Menopause. *Contemporary OB/GYN,* 17.

Hsia, J., et al. (2004). WHI: What Will the Estrogen Arm Show? *Women's Health Gynecology Edition,* 4, (2), 100.

Hudson, T. (2001). Natural Progesterone: Clinical Indications in Women's Health. *The Female Patient,* (26), 43-48.

Hudson, T. (2004). Nutritional Influences on Osteoporosis. *The Female Patient,* 29, 35-42.

Hudson, T. (2005). Hyperlipidemia: Nutritional, Botanical, and Lifestyle Influences. *The Female Patient,* 30, 42-46.

Humtley, A., et al. (2003). A Systematic Review of Herbal Medicinal Products for the Treatment of Menopausal Symptoms. *The Journal of the North American Menopause Society,* 10 (5), 465-476.

(2005) Infophase. *Internet.*

Israel, D., et al. (1997). Herbal Therapies for Perimenopausal and Menopausal Complaints. *Pharmacotherapy,* 17 (5), 970-984.

Jones, K. (2000). Menopause and Cognitive Function: Estrogens and Alternative Therapies. *Clinical Obstetrics and Gynecology,* 43 (1), 198-206.

Kagan, L. (June 2005). Osteoporotic Fractures and Falls: Reducing the Risk. *The Female Patient,* 7-8.

Kang, H., et al. (2002). Use of Alternative and Complementary Medicine in Menopause. *International Journal of Gynecology & Obstetrics,* 79, 195-207.

Kass-Annese, B. (2000). Alternative Therapies for Menopause. *Clinical Obstetrics and Gynecology,* 43 (1), 162-183.

Kaunitz, A. (2003). Treating Hot Flashes: Options to Estrogen. *The Female Patient,* 28, 52-54.

Kearns, A. (May 2004). Potential Anabolic Effects of Androgens on Bone. *OBG Management,* 11-14.

Kreisberg, R. (Sept/Oct 2002). HRT and Cardioprotection: Past, Present and Future. *Menopause Management,* 16-20.

Krystal, A. (2004). Depression and Insomnia in Women. *Clinical Cornerstone,* 6, S19-28.

Langer, R. (Nov. 2004). Strategies to Optimize the Safety of Hormone Therapy. *OBG Management,* 10-15.

Lewis, V. (2004). New Hormone Therapy Formulations and Routes of Delivery: Meeting the Needs of Your Patients in the Post-WHI World. *OBG Management Supplement,* 11-17.

Liu, J. (Jan. 2004). Use of Conjugated Estrogens After the Women's Health Initiative. *The Female Patient,* 1-6.

Lewiecki, E. (2004). Bone Density Testing in the Management of Postmenopausal Osteoporosis. *Women's Health,* 4 (4), 183-193.

Lobo, R. (2004). Cardiovascular Disease in Postmenopausal Women: Emerging Information About Hormone Therapy. *The Female Patient,* 29, 38-44.

Lowes, R. (Sept. 2004). A Field Guide to Alternative Healers. *Medical Economics,* 21-25.

Mahady, G., et al. (2002). Black Cohosh: An Alternative Therapy for Menopause? *Nutrition in Clinical Care,* 5 (6), 283-289.

McSweeney, J. et al., (Feb. 2005). Heart Disease in Women: Knowing the Risks, Recognizing the Symptoms. *The Female Patient,* 5-7.

Metric Conversion Chart. *Internet.*

(2005). Internet French Property Co.

References

Metric Prefixes. *Internet.*

(2005). Metric System Units. *Webdocs.*

(2005). Metric System. *Internet.*

(2005) Metric System Table. *Internet.* Miller, E. (2004). Women and Insomnia. *Clinical Cornerstone,* 6, S6-S18

Mugford, J., et al. (2007). Heart Disease in Women. *The Female Patient,* 32, 39-44.

Murray, M. (July 2004). Black Cohosh: Nature's Best Solution for Hot Flashes. *Alive,* 48-51.

Muto M. (Oct. 2004). Ovarian Cancer: Identifying and Managing High-risk Patients. *OBG Management,* 60-69.

(2005). The 2004 NAMS Position Statement on Hormone Therapy. *Women's Health Gynecology Edition,* 5 (1), 26-33.

Northrup, C. (1997). Menopause. *Primary Care,* 24 (4), 921-948.

Northrup, C. (2001). *The Wisdom of Menopause,* Bantam Dell Publishing Co., 2001

Notelovitz, M. (May 2004). Hot Flashes and Androgens. *OBG Management,* 6-10.

(2004). *PDR for Herbal Medicines, Third Edition* (Thompson) Montvale, NJ.

(2001). *PDR for Nutritional Supplements* (Thompson) Montvale, NJ.

Phillips, O. (Nov. 2002). SERMs in Preventive Healthcare. *The Female Patient,* S1-10.

Phillips, O. (2004). WHI In Perspective – Focus on Coronary Heart Disease. *The Forum,* 2 (1), 15-18.

(2005). *Physicians' Desk Reference, 59th Edition* (Thompson) Montvale, NJ.

Pradhan, A., et al. (2004). Today's Therapeutic Options for Hot Flashes. *Women's Health, Gynecology Edition,* 4 (2), 81-86

Prendergast, K. et al., (2005). Therapeutic Options in the Management of Osteoporotic Patients. *Women's Health, Gynecology Edition,* 5 (1), 43-48.

Rossouw, J., et al. (2007). Postmenopausal Hormone Therapy and Risk of Cardiovascular Disease by Age and Years Since Menopause. *JAMA,* 297, 1465-1477.

Roth, D. (1999). No It's Not Hot In Here, Ant Hill Press, 146-152.

(Jan/Feb 2003). Roundtable: Suspected CHD Risk. *Menopause Management,* 19-24.

Russell, L., et al. (2002). Phytoestrogens: A Viable Option? *American Journal Medical Society,* 324 (4), 185-188.

Sand, P., et al. (1990). Nonsurgical Treatment of Detrusor Overactivity in Postmenopausal Women. *Reproductive Medicine,* 35 (8), 758-764.

Sarrel, P. (Feb. 2004). Vasomotor and Vascular Considerations. *The Female Patient,* 10-18.

Shifren, J. (May 2004). The Role of Androgens in Female Sexual Dysfunction. *OBG Management,* 14-18.

Simetric.co.uk. *Internet.*

Simon, J. (2004). Assessing Risks and Benefits of Hormone Therapy for the Individual Patient: Breast Cancer, Osteoporosis, and Cognitive Decline. *OBG Management,* 7-10.

Speroff, L. (2007). Premenopausal Atherosclerosis. *Contemporary OB/GYN,* 84-49.

Stearns, V., et al, (2003). Controlled-Release Paroxetine Reduces Hot Flashe., *Journal of the American Medical Association,* 289, 2827-2834.

Sulak, P. (May 2004) Selecting the Option That Provides Maximum Health Benefits and Alleviates Menstrual Symptoms for the Perimenopausal Patient. *OBG Management,* 1-5.

Tapson, E. (2005). A Dictionary of Units. *Internet.*

Taylor, M. (1997). Alternatives to Conventional Hormone Replacement Therapy. *Comprehensive Therapeutics,* 23 (8), 514 -532.

Taylor, M. (2003). Alternatives to HRT: AN Evidence-Based Review. *International Journal of Fertility in Women's Medicine,* 48 (2), 64-68.

Thacker, H. (2005). Menopausal Hormone Therapy: The Symptomatic Patient. *The Female Patient,* 30, 16-21.

Thorncycroft, I. (2004). WHI in Perspective: Focus on the Estrogen –Only Study. *The Forum,* 2 (2), 4-6.

Thorneycroft, I. (Feb. 2004). Unopposed Estrogen and Cancer. *The Female Patient,* 19-26.

Utian, W. (2004). NAMS Publishes Hormone Therapy Recommendations. *The Female Patient,* 29, 54-56.

Utian, W. (May 2004). Update on Menopause: An Expert's Insight on Pivotal Studies. *OBG Management,* 60-68.

Utian, W. (2005). Postmenopausal Hormone Therapy: Clarifying the Role. *The Female Patient,* 30, 53-54.

Utian, W. (2005). Bio-identical Hormones: Separating Science From Marketing. *The Female Patient,* 30, 21-22.

References

Vankireddy, H. et al. (2004). Insomnia. *The Female Patient,* 29, 14-22.

Warren, M., et al. (2002). Use of Alternative Therapies in Menopause. *Best Practice & Research in Clinical Obstetrics & Gynecology,* 16 (3), 411-448.

Warren, M., et al. (2004). Custom-Compounded Hormone Therapy: Is There Science to Support the Claims? *Council on Hormone Education,* 2 (4), 3-8.

Watt, P., et al. (2003). A Holistic Programmatic Approach to Natural Hormone Replacement. *Family Community Health,* 26 (1), 53-63.

Whyte, J. (2003). Osteoporosis: Diagnosis and Treatment. *CME Resource,* 118(10), 27-46.

Willhite, L., et al. (2001). Urogenital Atrophy: Prevention and Treatment. *Pharm,* 21 (4), 464-480.

Wingert, P., et al. (2007, Jan.15). The New Prime Time. *Newsweek,* 38-60 (cover story).

Zacur, H. et al., (July 2004). Estrogen Therapy: Is Oral Superior to Transdermal for Endothelial Function? *OBG Management,* 12-14.

INDEX

A

Abnormal bleeding, 164-165, 391-392
Accutane (Isotretinoin)
    For management of acne, 288
Acetominophen
    For management of joint stiffness and joint pain, 231
Acid-base balance
    And douching, 259
    Urinary tract infections and, 257
    Vaginal dryness and, 252
Acne, 76, 77, 285-288, 439, 440
    As a side effect of medications, 151, 207, 283, 338, 407
    As a symptom of testosterone excess, 149
    Birth control pills and, 144
    Botanical and herbal options, 287
    Diet and lifestyle options, 286-287
    During puberty, 48, 49
    Hormonal medication options, 287-288
    Non-hormonal medication options, 288
    Sequence of events causing, 285
    Testosterone and, 68, 149, 151
    Vitamin and mineral options, 287
Activity level
    Effect on risk of breast cancer, 346, 352
    Effect on risk of osteoporosis, 318, 329
    For prevention of Alzheimer's disease, 403-404
Actonel (Risedronate), 133-134
    For prevention of osteoporosis, 341, 342, 343
Acupuncture, 86, 92, 105
    Acupuncturists, 92
    For management of urinary incontinence, 269

Adolescence,
> And acne, 285
> And depression, 217
> And sex drive, 250-251
> And sleep, 183
> And weight gain, 220
> Definition, 48
> Male perspective, 440, 443, 444
> Puberty in reverse, 48-50
> Similarities to menopause, 73, 76-77, 78, 438, 439, 440, 443, 444, 445

Adrenal glands, 68, 151, 277-278

Advil
> For management of joint stiffness and joint pain, 231
> For management of headaches, 294
> With aspirin, 312

Aerobic exercise
> For prevention of Alzheimer's disease, 403-404
> For prevention of osteoporosis, 329
> For weight control, 274-275

Affinity, 110-115

Age
> And balance, 329-330
> And bone density, 319, 322-324, 324-326
> And dehydroepiandrosterone (DHEA), 151
> And joint stiffness and joint pain, 223, 225
> And mammograms, 372, 373-376
> And skin, 233, 235
> And sleep, 183-185, 188
> At first full term pregnancy, 346, 394
> Effect on risk of Alzheimer's disease, 402
> Effect on risk of breast cancer, 345, 346, 351
> Effect on risk of ovarian cancer, 394
> Effect on risk of uterine cancer, 377, 381
> Of first period, 346, 350, 394
> Of menopause, 37, 73, 346, 350, 394
> Premature menopause, 64-65

Index

Aging
    And bone density scores, 324-326
    And calcium absorption, 335
    And depression, 211
    And dry skin, 233-235
    And forgetfulness, 207
    And joint stiffness and joint pain, 223-225
    And sleep, 183-185
    And urinary incontinence, 260
    And uterine cancer, 377
    And vitamin D, 331
    And Women's Health Initiative (WHI) findings, 427-429, 433
    Anti-aging, 118, 306
    Cultural differences, 87
    Benzodiazepines and, 190-191, 200
    Male aging, 441-443
    Male perspective, 444
    Premature menopause and, 64, 65
    Research, 415, 433-434
    Similarities to menopause, 76-77, 440-441
ALA (Alpha Lipoic Acid)
    For management of dry skin, 237
    For prevention of heart attack, 308
Alcohol
    Cravings for, 220
    Effect on forgetfulness, 205
    Effect on hot flashes, 168, 170
    Effect on insomnia, 186
    Effect on joint stiffness and joint pain, 227
    Effect on mood swings, irritability, and depression, 213
    Effect on risk of breast cancer, 347, 354
    Effect on risk of heart attack, 304
    Effect on risk of osteoporosis, 318, 332
    Effect on urinary incontinence, 263
    Effect on urinary tract infections, 257-258
    Effect on weight gain, 274
Alendronate (Fosamax), 133-134
    For prevention of osteoporosis, 341, 342

Aleve
> For management of headaches, 292
> For management of joint stiffness and joint pain, 231

Allopathic medicine, 80, 91, 91-93, 99

Aloe (*Aloe vera*)
> For management of joint stiffness and joint pain, 230

Alora, 253

Alpha Lipoic Acid (ALA)
> For management of dry skin, 237
> For prevention of heart attack, 308

Alternative and complementary medicine, 86, 91-94, 123, 140
> Guidance, 99
> Principles for use, 94

Alzheimer's disease, 401-407
> And Women's Health Initiative (WHI), 433
> Botanical and herbal options, 406
> Description, 401
> Diet and lifestyle options, 403-404
> Estrogen and, 402
> Figure 21, 401
> Hormonal medication options, 406
> Risk factors, 402-403
> Vitamin and mineral options, 404-405

Ambien (Zolpidem tartrate)
> For management of fatigue, 201
> For management of insomnia, 191-192

Amitriptyline (Elavil)
> For management of depression, 218
> For management of fatigue, 202
> For management of insomnia, 192

Anagen, 239

Anaprox (Naproxen sodium)
> For management of headaches, 292
> For management of joint stiffness and joint pain, 231
> With aspirin, 312

Anastrozole (Armidex)
> For management of breast cancer, 361

Anatomy
> Of endometrium, 53-54

Index

Of female reproductive organs, 51-57, 437
Figure 1, 51
Of female reproductive and urinary systems, 255-256, 260-261
Figure 11, 2575
Of skin, 233-234
Figure 8, 234
Of the vagina, 249-250
Figure 10, 249

Anorexia
Effect on risk of osteoporosis, 314, 318, 319

Antibiotics
And vaginal yeast infections, 288
For management of acne, 288

Anticholinergics
For management of urinary incontinence, 266

Antidepressants
SSRI (Selective Serotonin Reuptake Inhibitors)
Effect on sex drive, 175, 181-182, 218, 279
For management of depression, 218
For management of fatigue, 202
For management of hot flashes, 175
For management of insomnia, 192-193
For management of night sweats, 181-182
For management of urinary incontinence, 267
Tricyclic
Effect on sex drive, 279
For management of depression, 218
For management of fatigue, 202
For management of insomnia, 192
For management of urinary incontinence, 267

Antihistamines
For management of fatigue, 202
For management of insomnia, 193

Antihypertensive agents
For management of hair loss on the scalp, 243
For management of headaches, 292
For management of hot flashes, 176
For management of night sweats, 182

Antispasmodics
    For management of urinary incontinence, 267
Anxiety, 135, 185, 216
    As a symptom of progesterone deficiency, 135
    Relief of, 189, 198
Armidex (Anastrozole)
    For management of breast cancer, 361
Aromasin (Exemestane)
    For management of breast cancer, 361
Aromatase inhibitors
    Effect on blood clots, 361
    Effect on heart attack, 361
    Effect on hot flashes, 361
    Effect on osteoporosis, 361
    Effect on uterine cancer, 361
    For management of breast cancer, 361
Arthritis, *see* Joint stiffness and joint pain
Aspiration of the breast, 371, 372, 373, 376
Aspirin
    For prevention of heart attack, 312
Atorvastatin (Lipitor)
    For management of cholesterol and prevention of heart attack, 311
Axillary tail of the breast, 363-364
    Figure 16, 364

B

Balance
    Between estrogen and progesterone, 381-382
    For prevention of Alzheimer's disease, 404
    For prevention of osteoporosis, 329-330
    With age, 329-330
Balancing act, 83-89
Balding, see hair loss
Behavior modification
    For management of cravings, 220
    For management of urinary incontinence, 264-265

Index

Bellergal
    For management of hot flashes, 175
    For management of night sweats, 182
Benign breast disease
    Effect on risk of breast cancer, 347
Benzodiazepines
    For management of fatigue, 200-201
    For management of insomnia, 190-191
Benzoyl peroxide
    For management of acne, 288
Beta blockers
    For management of headache, 292
Bextra (valdecoxib)
    For management of joint stiffness and joint pain, 231-232
Bi-est, 124
Bilateral oophorectomy, 61, 62-63
Bilateral salpingectomy, 60, 62-63
Bilateral salpingo-oophorectomy, 62, 63
Binding, 104-105, 110-115
Bioflavonoids, 118
Bioidentical estrogen, 109, 123-125
    Estradiol, 123-125
    Estriol, 123-125
    Estrone, 123-125
Bioidentical hormones, 100-101, 102-105
    Association with heart attacks, 124-125
    Association with strokes, 124-125
    Compounding, 103-105, 124-125
Bioidentical progesterone, 138-139, 140
    Crinone, 139
    Oral micronized progesterone, 138
    ProGest, 139
    Progesterone cream, 139
    Progesterone gel, 139, 140
    Prometrium, 139
    U.S.P. Progesterone, 139
Bioidentical testosterone, 151
    Dehydroepiandrosterone (DHEA), 151
    Testosterone cream, 151

Biopsy
- Of the breast, 371, 372, 373, 376
- Of the uterus, 132, 147, 340, 361, 380, 392

Biotin
- For management of hair loss on the scalp, 241
- For management of mood swings, irritability, and depression, 213-214

Birth control, 141-146
- Pills, 142-145, 388
- Patches, 145-146
- During peri-menopause, 71-72

Birth control patches, 142, 145-146
- For management of headaches, 291
- For management of irregular vaginal bleeding, 165
- For prevention of uterine cancer, 387-389

Birth control pills, 142-146
- And breast cancer, 145, 348, 389
- And blood clots, 143, 145, 389
- And heart attack, 143, 145, 389
- And pregnancy, 389
- And smoking, 143, 145, 389
- And stroke, 143, 145, 391
- For management of acne, 287
- For management of hair loss on the scalp, 242
- For management of headaches, 291
- For management of hair growth in undesirable locations, 247
- For prevention of ovarian cancer, 144, 399
- For prevention of uterine cancer, 387-389, 391

Bisphosphonates, 133-134
- Actonel (Risedronate), 133-134
- Boniva (Ibandronate), 133-134
- Effect on risk of breast cancer, 133
- Effect on risk of heart attack, 133
- Effect on risk of uterine cancer, 133
- For prevention of osteoporosis, 133-134, 343-345
- Fosamax (Alendronate), 133-134

Black Cohosh (*Cimicifuga racemosa*), 119-121
- For management of hot flashes, 173
- For management of insomnia, 189

INDEX

    For management of mood swings, irritability, and depression, 216

    For management of night sweats, 179-180

    For management of vaginal dryness, 252

Bladder

    And incontinence, 260-269

    And urinary tract infections (UTIs), 256-259

    Figure 11, 255

Bladder drills

    For management of urinary incontinence, 265

Bladder irritants, 186, 263

Bloating

    As a symptom of estrogen excess, 109

    As a symptom of ovarian cancer, 395-396

Blood clots (thrombosis), 295, 296, 312

    And bioidentical hormones, 124-125

    And birth control pills, 143, 145, 389

    And heart attack and stroke, 295, 296, 300, 312

    And hormone eligibility, 94-95

    And Women's Health Initiative (WHI), 424, 425, 426, 428, 430, 433

    Effect of homocysteine on, 308

    With aromatase inhibitors, 361

    With aspirin, 312

    With birth control patches, 145

    With birth control pills, 143, 145, 389

    With estrogen, 124-125

    With estrogen pills, 126-127, 310-311

    With estrogen plus progesterone (HRT) patches, 148

    With estrogen skin patches, 128, 148

    With raloxifene (Evista), 132-133, 340-341

    With tamoxifen (Nolvadex), 131-132, 340, 360

    With tibolone, 134

    With vitamin E, 306

Blood pressure

    And alcohol, 304

    And antihistamines, 193

    And Black Cohosh, 120

    And tricyclic antidepressants, 267

And SSRI antidepressants, 192-193, 202
Effect on risk of Alzheimer's disease, 403
Effect on risk of heart attack, 298
Effect of soy on, 290
Medications for high blood pressure
    And risk of osteoporosis, 318
    Beta blockers, 292
    Clonidine, 176, 182
    For management of headaches, 292
    For management of hot flashes, 176
    For management of night sweats, 182
    Lefoxidine, 176, 182
    Methyldopa, 176, 182
    Minoxidil (Rogaine), 243
Side effect of medications, 120, 121

BMI (Body mass index), 264, 272-273, 298

Body habitus
    And risk of heart attack, 298, 302
    And risk of osteoporosis, 317

Body mass index, 264, 272-273, 298

Bone, see osteoporosis

Bone density testing, 321-327
    Guidelines for, 323-324
    T score, 324-326
    Z score, 326

Bone mass, *see* osteoporosis

Bone quality and quantity, 320-321, 328

Boniva (Ibandronate), 133-134
    For prevention of osteoporosis, 341, 342

Boron
    For prevention of osteoporosis, 336

Botanical and herbal estrogen, 118-123
    Bioflvonoids, 118
    Black Cohosh (*Cimicifuga racemosa*), 119-121
    Chai Hu Long Gu Muli Wang, 123
    Chasteberry (*Vitex agnus-castus*), 119
    Dong Quai (*Angelica sinensis*), 118-119
    False Unicorn Root (*Veratum luteum*), 122-123

Index

    Flaxseed, 117-118
    Hops (*Humulul lupulus*), 122
    Joyful Change, 123
    Licorice Root (*Glycyrrhiza glabra*), 121
    Motherwort (*Leonurus cardiaca*), 123
    Phytoestrogens, 109-118
    Soy, 116-117
    St. John's Wort (*Hypericum perforatum*), 121
    Valerian (*Valeriana officinalis*), 121-122

Botanical and herbal options, 92,
    See also Botanical and herbal estrogen,
    See also Botanical and herbal progesterone,
    See also Botanical and herbal testosterone
    Definitions, 95-96
    Estrogen, 118-123
    For management of acne, 287
    For management of decreased sex drive, 280-281
    For management of dry skin, 237
    For management of fatigue, 197-198
    For management of forgetfulness, 206
    For management of hair loss on the scalp, 242
    For management of headaches, 290
    For management of hot flashes, 171-173
    For management of insomnia, 188-189
    For management of joint stiffness and joint pain, 229-230
    For management of mood swings, irritability, depression, 215-216
    For management of night sweats, 178-180
    For management of vaginal dryness, 254
    For prevention of Alzheimer's disease, 406
    For prevention of heart attack, 309
    For prevention of osteoporosis, 336-337
    For prevention of uterine cancer, 383-384
    Manufacture and regulation, 97-99
    Phytoestrogens, 109-118
    Progesterone, 137-139
    Soy, 116-117
    Testosterone, 149-150

Botanical and herbal progesterone, 137-139
- Chasteberry (*Vitex agnus-castus*), 137
- Wild Yam (*Dioscorea villosa*), 137-138

Botanical and herbal testosterone, 149-150
- Cayenne (*Capsicum species*), 149-150
- Cubeb (*Piper cubeba*), 150
- Damiana (*Turnera diffusa*), 150

Botanical and herbal therapy, 95-99
- Manufacture and regulation, 97-99

Botanicals
- As a category of options for managing menopause, 86, 93-94, 95-96, 446
- As a source of unopposed estrogen, 378, 383, 385-386
- Definitions, 95-96
- Dosages, 153, 154-157
- Manufacture and regulation, 97-99
- Principles for use, 94
- Purity, 95, 97-99

Botanists, 92, 99

BRCA-1 and BRCA-2
- Effect on risk of breast cancer, 346
- Effect on risk of ovarian cancer, 393-394, 399

Breakfast
- For management of forgetfulness, 204
- For management of weight gain, 273-274

Breast aspiration, 371, 372-373, 376

Breast biopsy, 371, 372-373, 376

Breast cancer, 345-376
- And birth control pills, 145, 348, 389
- And Women's Health Initiative (WHI), 422-428, 433
- Diet and lifestyle options, 351-354
- Effect of raloxifene (Evista) on, 132-133, 340-341
- Effect of tamoxifen (Nolvadex) on, 131-132, 340, 360-361
- Family history, 346, 349-350
- Genetics, 346, 349-350
- Hormonal medication options, 354-360
- Mammograms, 372-376
- Non-hormonal medication options, 360-361

INDEX

    Risk factors, 345-351

    Self breast examination, 362-372

    Statistics, 345

Breastfeeding

    And breast density, 347, 373-376

Breast "lumps," 369-371-373-376

Breast MRI (magnetic resonance imaging), 372-373, 376

Breast pain, 221-222

    As a side effect of medications, 134, 173, 180

    As a symptom of estrogen excess, 108, 222

    As a symptom of menopause, 76, 77, 439, 440

Breast self exam, *see* self breast exam

Breast ultrasound, 372-373, 373-375, 378

Breathing

    During hot flashes, 171

Bulimia

    Effect on risk of osteoporosis, 314, 318, 319

C

CA-125, 396-397

Caffeine

    Cravings, 220

    Effect on hot flashes, 168, 170

    Effect on insomnia, 186

    Effect on joint stiffness and joint pain, 226-227

    Effect on mood swings, irritability, and depression, 213

    Effect on risk of osteoporosis, 318, 331

    Effect on urinary incontinence, 263

    Effect on urinary tract infections (UTIs), 259

Calcitonin (Miacalcin, Fortical)

    For prevention of osteoporosis, 338-339

Calcium

    And bone, 320-321

    Deficiency, 109

    For bone strengthening, 320-321, 334-335, 343

For management of joint stiffness and joint pain, 226
For management of mood swings, irritability, and depression, 213-214
For management of urinary incontinence, 263
For prevention of heart attack, 305

California Poppy (*Eschscholtzia californica*)
For management of mood swings, irritability, and depression, 216

CapSure shield
For management of urinary incontinence, 268

Carbohydrates
Cravings for, 48, 76-77, 219-220, 439-440
Effect on mood swings, irritability, and depression, 213
Effect on risk of breast cancer, 353
Effect on risk of heart attack, 300-301
Effect on weight gain, 274
Refined, 353

Cartilage, 224, 227, 228
Catagen, 239
Categories of hormones
Estrogen, 107, 108-134
Estrogen plus progesterone, 107, 141-148
Estrogen plus testosterone, 107, 152
Progesterone, 107, 135-141
Testosterone, 107, 149-151, 152

Causative agent test
For breast cancer, 354-359
For uterine cancer, 385-386

Cayenne (*Capsicum species*), 149-150
For management of decreased sex drive, 280-281

Celebrex (Celecoxib)
For management of joint stiffness and joint pain, 231-232

Cenestin, 99-100, 101, 420
Cervix, 51-52
Figure 2, 52

Chai Hu Long Gu Muli Wang, 123
For management of insomnia, 189
For management of mood swings, irritability, and depression, 216

INDEX

Chasteberry (*Vitex agnus-castus*), 119, 137
    For management of decreased sex drive, 281
    For management of insomnia, 189
    For management of mood swings, irritability, and depression, 216
    For management of vaginal dryness, 252
    For prevention of uterine cancer, 383-384

Chemotherapy
    And premature menopause, 64-65, 430
    And surgical menopause, 64-65
        Hot flashes, 167
    And testosterone levels, 68

Cholesterol, 295-297
    And phytoestrogens, 309
    Arterial build-up of, 295-297
    Effect on risk of Alzheimer's disease, 403
    Figure 12, 296
    Low cholesterol diet, 300-301

Chondroitin sulfate
    For management of joint stiffness and joint pain, 228

Cialis (Tadalafil)
    For management of decreased sex drive, 284, 442

Climara, 253

Clonidine
    For management of hot flashes, 176
    For management of night sweats, 182

Cobalmin, *see* Vitamin B12

Coenzyme Q 10
    For management of dry skin, 237
    For prevention of breast cancer, 353
    For prevention of heart attack, 307

Collagen
    Injectable substance for urinary incontinence, 268
    In skin, 233-234, 237, 238
    Urine testing for osteoporosis, 326-327

Colon cancer
    And WHI, 425, 426, 428

Compounding, 103-105, 124-125, 311

Compounding pharmacies, 104, 124, 125, 311
Continuous estrogen plus progesterone, 147-148
    For prevention of uterine cancer, 381-382, 386-387, 391-392
Conventional medicine, *see* allopathic medicine
Cool Sets, 178
Copper
    For management of mood swings, irritability, and depression, 213-214
    For prevention of osteoporosis, 336
CoQ10 (Coenzyme Q 10)
    For management of dry skin, 237
    For prevention of breast cancer, 353
    For prevention of heart attack, 307
Cortical bone, 316-317
    Figure 15, 316
Coumestans, 109-110
    For management of hot flashes, 172
    For management of night sweats, 179
COX 1 and COX 2 (Cyclooxygenase inhibitors)
    For management of joint stiffness and joint pain, 231-232
Cranberry juice, 258
Cravings 219-220
    And hormones, 219-220
    During adolescence, 48, 76-77, 219, 440
    During menopause, 76, 220, 439
    During pregnancy, 77, 219-220, 440, 444
    With estrogen excess, 108
    With PMS, 219-220
Crinone, 139
Cubeb (*Piper cubeba*), 150
    For management of decreased sex drive, 281
Custom-compounded medications, 104-105
Cyclic estrogen plus progesterone, 146-147
    For prevention of uterine cancer, 386-387, 389-391
Cycling, 225
Cyclooxygenase inhibitors
    For management of joint stiffness and joint pain, 231-232

Index

D

Dalmane (Flurazepam)
    For management of fatigue, 200-201
    For management of insomnia, 190-191
Damiana (*Turnera diffusa*), 150
    For management of decreased sex drive, 281
Decoctions, 96
Dehydroepiandrosterone, 151
    Effect on acne, 285
    For management of decreased sex drive, 283
    For management of forgetfulness, 207
    For prevention of Alzheimer's disease, 407
Dense breasts
    Effect on risk of breast cancer, 347, 373-376
    Figure 18, 374
Dental hygiene, 3064
Depression, 209-218
    As a side effect of medications, 182
    As a symptom of estrogen excess, 109
    As a symptom of progesterone excess, 135
    As a symptom of menopause, 76, 77, 439, 440
    Botanical and herbal options, 215-216
    Consequences, 211-212
    Description, 210
    Diet and lifestyle options, 213
    Effect on risk of heart attack, 299
    Hormonal medication options, 217
    Hot flashes and, 175, 210
    Incidence, 210
    Insomnia and, 185-186, 211
    Mechanisms, 210-212
    Non-hormonal medication options, 217-218
    Vitamin and mineral options, 213-215
Derma Therapy Bedding, 178
DES (Diethylstilbesterol), 415
Detrol (Tolterodine)

For management of urinary incontinence, 266
DEXA (Dual energy x-ray absorption), 321-323, 326-326
Dexamethasone
    For management of hair loss on the scalp, 242
    For management of hair growth in undesirable locations, 247-248
DHEA (Dehydroepiandrosterone), 151
    Effect on acne, 285
    For management of decreased sex drive, 282-283
    For management of forgetfulness, 207
    For prevention of Alzheimer's disease, 407
Diabetes
    Effect on risk of heart attack, 298-299
    Effect on risk of osteoporosis, 318
Diet
    Effect on headaches, 290
    Effect on risk of breast cancer, 346
    Effect on risk of ovarian cancer, 395
    For management of acne, 286
    For management of forgetfulness, 204-205
    For management of headache, 290
    For management of hot flashes, 168
    For management of joint stiffness and joint pain, 226-227
    For management of mood swings, irritability, and depression, 213
    For management of urinary incontinence, 263
    For management of vaginal dryness, 251
    For management of weight gain, 273-274
    For prevention of Alzheimer's disease, 403
    For prevention of breast cancer, 353
    For prevention of heart attack, 300-301
    For prevention of ovarian cancer, 398
    For prevention of uterine cancer, 383
Diet and lifestyle options, 86, 91
    For management of acne, 286-287
    For management of breast pain, 221
    For management of cravings for sweets, carbohydrates, alcohol, 220

INDEX

    For management of decreased sex drive, 280
    For management of dry skin, 235-237
    For management of fatigue, 196-197
    For management of forgetfulness, 204-205
    For management of hair growth in undesirable locations, 246-247
    For management of hair loss on the scalp, 240-241
    For management of headaches, 290
    For management of hot flashes, 170-171
    For management of insomnia, 186-187
    For management of joint stiffness and joint pain, 225-227
    For management of mood swings, irritability, depression, 213
    For management of night sweats, 177-178
    For management of urinary incontinence, 262-265
    For management of urinary tract infections, 257-259
    For management of vaginal dryness, 250-251
    For management of weight gain, 273-275
    For prevention of Alzheimer's disease, 403-404
    For prevention of breast cancer, 351-354
    For prevention of heart attack, 300-304
    For prevention of osteoporosis, 327-334
    For prevention of ovarian cancer, 398-399
    For prevention of uterine cancer, 382-383

Dietary fat,
    And vitamin C, 306
    Effect on forgetfulness, 204-205
    Effect on homocysteine, 308
    Effect on joint stiffness and joint pain, 232
    Effect on mood swings, irritability, and depression, 213
    Effect on risk of breast cancer, 346, 353
    Effect on risk of heart attack, 300-301, 308
    Effect on risk of ovarian cancer, 395, 398
    Effect on weight gain, 274

Dietary supplements, 97

Diethylstilbesterol (DES), 415

Dieting, 273-274

Ditropan (Oxybutinin)
    For management of urinary incontinence, 267

Doloxetine
    For management of stress urinary incontinence, 267
Dong Quai (*Angelica sinensis*), 118-119
    For management of fatigue, 198
    For management of hot flashes, 173
    For management of night sweats, 180
    For management of vaginal dryness, 252
Doral (Quazepam)
    For management of fatigue, 200-201
    For management of insomnia, 190-191
Douching, 259
Dry skin, 233-238
    Anatomy, 233-234
    As a symptom of estrogen deficiency, 108
    As a symptom of menopause, 76, 77, 439, 440
    Botanical and herbal options, 237
    Description, 233
    Diet and lifestyle options, 235-237
    Figure 8, 234
    Hormonal medication options, 238
    Vitamin and mineral options, 237
Dual energy x-ray absorption (DEXA), 321-323, 324-326

E

Ecslim, 253
Educational level
    And use of alternative and complementary medicine, 93
    Effect on risk of Alzheimer's disease, 403
Effexor (venlafaxine)
    For management of hot flashes, 175
    For management of night sweats, 181
Eflornithine hydrochloride (Vaniqa cream), 248
Elavil (Amitriptyline)
    For management of depression, 218
    For management of fatigue, 202
    For management of insomnia, 192

Index

Electrical stimulation
    For management of urinary incontinence, 269
Electrolysis
    For management of hair growth in undesirable locations, 246
Emepromium bromide
    For management of urinary incontinence, 266
Emerita's personal lubricant
    For management of vaginal dryness, 251
Endometrial cancer, *see* uterine cancer
Endometrium, 53-54
    Figure 3, 53
    Figure 4, 54
    In uterine cancer, 377-378
Energy level, *see* fatigue
ERT (Estrogen Replacement Therapy), 141
    Effect on risk of breast cancer, 348
    Effect on risk of uterine cancer, 378-380, 385-386
Estazolam (ProSom)
    For management of fatigue, 200-201
    For management of insomnia, 190-191
Estraderm, 253
Estradiol, 67, 103, 123-124, 271, 278
Estratest, 152
    For management of decreased sex drive, 282
Estratest HS, 152
    For management of decreased sex drive, 282
Estriol, 123-124
Estrogen, 67, 438
    And wild yam, 384
    Bioidentical, 109, 123-125
    Botanical and herbal, 109-123
    Categories, 109
    Creams, 128-129, 250, 253, 282, 433
    Deficiency, 108
    Effect on risk of Alzheimer's disease, 401, 402, 406-407
    Effect on risk of breast cancer, 346-348, 354-359
    As a causative agent, 354-359
    Effect on risk of uterine cancer, 378-380, 385-386

Excess, 108-109, 378-380
    And uterine cancer, 378-381, 383-382, 385-386
    Figure 20, 379
For management of acne, 288
For management of decreased sex drive, 281-282
For management of dry skin, 238
For management of forgetfulness, 206-207
For management of hair growth in undesirable locations, 247
For management of hair loss, 242
For management of hot flashes, 174
For management of joint stiffness and joint pain, 230-231
For management of mood swings, irritability, and depression, 217
For management of night sweats, 180
For management of urinary incontinence, 266
For management of vaginal dryness, 252-253
For prevention of Alzheimer's disease, 406-407
For prevention of heart attack, 310-311, 422-433
For prevention of osteoporosis, 321-323, 337-338
Gels, 124, 129-130, 174, 180, 217, 337
Pellets, 130
Phytoestrogens, 109-118
Pills, 126-127, 128, 174, 180, 217, 281-282, 337
Shots, 127, 174, 180, 217, 337
Skin patches, 127-128, 174, 180, 213, 255, 337
Synthetic, 109, 126-130
Tibolone, 134-135
Unopposed, 378-380, 385-386
Vaginal creams, 128-129, 253, 282, 360, 433
Vaginal rings, 127, 174, 180, 217, 253, 337, 433
Vaginal suppositories, 255
Vaginal tablets, 130, 255

Estrogen alone
    Effect on risk of ovarian cancer, 394-395
    Effect on risk of uterine cancer, 385-386
    Women's Health Initiative (WHI) study, 423, 427-428, 433

Estrogen plus progesterone
    Birth control patches, 145-146, 387-389

Index

　　Birth control pills, 141-145, 387-389
　　Continuous regimen, 147-148, 391-392
　　Cyclic regimen, 146-147, 386-391
　　Dosages, 141-148
　　Effect on risk of breast cancer, 356, 360
　　Effect on risk of ovarian cancer, 394-395
　　For birth control, 141-146, 387-389
　　For prevention of uterine cancer, 385-392
　　HRT skin patches, 148
　　In HRT (hormone replacement therapy), 141-142, 146-148
　　WHI study, 423-427, 429-430, 432-433
Estrogen Replacement Therapy (ERT), 126, 141
　　Effect on risk of breast cancer, 348
　　Effect on risk of uterine cancer, 378-380, 385-386
Estrone, 123-124, 271, 415
Eszopiclone (Lunesta)
　　For management of fatigue, 201
　　For management of insomnia, 191-192
Evening Primrose (*Oenothera biennis*)
　　For management of breast pain, 221
　　For management of hot flashes, 173
　　For management of night sweats, 180
Everything You Always Wanted to Know About Sex (Rueben), 417
Evista (Raloxifene), 102, 133
　　Effect on risk of breast cancer, 132-133
　　Effect on risk of heart attack, 132-133
　　Effecton risk of uterine cancer, 132-133
　　For prevention of osteoporosis, 132, 340-341, 342-343
Exemestane (Aromasin)
　　For management of breast cancer, 361
Exercise
　　Aerobic, 274-275, 301-302, 329
　　Excessive
　　　　Effect on risk of osteoporosis, 314, 318
　　For management of cravings, 220
　　For management of fatigue, 196
　　For management of headaches, 290
　　For management of hot flashes, 170-171

493

For management of insomnia, 188
For management of joint stiffness and joint pain, 225
For management of mood swings, irritability, and depression, 213
For management of weight gain, 271, 274-275
For prevention of Alzheimer's disease, 403-404
For prevention of breast cancer, 352
For prevention of heart attack, 301-302, 303
For prevention of osteoporosis, 330
For weight loss, 275, 302-303
For weight maintenance, 275
Quantity, 275, 302-303
Resistance training, 274-275, 329
Type of, 196-197
Weight-bearing, 329

F

Facial hygiene
    For management of acne, 287
Falling
    Effect on risk of osteoporosis, 317-318, 322
    Prevention of, 327-328
Fallopian tubes, 55
    Figure 5, 55
False Unicorn Root (*Veratum luteum*), 122-123
Family history
    Effect on risk of breast cancer, 346, 349-350
    Effect on risk of heart attack, 299
    Effect on risk of osteoporosis, 317
Fat (body fat)
    As a source of estrogen, 271-272, 379-380, 381
Fatigue, 195-202
    As a side effect of medications, 182
    As a symptom of estrogen deficiency, 108
    As a symptom of menopause, 76, 77, 439, 440

Index

    As a symptom of progesterone excess, 135
    Botanical and herbal options, 197-198
    Consequences, 212
    Description, 195
    Diet and lifestyle options, 196-197
    During menarche, 195-196
    During pregnancy, 195-196
    Energy level, 149, 195
    Hormonal medication options, 199
    Non-hormonal medication options, 199-202
    Vitamin and mineral options, 197

Fatty breasts, 375-376
    Figure 19, 375

Fatty fish, 226, 236

Feedback, 69-70, 79-80

Female reproductive organs, 51-57
    Figure 1, 51
    Figure 11, 255

Female urinary system, 255-269
    Figure 11, 255

Femara (Letrozole)
    For management of breast cancer, 361

Fem-Assist
    For management of urinary incontinence, 268

Feminine Forever (Wilson), 416, 417

Feverfew (*Tanacetum parthenium*)
    For management of headaches, 290
    For management of joint stiffness and joint pain, 229-230

Fiber
    Effect on risk of ovarian cancer, 395, 398
    Flaxseed, 117-118, 353
    For management of acne, 286
    For management of dry skin, 236
    For management of forgetfulness, 205
    For management of mood swings, irritability, and depression, 213
    For management of weight gain, 274
    For prevention of breast cancer, 353

       For prevention of heart attack, 301
       For prevention of ovarian cancer, 398
       Soy, 116-117
Fibrocystic breasts, 369-371, 373-376
Flavonoids, 116, 118
       For management of joint stiffness and joint pain, 227
Flaxseed, 110, 117-118
       For prevention of osteoporosis, 333
Fluoxetine (Prozac)
       For management of depression, 218
       For management of hot flashes, 175
       For management of night sweats, 181
       With aspirin, 312
Fluoxetine hydrochloride (Serafem)
       For management of depression, 218
Flurazepam (Dalmane)
       For management of fatigue, 200-201
       For management of insomnia, 190-191
Folate, *see* Vitamin B9
Follicle Stimulating Hormone (FSH), 69-70
       For diagnosis of menopause, 79-80
Forgetfulness, 203-207
       As a symptom of estrogen deficiency, 108
       As a symptom of menopause, 76, 77, 439, 440
       Botanical and herbal options, 206
       Consequences, 212
       Description, 203-204
       Diet and lifestyle options, 204-205
       Hormonal medication options, 206-207
       Vitamin and mineral options, 205-206
Forteo (Teriparatide)
       For management of osteoporosis, 339
Fortical
       For management of osteoporosis, 338-339
Fosamax (Alendronate), 133-134
       For prevention of osteoporosis, 341, 342
Framingham Heart Study, 418
FSH (Follicle Stimulating Hormone), 69-70
       For diagnosis of menopause, 79-80

Index

G

GABA (Gamma Aminobytyric Acid), 185, 216
Gabapentin (Neurontin)
    For management of hot flashes, 175
    For management of night sweats, 182
Gamma Aminobytyric Acid (GABA), 185, 216
Gambrell, Ben R., 418
Gender
    Effect on risk of Alzheimer's disease, 402-403
Genetics
    Effect on risk of Alzheimer's disease, 403
    Effect on risk of breast cancer, 346, 349-350
    Effect on risk of heart attack, 299
    Effect on risk of ovarian cancer, 393-394
GH (Growth Hormone), 184
Ginkgo (*Ginkgo biloba*)
    For management of forgetfulness, 206
    For prevention of Alzheimer's disease, 406
Glucosamine
    For management of joint stiffness and joint pain, 228
Glucosamine chondroitin sulfate
    For management of joint stiffness and joint pain, 228-230
Gotu Kola (*Centella asiatica*)
    For management of forgetfulness, 206
Green tea (*Camellia sinensis*)
    For management of dry skin, 237
    For prevention of heart attack, 301
    For prevention of osteoporosis, 337
Greer, Germaine, 421
Growth Hormone (GH), 184
Guidelines
    Economic, 323-324
    For bone density testing, 323-324
    For mammograms, 372-373
Gum disease
    Effect on risk of heart attack, 298, 304

H

Habit retraining
    For management of urinary incontinence, 265
Hair color
    Effect on risk of osteoporosis, 317
Hair growth in undesirable locations 245-248
    As a symptom of menopause, 76, 77, 439, 440
    As a symptom of testosterone excess, 149
    Description, 245
    Estrogen and, 245
    Hormonal medication options, 247
    Mechanical options, 246
    Non-hormonal medication options, 247-248
    Testosterone and, 207, 245, 283, 338, 407
Hair loss on the scalp, 239-243
    As a symptom of menopause, 76, 77, 439, 440
    As a symptom of estrogen deficiency, 108
    Botanical and herbal options, 242
    Diet and lifestyle options, 240-242
    Effect of testosterone on, 207
    Figure 9, 240
    Hair manipulation, 241
    Hair phases, 239-240
    Hormonal medication options, 242
    Non-hormonal medication options, 242-243
    Pubic hair, 149
    Vitamin and mineral options, 241-242
Hair manipulation, 241
Halcion (Triazolam)
    For management of fatigue, 200-201
    For management of insomnia, 190-191
Hawthorne
    For prevention of heart attack, 309
HDL (High Density Lipoproteins), 296-297
    Effect of alcohol on, 304
    Effect of birth control pills on, 145, 387-388

INDEX

Effect of DHEA on, 151
Effect of estrogen on, 310
Effect of estrogen gels on, 129
Effect of estrogen pills on, 126, 310
Effect of estrogen skin patches on, 310
Effect of flaxseed on, 118
Effect of L-Carnitine on, 308
Effect of raloxifene (Evista) on, 132, 341
Effect of soy on, 117
Effect of testosterone on, 151, 283
Effect of vitamin B3 on, 307
Effect on risk of heart attack, 298, 299

Headaches, 291-294
    As a side effect of medications, 173, 180, 182, 192, 201, 218, 267
    As a symptom of estrogen excess, 109
    As a symptom of menopause, 76, 77, 439, 440
    Botanical and herbal options, 290
    Description, 289-290
    Diet and lifestyle options, 290
    Hormonal medication options, 291
    Migraines, 289, 291
    Non-hormonal medication options, 292

Head injury
    Effect on risk of Alzheimer's disease, 403

Heart and Estrogen/Progestin Replacement Study (HERS), 421

Heart Attack, 295-312
    And bioidentical hormones, 124-125
    And birth control pills, 145, 389
    And Women's Health Initiative (WHI), 422-434
    Botanical and herbal options, 309
    Causes, 295-297
    Diet and lifestyle options, 300-304
    Effect of raloxifene (Evista) on, 132-133, 340-341
    Effect of tamoxifen (Nolvadex) on, 131-132, 340, 361
    Hormonal medication options, 309-311
    Male-female differences, 295, 297-298
    Non-hormonal medication options, 311-312
    Risk factors, 298-299

    Statistics, 295
    Symptoms, 297-298
    Vitamin and mineral options, 305-308
Heart palpitations,
    As side effect of medications, 218
    In menopause, 297
    With hot flashes, 168
    With night sweats, 177
Heat
    As a trigger for hot flashes, 170
    During hot flashes, 167-168
    For management of joint stiffness and joint pain, 226
    Intolerance, 169
Herbalists, 92, 99
Herbs
    As a category of options for managing menopause, 86, 92, 93-94, 95-96, 446
    As a source of unopposed estrogen, 378, 378-380
    Definitions, 95-96
    Dosages, 153-157
    Manufacture and regulation of, 97-99
    Principles for use, 94
    Purity, 95, 97-99
HERS (Heart and Estrogen/Progestin Replacement Study), 421
High blood pressure
    Effect on risk of Alzheimer's disease, 403
    Effect on risk of heart attack, 298
High Density Lipoproteins (HDL), 296-297
    Effect of alcohol on, 304
    Effect of birth control pills on, 145, 387-388
    Effect of dehydroepiandrosterone (DHEA) on, 151
    Effect of estrogen on, 310
    Effect of estrogen gels on, 129
    Effect of estrogen pills on, 126, 310
    Effect of estrogen skin patches on, 310
    Effect of flaxseed on, 118
    Effect of L-Carnitine on, 308

Index

Effect of raloxifene (Evista) on, 132, 341
Effect of soy on, 117
Effect of testosterone on, 151, 283
Effect of vitamin B3 on, 307
Effect on risk of heart attack, 298, 299

Hip
- Bone density tests and, 321-323
- Effect of bisphosphonates on hip fracture, 133-134
- Effect of raloxifene (Evista) on hip fracture, 132-133
- Effect of tamoxifen (Nolvadex) on hip fracture, 131-132
- Fractures and birth control pills, 145
- Fractures and soy, 332
- Fractures in Women's Health Initiative (WHI) study, 425, 428
- Osteoporosis, 314-316, 319, 322, 325-326
- SERMS and hip fracture, 130-131, 340, 342-343
- Waist : hip ratio, 298, 302

History of Postmenopausal hormones, 414-422

Homocysteine
- Effect on risk of heart attack, 299
- For prevention of blood clots, 308
- For prevention of heart attack, 308
- For prevention of stroke, 308

Hoover, Robert, 418

Hops (*Humulus lupulus*)
- For management of fatigue, 198
- For management of insomnia, 189

Hormonal medication options, 87
- Basic principles for using, 94-95
- Bioidentical estrogen, 123-125
- Bioidentical hormones, 102-105
- Bioidentical progesterone, 138-139
- Bioidentical testosterone, 151
- Estrogen, 123-130
- Estrogen plus progesterone, 141-148
- For management of acne, 287-288
- For management of breast pain, 221-222
- For management of decreased sex drive, 281-284

For management of dry skin, 238
For management of fatigue, 199
For management of forgetfulness, 206-207
For management of hair growth in undesirable locations, 247
For management of hair loss on the scalp, 242
For management of headaches, 291
For management of hot flashes, 174
For management of insomnia, 189-190
For management of joint stiffness and joint pain, 230-231
For management of mood swings, irritability, depression, 217
For management of night sweats, 180-181
For management of periods with a personality change, 165
For management of urinary incontinence, 266
For management of vaginal dryness, 252-254
For prevention of Alzheimer's disease, 406-407
For prevention of breast cancer, 354-360
For prevention of heart attack, 309-311
For prevention of osteoporosis, 337-339
For prevention of ovarian cancer, 399
For prevention of uterine cancer, 385-392
Synthetic estrogen, 126-130
Synthetic Progesterone, 139-141
Synthetic Testosterone, 152
Hormone Replacement Therapy (HRT), 141-142
    And weight gain, 272
    Continuous estrogen plus progesterone, 147-148, 386, 391-392
    Cyclic estrogen plus progesterone, 146-147, 386, 387-391
    Effect on risk of breast cancer, 360
    Effect on risk of ovarian cancer, 394-395
    Estrogen plus progesterone skin patches, 148
    For management of headaches, 291
    For management of uterine cancer, 385-392
    Versus birth control pills, 141-142, 388
Hot flashes, 167-176
    And depression, 210
    And surgical menopause, 167
    As a symptom of estrogen deficiency, 108
    As a symptom of menopause, 75, 77, 439, 440

INDEX

    Botanical and herbal options, 171-173
    Causes, 169-170
    Description, 167-168
    Diet and lifestyle options, 170-171
    Hormonal medication options, 174
    Incidence, 167
    Non-hormonal medication options, 175-176
    Triggers, 168, 170
    Variables affecting, 168-169
    Vitamin and mineral options, 171
    With raloxifene (Evista), 341
HRT (Hormone Replacement Therapy), 141-142
    Continuous, 147-148
        For prevention of uterine cancer, 391-392
    Cyclic, 146-147
        For prevention of uterine cancer, 389-391
    Effect on risk of breast cancer, 360
    Effect on risk of ovarian cancer, 394-395
    For management of uterine cancer, 385-392
    For management of headaches, 291
    Versus birth control pills, 141-142, 388
5-HTP (5-Hydroxytryptophan)
    For management of fatigue, 197
    For management of insomnia, 188
    For management of mood swings, irritability, and depression, 214
Hygiene
    Dental hygiene, 304
    Facial hygiene and acne, 285, 287, 288
    Pelvic hygiene, 259
    Sleep hygiene, 186-187, 190, 199
Hypnosis, 86, 92, 105
    For management of cravings, 220
    For management of urinary incontinence, 269
    Hypnotists, 92
Hysterectomy, 57-59
    Subtotal or partial hysterectomy, 59, 62-63
    Total hysterectomy, 58-59, 62

I

Ibandronate (Boniva), 133-134
    For prevention of osteoporosis, 341, 342
Ibuprofen
    For management of headaches, 292
    For management of joint stiffness and joint pain, 231
    With aspirin, 312
Imidazopyridines
    For management of fatigue, 201
    For management of insomnia, 191-192
Imipramine (Tofranil)
    For management of depression, 218
    For management of urinary incontinence, 267
Imperial system, 155-156
Impress softpatch
    For management of urinary incontinence, 268
Incontinence devices, 267-268
Incontinence dish
    For management of urinary incontinence, 268
Incontinence ring
    For management of urinary incontinence, 268
Infertility
    Effect on risk of ovarian cancer, 394
Infertility drugs
    Effect on risk of ovarian cancer, 394
Infusions, 96
Injectable substances for urinary incontinence, 268
Inositol
    For management of mood swings, irritability, and depression, 214
Insomnia, 183-193
    And depression, 211
    As a symptom of estrogen deficiency, 108
    As a symptom of menopause, 75, 77, 439, 440
    Botanical and herbal options, 188-189
    Consequences, 185-186, 212
    Description, 183

Index

    Diet and lifestyle options, 186-187
    Hormonal medication options, 189-190
    Hormones and aging, 183-185
    Non-hormonal medication options, 190-193
    Vitamin and mineral options, 188
Introl's bladder neck support prosthesis
    For management of urinary incontinence, 268
Irregular periods (periods with a personality change), 163-165
    As a symptom of progesterone deficiency, 135
    Hormonal medication options, 165
Irregular vaginal bleeding, 380. See also uterine cancer
    As a side effect of medications, 174
Irritability, 211-220
    As a symptom of estrogen deficiency, 108
    As a symptom of menopause, 76, 77, 439, 440
    Botanical and herbal options, 215-216
    Consequences, 212
    Description, 209-210
    Diet and lifestyle options, 213
    Hormonal medication options, 217
    Non-hormonal medication options, 217-218
    Vitamin and mineral options, 213-215
Isoflavones, 109-110, 115-118, 121
    For management of hot flashes, 172
    For management of night sweats, 179
Isoretinoin (Accutane)
    For management of acne, 288

J

Joint stiffness and joint pain, 223-232
    As a symptom of estrogen deficiency, 108
    As a symptom of menopause, 76, 77, 439, 440
    Botanical and herbal options, 229-230
    Description, 223-225
    Diet and lifestyle options, 225-227
    Figure 7, 224

Heat, 226
Hormonal medication options, 230-231
Non-hormonal medication options, 231-232
Vitamin and mineral options, 228-229
Joyful Change, 123
For management of insomnia, 189
For management of vaginal dryness, 252

K

Kava Kava (Piper methysticum)
For management of fatigue, 197, 198
For management of insomnia, 188
Kegel exercises, 262-263
K-Y Jelly
For management of vaginal dryness, 251

L

Laser
For management of hair growth in undesirable locations, 247
L-Carnitine
For prevention of heart attack, 308
LDL (Low Density Lipoproteins), 296-297
Effect of birth control pills on, 145, 388-389
Effect of DHEA on, 151
Effect of estrogen on, 310-311
Effect of estrogen pills on, 310-311
Effect of exercise on, 301
Effect of flaxseed on, 117-118
Effect of raloxifene (Evista) on, 132-133, 340-341
Effect of soy on, 117, 301, 309
Effect of sugar on, 300-301
Effect of tamoxifen (Nolvadex) on, 131-132, 360-361

Index

    Effect of testosterone on, 152
    Effect of vitamin B3 on, 307
    Effect on risk of heart attack, 296, 298

Lecithin
    For prevention of Alzheimer's disease, 403, 405

Lefoxidine
    For management of hot flashes, 176
    For management of night sweats, 182

Leg cramps
    As a symptom of calcium deficiency, 109
    As a symptom of estrogen excess, 109

Letrozole (Femara)
    For management of breast cancer, 361

Levitra (Vardenafil)
    For management of decreased sex drive, 284, 442

LH (Luteinizing Hormone), 70

Libido, *see* sex drive

Licorice Root (*Glycyrrhiza glabra*), 121
    For management of fatigue, 198

Lignans, 109-110, 115, 117-118, 121
    For management of hot flashes, 172
    For management of night sweats, 179
    For prevention of breast cancer, 353

Lipids
    And statin drugs, 311
    Effect on risk of heart attack, 295-297
    Figure 12, 296
    Heart attack and, 295-297
    Progesterone and, 311
    Ratios, 297
    Vitamin B3 and, 307

Lipitor, (Atorvastatin)
    For management of cholesterol and prevention of heart attack, 311

Lotion
    For management of dry skin, 236-237

Lovastatin (Mevacor)
    For management of cholesterol and prevention of heart attack, 311

Low Density Lipoproteins (LDL), 296-297
>   Effect of birth control pills on, 145, 388-389
>   Effect of dehydroepiandrosterone (DHEA) on, 151
>   Effect of estrogen on, 310-311
>   Effect of estrogen pills on, 310-311
>   Effect of exercise on, 301
>   Effect of flaxseed on, 117-118
>   Effect of raloxifene (Evista) on, 132-133, 340-341
>   Effect of soy on, 117, 301, 309
>   Effect of sugar on, 300-301
>   Effect of tamoxifen (Nolvadex) on, 131, 132, 360-361
>   Effect of testosterone on, 152
>   Effect of vitamin B3 on, 307
>   Effect on risk of heart attack, 296, 298

Low dose birth control pills, 142-145
>   For prevention of uterine cancer, 387-389

Low dose birth control skin patches, 145-146
>   For prevention of uterine cancer, 387-389

Lubricants
>   For management of vaginal dryness, 251

Lunesta (Eszopiclone)
>   For management of fatigue, 201
>   For management of insomnia, 191-192

Luteinizing Hormone, (LH), 70

Lymph, 301

M

Magnesium
>   Deficiency, 305
>   For management of mood swings, irritability, and depression, 213-214
>   For prevention of Alzheimer's disease, 405
>   For prevention of heart attack, 305
>   For prevention of osteoporosis, 335

Magnetic Resonance Imaging (MRI) of the breast, 372-373, 376

Male aging, 441-442
Male menopause, 441-443
    Emotional and psychological issues, 442
    Male aging, 441-442
    Mid-life crisis, 442-443
Male pattern baldness, 239-240, 245-246
    Figure 9, 240
Male perspective, 443-447
    Knowledge and preparation, 444-445
    Male role, 443-444
    Sex and romance, 445-446
    Support, 443-447
Male reproduction, 441
Mammograms, 372-376
    And dense breasts, 373-376
    Guidelines, 372-373
Management options
    Categories, 86-87
Manganese
    For prevention of osteoporosis, 336
Mechanical options
    For management of hair growth in undesirable locations, 246-247
    For management of vaginal dryness, 251-252
Melatonin
    For management of fatigue, 197
    For management of insomnia, 188
Menarche, 48, 197-198
    And fatigue, 195-196
Menopause, 37-38, 47-48
    Brief overview ("In a flash"), 437-441
    Diagnosis of, 78-80
    Premature, 63, 64
    Surgical, 64-66
    Surgical procedures resulting in, 57-58, 61, 62-63
    Symptoms, 75-77
Menstrual cycle, 47-49, 53,
    After surgery, 58-63

And breast checking, 366-368
And estrogen, 68
And mood swings, 209
And puberty, 48
And mammograms, 373
And menopause, 49
Basic overview ("For the Guys"), 437-438
Birth control pills and, 142-143
Blood FSH levels and, 79
Cyclic hormone replacement therapy (HRT) and, 146-147
Effect on risk of breast cancer, 346-348, 350, 357
Effect on risk of ovarian cancer, 394
Effect on risk of uterine cancer, 377-378, 381, 385-392
Estrogen and progesterone and, 53-54, 141-142
Figure 4, 54
Frequency, 75, 77, 108, 439, 440
FSH levels and, 70
Headaches and, 289
LH levels and, 70
Ovulation, 47, 55-56
Puberty and, 48-50
Requirements for "post-menopause," 72
Symptoms in peri-menopause, 75, 163-164
Timing of diagnosis of menopause, 80
Uterus and, 53-54

Menstrual life, 347-348
    Effect on risk of breast cancer, 347-348
    Effect on risk of ovarian cancer, 394

Metabolism / metabolic rate, 271, 274-274, 275

Methanteline bromide
    For management of urinary incontinence, 266

Methyldopa
    For management of hot flashes, 176
    For management of night sweats, 182

Methylsulfonylmethane (MSM)
    For management of hair loss on the scalp, 241-242
    For management of joint stiffness and joint pain, 229

Metric system, 154-155

INDEX

Mevacor (Lovastatin)
    For management cholesterol and prevention of heart attack, 311
Miaclcin
    For prevention of osteoporosis, 338-339
Micronized progesterone, 138
Migraine headaches, 289-290
    And birth control pills, 291
    As a symptom of progesterone deficiency, 135
Mind games
    For prevention of Alzheimer's disease, 404
Minoxidil (Rogaine),
    For management of hair loss on the scalp, 243
Mirtazapine
    For management of fatigue, 202
    For management of insomnia, 192-193
Moisturizers
    For management of vaginal dryness, 252
Mood swings, 209-218
    And birth control pills, 144
    As a symptom of estrogen deficiency, 108
    As a symptom of menopause, 76, 77, 439, 440
    As a symptom of testosterone excess, 149
    Botanical and herbal options, 215-216
    Consequences, 212
    Description, 209
    Diet and lifestyle options, 213
    Hormonal medication options, 217
    Non-hormonal medication options, 217-218
    Vitamin and mineral options, 213-214
Motherwort (*Leonurus cardiaca*), 123
Motrin
    For management of headache, 292
    For management of joint stiffness and joint pain, 231
    With aspirin, 312
MRI (magnetic resonance imaging) of the breast, 372-373, 376
MSM (Methylsulfonylmethane)
    For management of joint stiffness and joint pain, 229

For management of hair loss on the scalp, 241-242
Multivitamins, 205, 241, 306, 336, 404, 405
Muscle
- Aging and, 325-326
- And balance, 329-330
- And protein, 263
- And vitamin C, 265
- And zinc, 265
- Atrophy of vaginal muscles, 250, 256
- Decrease in mass, as a symptom of testosterone deficiency, 149
- Kegel exercises, 262-263
- Medication side effects, 216, 229, 361
- Osteoporosis and, 317-318
- Resistance training, 275, 329
- Tension, 189, 198
- Tone, 256
- Urethral, 260-261
- Uterine, 54-55
- Water content of, 235
- Weight control, 275

N

Naproxen sodium (Anaprox)
- For management of headaches, 292
- For management of joint stiffness and joint pain, 231
- With aspirin, 312

National Institutes of Health (NIH), 420, 422

"Natural" hormones, 99-101
- Bioidentical hormones, 100-101, 102-105

Naturopathic medicine, 80, 92

Nausea
- As a side effect of medications, 173, 175, 180, 182, 192, 201, 218, 267
- As s symptom of estrogen excess, 108

Neurontin (Gabapentin)

Index

    For management of hot flashes, 175
    For management of night sweats, 182

Niacin, *see* Vitamin B3

NIH (National Institutes of Health), 420, 422

Night sweats, 177-183
    As a symptom of estrogen deficiency, 108
    As a symptom of menopause, 75, 77, 439, 440
    Botanical and herbal options, 178-180
    Consequences, 212
    Description, 177
    Diet and lifestyle options, 177-178
    Hormonal medication options, 180-181
    Non-hormonal medication options, 181-182
    Vitamin and mineral options, 178

Nolvadex (Tamoxifen), 131-132
    For prevention of breast cancer, 131-132, 360-361
    For prevention of osteoporosis, 132, 340

Non-hormonal medication options, 87
    For management of acne, 288
    For management of decreased sex drive, 284
    For management of fatigue, 199-202
    For management of hair growth in undesirable locations, 247-248
    For management of hair loss on the scalp, 242-243
    For management of headaches, 292
    For management of hot flashes, 175-176
    For management of insomnia, 190-193
    For management of joint stiffness and joint pain, 231-232
    For management of mood swings, irritability, depression, 217-218
    For management of night sweats, 181-182
    For management of urinary incontinence, 266-267
    For management of weight gain, 276
    For prevention of breast cancer, 360-361
    For prevention of heart attack, 311-312
    For prevention of osteoporosis, 339-343

Nonsteroidal anti-inflammatory drugs (NSAIDs)

For management of headaches, 292
For management of joint stiffness and joint pain, 231-232
With aspirin, 312
Nurses Health Study, 418-419

O

Obesity
> BMI and, 272-273
> Effect on joint stiffness and joint pain, 227, 232
> Effect on risk of breast cancer, 346, 352-353
> Effect on risk of heart attack, 298
> Effect on risk of ovarian cancer, 394, 398
> Effect on risk of uterine cancer, 381

Oils, 96
Oligomeric proanthocyanidins (OPCs)
> For management of dry skin, 237
> For management of joint stiffness and joint pain, 227

Omega 3 fatty acids
> Flaxseeds, 118
> For management of dry skin, 236
> For management of joint stiffness and joint pain, 226
> For prevention of breast cancer, 353
> Sources, 118

Omega 6 fatty acids
> For management of mood swings, irritability, and depression, 213-214

Oophorectomy, 60-63
OPCs (Oligomeric proanthocyanidins)
> For management of dry skin, 237
> For management of joint stiffness and joint pain, 227

Orgasm
> And sex drive, 278
> Effect of medications on, 149, 175, 182, 218
> Difficulty, as a symptom of testosterone deficiency, 149

Osteoarthritis, see joint stiffness and joint pain

Index

Osteopathic medicine, 80, 91, 92, 99
Osteopenia, 325-326
Osteoporosis, 313-343
    And estrogen, 313, 320-321
    And estrogen dosage, 126
    And WHI, 425, 426, 428
    As a symptom of testosterone deficiency, 149
    Bone architecture, 316-317
    Bone density, 321-327
    Bone loss, 313-314, 320-321
    Bone maintenance, 320-321
    Bone strengthening, 320-321
    Botanical and herbal options, 336-337
    Calcium and, 320-321
    Definition, 313-314, 325
    Diet and lifestyle options, 327-334
    Effect of raloxifene (Evista) on, 133, 342-343
    Effect of tamoxifen (Nolvadex) on, 132, 342, 362
    Epidemiology, 315
    Estrogen loss and, 315-316, 319, 321, 322, 322-323
    Figure 13 (Normal vs. osteoporotic bone), 314
    Figure 14 (Postural changes), 315
    Hormonal medication options, 337-339
    Non-hormonal medication options, 339-343
    Prognosis, 315
    Rates of bone loss, 314
    Risk factors, 317-320
    Symptoms, 314-315
    Types of bone, 316-317
        Figure 15 (Trabecular vs. cortical bone), 316
    Vitamin and mineral options, 334-336
Ovarian cancer, 393-400
    Diagnosis, 396-398
    Diet and lifestyle options, 398-399
    Effect of birth control pills on, 144
    Hormonal medication options, 399
    Incidence, 393
    Preventive surgery for, 399-400

Risk factors, 393-395
Symptoms, 395-396
Ovaries, 56-57, 437
Figure 6, 56
Ovulation, 56-57
Oxybutinin (Ditropan)
For management of urinary incontinence, 267

P

Paced respiration, 171
Palpitations
As a side effect of medications, 218
In menopause, 297
With hot flashes, 168
With night sweats, 177
Pantothenic acid, *see Vitamin* B5
Paroxetine (Paxil)
For management of depression, 218
For management of hot flashes, 175
For management of night sweats, 181
With aspirin, 312
Partial hysterectomy, 59, 62-63
Partial hysterectomy, bilateral salpingo-oophorectomy, 62-63
Passion Flower (*Passiflora incarnata*)
For management of fatigue, 198
For management of insomnia, 189
Paxil (Paroxetine)
For management of depression, 218
For management of hot flashes, 175
For management of night sweats, 181
With aspirin, 312
"Pebbles," 369-371
On mammogram, 372-373
Pelvic hygiene
And UTIs, 259
PEPI (Postmenopausal Estrogen/Progesterone Intervention) Trial, 419

INDEX

Peri-menopause 71-72, 438
    And mood swings, 209
Periods, *see* vaginal bleeding. *See also* menstrual cycle
Periods with a personality change, 163-165
    As a symptom of progesterone deficiency, 135
    Hormonal medication options, 165
Personal history
    Effect on risk of breast cancer, 346
    Effect on risk of heart attack, 298
    Effect on risk of ovarian cancer, 393-394
Pharmacists, 92
Phases of menopause, 70-73, 438
pH balance (acid-base balance)
    And calcium absorption, 335
    And douching, 259
    And urinary tract infections (UTIs), 259
    And vaginal dryness, 252
Phytoestrogens, 109-118
    Affinity, 110-116
    Bioflavonoids, 118
    Coumestans, 109, 110
    Flaxseed, 117-118
    For management of hot flashes, 172
    For management of night sweats, 179
    For management of vaginal dryness, 252
    For prevention of heart attack, 309
    For prevention of osteoporosis, 336-337
    Isoflavones, 109-110
    Lignans, 109-110
    Soy, 116-117
Pilates
    For management of fatigue, 197
    For management of joint stiffness and joint pain, 225
    For prevention of osteoporosis, 329, 330
PMS (premenstrual syndrome)
    And breast pain, 221
    And cravings, 219-220
    And forgetfulness, 204
    As a symptom of progesterone deficiency, 135

Black Cohosh and, 120
Chasteberry and, 119
Effect of birth control pills on, 144
Effect of Evening Primrose on, 173
Hormone cycles and, 443
Male perspective, 443
Progesterone and, 135, 174, 181
Postmenopausal Estrogen/Progesterone Intervention (PEPI) Trial, 419
Post-menopause, 72-73, 438
Average age of, 73
Potassium
For prevention of heart attack, 305
Pranayama, 171
Pravachol (Pravastatin)
For management cholesterol and prevention of heart attack, 311
Pregnancy
And breast pain, 221
And cravings, 219-220
And fatigue, 195-196
And forgetfulness, 204
And hair loss, 239
And mood changes, 209, 217
And sleep, 183-185
After surgery, 59-63
Birth control pills and, 389
During peri-menopause, 71-72
Effect on risk of breast cancer, 346-348, 349, 350-351, 373-376
Effect on risk of ovarian cancer, 394
Effect on risk of urinary incontinence, 260-261
Endometrium and, 53-54
Estrogen during, 123-124
Fertilization and, 55-56
HRT (hormone replacement therapy) and, 146-148, 291, 388, 390
Irregular vaginal bleeding and, 380
Male perspective, 443, 444-446
Prevention, 142-146, 390
Progesterone and, 67-68, 189-190, 199

Index

    Similarities to menopause, 76-77, 440-441, 443
Premature menopause, 64-65
    Effect on risk of Alzheimer's disease, 402
    Effect on risk of osteoporosis, 317
    And Women's Health Initiative (WHI), 430, 433
Premarin, 100, 101, 126, 415, 417, 420, 421, 429
Pre-menopause, 70, 438
Premenstrual syndrome (PMS)
    And breast pain, 221
    And cravings, 219-220
    And forgetfulness, 204
    As a symptom of progesterone deficiency, 135
    Black Cohosh and, 120
    Chasteberry and, 119
    Effect of birth control pills on, 144
    Effect of Evening Primrose on, 173
    Hormone cycles and, 443
    Male perspective, 443
    Progesterone and, 135, 141, 174, 181
Prempro, 420, 429
Primrose oil, *see* Evening Primrose
Proanthocyanidins
    For management of dry skin, 237
    For management of joint stiffness and joint pain, 227
    For prevention of heart attack, 309
ProGest, 139, 360
Progesterone 67-68
    Bioidentical, 136, 138-139
    Birth control pills, 140-141
    Botanical and herbal, 136, 137-138
    Categories, 136-148
    Creams, 137, 138, 139, 174, 181, 207, 384
    Deficiency, 135
    Effect on risk of breast cancer, 356, 358, 360, 361
    Excess, 135
    For management of decreased or increased sex drive, 284
    For management of dry skin, 238
    For management of fatigue, 199

For management of forgetfulness, 207
For management of headaches, 291
For management of hot flashes, 174
For management of insomnia, 189-190
For management of night sweats, 181
For prevention of heart attack, 309-310, 311
For prevention of osteoporosis, 338
For prevention of uterine cancer, 378-380, 381-382, 383-384, 385-392, 433
Gels, 137, 138, 139, 207, 383, 384
IUD (intrauterine device), 141
Micronized progesterone, 138
Pills, 140, 207, 360
Shots, 140
Skin patches, 137
Synthetic, 136, 139-141
Progesterone cream, 139
Promensil
For management of hot flashes, 172
For management of night sweats, 179
Prometrium, 139, 311, 360
Prompted voiding
For management of urinary incontinence, 265
Propantheline bromide
For management of urinary incontinence, 266
ProSom (Estazolam)
For management of fatigue, 200-201
For management of insomnia, 190-191
Protein
For management of forgetfulness, 204-205
For management of mood swings, irritability, and depression, 213
For management of urinary incontinence, 263
For prevention of heart attack, 308, 309
For prevention of osteoporosis, 332-333
For weight control, 274
Soy protein, 116, 205, 332
Prozac (Fluoxetine)

INDEX

    For management of hot flashes, 175
    For management of night sweats, 181
    With aspirin, 312
Puberty, 48-50
    And fatigue, 195-196
    Definition of, 48
    Puberty in reverse, 48-50, 438 439, 440
Pubic hair
    Thinning, as a symptom of testosterone deficiency, 149
Pyridoxine, *see* Vitamin B6

Q

Quazepam (Doral)
    For management f fatigue, 200-201
    For management of insomnia, 190-191

R

Race
    Effect on risk of osteoporosis, 317, 318-319
Radiation exposure
    And premature menopause, 64-65, 430
    And surgical menopause, 64-65
        Hot flashes, 167
    And testosterone levels, 68
    Effect on risk of breast cancer, 347, 349
    With bone density testing, 321, 322
Raloxifene (Evista), 102, 133
    Effect on risk of breast cancer, 132-133
    Effect on risk of heart attack, 132-133
    Effect on risk of uterine cancer, 132-133
    For prevention of osteoporosis, 132, 340-341, 342-343
Ramelteon (Rozarem)

   For management of fatigue, 200-201
   For management of insomnia, 190-191
Ratios
   Calcium : Magnesium, 305
   Estrogen : Progesterone, 379-380, 381-382, 384, 385-392
   Potassium : Sodium, 305
   Testosterone : Estrogen, 245-246, 277-279
   Total cholesterol : HDL, 297, 298
   Waist : Hip, 298, 302
Receptors, 104-105, 110
   Affinity and, 110-116
   Binding, 104-105
   Bioidentical hormones and, 102-103
   Estrogen receptors, 120, 131, 150, 402
   Estrogen receptor status in breast cancer, 360
   Progesterone receptors, 150
   SERMs (Selective Estrogen Receptor Modulators), 131-133, 253, 340
Refecoxib (Vioxx)
   For management of joint stiffness and joint pain, 231-232
Regimen for hormones, 141-142
Relaxation, 187
Reliance urinary control insert
   For management of urinary incontinence, 268
Remifemin, 173, 179
Renova (Tretinoin)
   For management of acne, 288
Replens vaginal moisturizer
   For management of vaginal dryness, 252
Research studies, 411-434
   Factors, 414
   On estrogen as a cause of breast cancer
      Tests for cancer-causing agents, 356-361
   Significance, 412-414
   Types, 411
   Women's Health Initiative (WHI), 420, 423-434

Resistance exercises
    For prevention of osteoporosis, 329
    For weight control, 275
Restoril (Temazepam)
    For management of fatigue, 200-201
    For management of insomnia, 190-191
Retin A (tretinoin)
    For management of acne, 288
    In combination with minoxidil (Rogaine), 243
Riboflavin, *see* Vitamin B2
Rimostil
    For management of hot flashes, 172
    For management of night sweats, 179
Risedronate (Actonel), 133-134
    For prevention of osteoporosis, 342, 343
Risk factors
    For Alzheimer's disease, 402-403
    For breast cancer, 345-348
    For heart attack, 298-299
    For osteoporosis, 317-320
    For ovarian cancer, 393-395
    For uterine cancer, 381-382
"Rocks," 369-371
    On mammogram, 372, 373-376
Rogaine (Minoxidil)
    For management of hair loss, 243
Rozarem (Ramelteon)
    For management of fatigue, 200-201
    For management of insomnia, 190-191
Rueben, David, 419
Rugae, *see* vaginal rugae

S

S-adenosyl-L-methionine (SAMe)
    For management of joint stiffness and joint pain, 229
    For management of mood swings, irritability, and depression, 214-215

Salpingectomy, 59-60, 61-63

Salivary hormones, 80

SAMe (S-adenosyl-L-methionine)
    For management of joint stiffness and joint pain, 229
    For management of mood swings, irritability, and depression, 214-215

Saturated fats
    Effect on risk of heart attack, 300
    Effect on risk of ovarian cancer, 398

Screening tests
    For osteoporosis, 321-327
    For ovarian cancer, 396-398

Sedatives, 67, 189, 190-192, 199, 200-202, 213, 215, 216

Sedentary lifestyle
    Effect on risk of breast cancer, 346
    Effect on risk of heart attack, 298
    Effect on risk of osteoporosis, 318

Selective Estrogen Receptor Modulators (SERMs), 130-134
    And vaginal dryness, 255
    Bisphosphonates, 133-134
    For prevention of osteoporosis, 341-345
    Raloxifene (Evista), 132-133
    Tamoxifen (Nolvadex), 131-132
    Tibolone, 134-135, 174, 181, 256

Selective Serotonin Reuptake Inhibitors (SSRIs)
    Effect on sex drive, 175, 181-182, 218, 279
    For management of depression, 217-218
    For management of fatigue, 202
    For management of hot flashes, 175
    For management of insomnia, 192-193
    For management of night sweats, 182

Index

    For management of urinary incontinence, 267
Selenium
    For management of forgetfulness, 205-206
Self breast exam, 362-372
    Figure 16, 364
    Figure 17, 365
    Target (What), 369-370
    Technique (How), 363-366
    Timing (When), 366-369
Self control
    For management of cravings, 220
Serafem (Fluoxetine hydrochloride)
    For management of depression, 218
SERMs (Selective Estrogen Receptor Modulators), 130-134
    And vaginal dryness, 253
    Bisphosphonates, 133-134
    For prevention of osteoporosis, 339-343
    Raloxifene (Evista), 132-133
    Tamoxifen (Nolvadex), 131-132
    Tibolone, 134, 174, 181, 254
Serotonin, 211, 214
Sertraline, (Zoloft)
    For management of depression, 218
    With aspirin, 312
Sexual activity
    For management of vaginal dryness, 250-251
Sex drive, 277-284
    As a symptom of menopause, 76, 77, 439, 440, 445-446
    Botanical and herbal options, 280-281
    Categories of decreased sex drive, 279
    Changes in, 277-279, 442, 445-446
    Decreased, as a symptom of estrogen deficiency, 108
    Decreased, as a symptom of testosterone deficiency, 149
    Description, 277-279
    Diet and lifestyle options, 280
    Hormonal medication options, 281-284
    Increased, as a symptom of testosterone excess, 149
    Mental aspect, 279

Non-hormonal medication options, 284
Physical/genital aspect, 279
Testosterone and, 149, 277-279, 282-283
Sex Hormone Binding Globulin (SHBG), 115, 126-127, 353
Sheehy, Gail, 421
Sildenafil (Viagra)
- For management of decreased sex drive, 284, 442

Silicon
- For prevention of osteoporosis, 336

Simvastatin (Zocor)
- For prevention of heart attack, 311

Skin
- Anatomy, 233-234
- Figure 8, 234

Skin patches
- Birth control, 145-146, 387-389
- Estrogen, 124, 127-128, 174, 180, 217, 253, 281-282, 310, 337-338
- Estrogen plus progesterone, 148
- Progesterone, 137
- Testosterone, 152, 282-283

Sleep apnea, 185-186
Sleep environment, 177-178
Sleep hygiene, 186-187
- Sleep restriction, 187
- Sleep routines, 187
- Stimulus control measures, 186-187

Slide chart, 408

Smoking
- And birth control pills, 143, 145, 389
- And weight gain, 276
- Effect on forgetfulness, 205
- Effect on hot flashes, 168, 170
- Effect on risk of breast cancer, 346, 351-352
- Effect on risk of heart attack, 298, 303
- Effect on risk of osteoporosis, 318, 330-331
- Effect on timing of menopause, 300, 303

INDEX

Effect on urinary incontinence, 263-264
Sodium
    For prevention of heart attack, 305
Soft drinks
    Effect on mood swings, irritability, and depression, 213
    Effect on risk of osteoporosis, 333
    Effect on urinary tract infections, 259
Sonata (Zalephon)
    For management of fatigue, 201
    For management of insomnia, 191-192
Soy, 116-117
    Effect on calcium, 117
    Effect on colon cancer, 117
    Effect on dry skin, 117
    Effect on hair loss on the scalp, 117
    Effect on hot flashes, 117
    Effect on mood swings and irritability, 117
    Effect on nails, 117
    Effect on night sweats, 117
    Effect on periods, 117
    Effect on PMS (premenstrual syndrome), 117
    Effect on weight gain, 117
    For management of forgetfulness, 205
    For management of headaches, 117, 290
    For management of vaginal dryness, 251
    For prevention of breast cancer, 117, 353
    For prevention of heart attack, 117, 301, 309
    For prevention of osteoporosis, 117, 332
    For prevention of uterine cancer, 117, 383
    Soy foods, 116-118, 172, 179
    Soy supplements, 172, 179
Spine
    Bone density tests and, 321-323
    Calcitonin and, 338-339
    Fractures, 315, 316, 340, 342-343
    Fractures and soy, 332
    Fractures and Women's Health Initiative (WHI), 425, 428

Osteoporosis and, 314-316, 319, 322, 325-326
   Selective Estrogen Receptor Modulators (SERMs) and, 132-134, 344
Spironolctone
   For management of hair loss, 243
   For management of unwanted hair growth, 247
SSRI (Selective Serotonin Reuptake Inhibitor) antidepressants
   Effect on sex drive, 175, 181-182, 218, 279
   For management of depression, 217-218
   For management of fatigue, 202
   For management of hot flashes, 175
   For management of insomnia, 192-193
   For management of night sweats, 182
   For management of urinary incontinence, 267
Standard of care, 40-41
Statin drugs
   For management of cholesterol and prevention of heart attack, 311
Steroids
   Effect on risk of osteoporosis, 318
   For management of joint stiffness and joint pain, 232
Stimulants, 213
St. John's Wort (*Hypericum perforatum*), 121
   For management of mood swings, irritability, and depression, 215-216
Stress
   Effect on headaches, 289, 290
   Effect on hot flashes, 171
Stress urinary incontinence (SUI), 261, 262-269. See also urinary incontinence
Stroke, 295, 296, 312
   And bioidentical hormones, 124-125
   And birth control pills, 143, 145, 389
   And homocysteine, 308
   And Women's Health Initiative (WHI), 424, 425, 426, 428
Subtotal hysterectomy, 59, 62-63
Subtotal hysterectomy, bilateral salpingo-oophorectomy, 62-63

Index

Sugar
- Cravings, 219-220
- Effect on acne, 286
- Effect on headaches, 289
- Effect on joint stiffness and joint pain, 227
- Effect on moods swings, irritability, and depression, 213
- Effect on risk of breast cancer, 353
- Effect on risk of heart attack, 300-301
- Effect on weight gain, 274
- Exercise and breast cancer, 352

SUI (Stress urinary incontinence), 261-262, 262-269. See also urinary incontinence

Sun exposure
- Effect on risk of osteoporosis, 318
- For prevention of osteoporosis, 331

Sun protection
- For management of dry skin, 235

Surgical menopause, 64-65
- Effect on risk of Alzheimer's disease, 402
- Effect on risk of headaches, 289
- Effect on risk of hot flashes, 167
- And Women's Health Initiative (WHI), 430
- Procedures resulting in, 61-63

Surgical procedures, 57-64
- Bilateral oophorectomy, 61
- Bilateral salpingectomy, 60
- Bilateral salpingo-oophorectomy, 62
- For management of stress urinary incontinence (SUI), 268
- For prevention of ovarian cancer, 399-400
- Oophorectomy, 60, 61, 62, 63
- Partial hysterectomy, 59
- Partial hysterectomy, bilateral salpingo-oophorectomy, 62-63
- Salpingectomy, 60, 61, 62, 63
- Subtotal hysterectomy, 59
- Subtotal hysterectomy, bilateral salpingo-oophorectomy, 62-63
- Total hysterectomy, 58-59

    Total hysterectomy, bilateral salpingo-oophorectomy, 62
    Unilateral oophorectomy, 60
    Unilateral salpingectomy, 59
    Unilateral salpingo-oophorectomy, 61-62
Swimming, 225, 329
    For management of joint stiffness and joint pain, 225
    For prevention of osteoporosis, 329
Sylk
    For management of vaginal dryness, 251
Symptoms of menopause, 75-77, 439-441
Synovial fluid, 229
Synthetic estrogen, 126-130
    Gels, 129
    Pellets, 130
    Pills, 126-127
    Skin patches, 127-128
    Shots, 127
    Vaginal creams, 128-129
    Vaginal rings, 127
    Vaginal tablets, 130
Synthetic estrogen plus progesterone, 141-148
    Continuous estrogen plus progesterone, 147-148
    Cyclic estrogen plus progesterone, 146-147
    Dosages, 141-142
    Low dose birth control pills, 142-145
    Low dose birth control skin patches, 145-146
    Regimens, 141-142
    Skin patches, 148
"Synthetic" hormones, 101-102
Synthetic progesterone, 139-141
    Gel, 139
    Pills, 140
    Progesterone only birth control pills, 140-141
    Shots, 140
    Intrauterine device (IUD), 141
Synthetic testosterone, 152
Systeme International (SI), 154-155

INDEX

T

Tables of options, 19-27
    Botanical and herbal options, 23
    Diet and lifestyle options, 19
    Hormonal medication options, 27
    Non-hormonal medication options, 25
    Vitamin and mineral options, 21
Tadalafil (Cialis)
    For management of decreased sex drive, 284, 442
T'ai chi, 225
Talcum powder
    Effect on risk of ovarian cancer, 395, 400-401
Tamoxifen (Nolvadex), 131-132
    For prevention of breast cancer, 131-132, 360-361
    For prevention of osteoporosis, 340
Target heart rate, 302
Teas, 96
Tea Tree Oil (*Medaleuca alternifolia*)
    For management of acne, 287
Telogen, 239
Temazepam (Restoril)
    For management of fatigue, 200-201
    Fr management of insomnia, 190-191
Teriparatide (Forteo)
    And bisphosphonates, 341
    For prevention of osteoporosis, 339
Testosterone, 68
    And acne, 68, 149, 152, 207, 283, 338, 407
    And hair growth in undesirable locations, 149, 151, 245-246, 407
    Bioidentical, 151
    Botanical and herbal, 149-150
    Categories, 149-150
    Cream, 151, 254, 283
    Deficiency, 149
    Effect of surgical menopause on, 68

Effect on risk of breast cancer, 358
Excess, 149, 151
For management of decreased sex drive, 68, 282-283
For management of forgetfulness, 207
For management of mood swings, irritability, and depression, 217
For management of vaginal dryness, 254
For prevention of osteoporosis, 338
Gel, 283
In males, 442
Pills, 152
Shots, 152
Skin patches, 152
Skin patches, 152, 283
Sublingual, 283
Synthetic, 152

Testosterone cream, 151, 254, 283
The Change (Greer), 421
The Golden Rule, 40-41
The Silent Passage (Sheehy), 421
Thiamine, *see* Vitamin B1
Thrombosis (blood clots), 312
    And heart attack and stroke, 295, 296, 300, 312
    And hormone eligibility, 94-95
    And Women's Health Initiative (WHI), 424, 425, 426, 428, 430, 433
    With aromatase inhibitors, 361
    With aspirin, 312
    With birth control patches, 145
    With birth control pills, 143, 145, 389
    With estrogen, 124-125
    With estrogen pills, 126-127, 310-311
    With estrogen plus progesterone patches (HRT), 148
    With estrogen skin patches, 128, 148
    With homocysteine, 308
    With raloxifene (Evista), 132-133, 340-341
    With tamoxifen (Nolvadex), 131-132, 340, 360
    With tibolone, 134
    With vitamin E, 306

Index

Thyroid disease
    Effect on risk of osteoporosis, 318
    Similarities to symptoms of menopause, 78, 169
Tibolone, 134
    For management of hot flashes, 174
    For management of night sweats, 181
    For management of vaginal dryness, 254
Timed voiding
    For management of urinary incontinence, 265
Tinctures, 95-96
Tobacco, *see* smoking
Tofranil (Imipramine)
    For management of depression, 218
    For management of urinary incontinence, 267
Tolterodine (Detrol)
    For management of urinary incontinence, 266
Total hysterectomy, 58-59, 62
Total hysterectomy, bilateral salpingo-oophorectomy. 62
Trabecular bone, 316-317
    Figure 15, 316
Traumatic head injury, 403
    Effect on risk of Alzheimer's disease, 403
Trazodone
    For management of fatigue, 202
    For management of insomnia, 192-193
Tretinoin (Retin A, Renova)
    For management of acne, 288
    For management of hair loss on the scalp, 243
Triazolam (Halcion)
    For management of fatigue, 200-201
    For management of insomnia, 190-191
Tricyclic antidepressants
    Effect on sex drive, 279
    For management of depression, 218
    For management of fatigue, 202
    For management of insomnia, 192
    For management of urinary incontinence, 267

Tri-est, 124
Triglycerides, 296-297
    Effect of testosterone on, 152
    Effect on risk of heart attack, 298, 299
Tropsium chloride
    For management of urinary incontinence, 267
Truncal obesity, 298, 302
T score, 324-326
Tylenol
    For management of joint stiffness and joint pain, 231

U

Ultrasound
    For bone density testing, 321-322
    For diagnosis of ovarian cancer, 397
    For diagnosis of thickened endometrium, 132, 340, 361, 380, 383, 392
    For diagnosis of uterine cancer, 132, 340, 361, 380, 383, 392
    For evaluating dense breasts, 371, 372-373, 374-376
    For evaluating unexpected vaginal bleeding, 147, 392
Unilateral oophorectomy, 60
Unilateral salpingectomy, 59-60
Unilateral salpingo-oophorectomy, 61
Unopposed estrogen, 378-380, 385-386.
    See also uterine cancer.
    See also estrogen alone.
    See also estrogen excess.
    Figure 20, 379
Unsaturated fats, 205, 300
Urethra, 256
    And incontinence devices, 267-268
    And urinary incontinence, 260-267
    And urinary tract infections (UTIs), 256-259
    And Kegel exercises, 262-263
    Figure 11, 255

Index

Urge incontinence, 261-269. See also urinary incontinence
Urine bone density testing, 326-327
Urinary incontinence, 260-269
    Acupuncture, 269
    As a symptom of estrogen deficiency, 108
    As a symptom of menopause, 76, 77, 439, 440
    Causes, 260-261
    Diet and lifestyle options, 262-265
    Effect of pregnancy on, 260-261
    Electrical stimulation techniques, 269
    Hormonal medication options, 266
    Hypnosis, 269
    Incidence, 260
    Incontinence devices, 267-268
    Non-hormonal medication options, 266-267
    Surgical procedures, 268-269
    Types, 261-262
    Vitamin and mineral options, 265
Urinary incontinence surgery, 268-269
Urinary system, 255-269
    Figure 11, 255
Urinary tract infections (UTIs)
    As a symptom of estrogen deficiency, 108
    As a symptom of menopause, 76, 77, 439, 440
    Cause, 256-257
    Diet and lifestyle options, 257-259
    Symptoms, 257
Urination
    After intercourse, 258-259
    Effect on urinary tract infections (UTIs), 258-259
    Frequent, 258
U.S. System, 155-156
Uterine cancer, 377-392
    Anatomy, 377-378
    Botanical and herbal options, 383-384
    Diet and lifestyle options, 382-383
    Effect of estrogen on the uterus, 378-380
    Effect of raloxifene (Evista) on, 132-133, 340-341

Effect of tamoxifen (Nolvadex) on, 131-132, 340, 360-361
Figure 20, 379
Hormonal medication options, 385-392
Incidence, 377
Irregular vaginal bleeding and, 380
Risk factors, 381-382
Uterine ultrasound,
    For diagnosis of thickened uterine lining, 132, 340, 361, 380, 383, 392
Uterus, 53-55
    Figure 3, 53
UTIs (Urinary tract infections), 256-259
    As a symptom of estrogen deficiency, 108
    As a symptom of menopause, 76, 77, 439, 440
    Cause, 256-257
    Diet and lifestyle options, 257-259
    Symptoms, 257

V

Vagina
    Anatomy, 249-250
    And Kegel exercises, 263
    Figure 10, 249
Vaginal atrophy, 250
Vaginal bleeding
    Abnormal, 108, 164-165
    And birth control pills, 94, 142-143, 144
    And hormones, 94
    As a symptom of estrogen excess, 108
    As a symptom of progesterone excess, 135
    Evaluation of, 147-148
    Irregular, 135, 380
    Side effect of medications, 134, 174, 181
    Unexpected, 94, 147-148, 380
    With continuous HRT, 147-148

INDEX

Vaginal dryness, 249-254
    And sex drive, 278
    As a symptom of estrogen deficiency, 108
    As a symptom of menopause, 76, 77, 439, 440
    Botanical and herbal options, 252
    Diet and lifestyle options, 250-251
    Hormonal medication options, 252-254
    Mechanical options, 251-252
    Vaginal anatomy, 249-250
    Vitamin and mineral options, 252
Vaginal itching, see vaginal dryness
Vaginal rugae, 249-250
    Figure 10, 249
Valdecoxib (Bextra)
    For management of joint stiffness and joint pain, 231-232
Valerian (*Valeriana officinalis*), 121-122
    For management of fatigue, 198
    For management of insomnia, 188
    For management of mood swings, irritability, and depression, 216
Vaniqa cream (eflornithine hydrochloride)
    For management of hair growth in undesirable locations, 248
Vardenafil (Levitra)
    For management of decreased sex drive, 284, 442
Vasoconstrictors
    For management of headaches, 292
Vasomotor symptoms, 169. *See also* Hot flashes
Venlfaxine (Effexor)
    For management of hot flashes, 175
    For management of night sweats, 181
Veralipride
    For management of hot flashes, 176
    For management of night sweats, 182
Viagra (Sildenafil)
    For management of decreased sex drive, 284, 442
Vioxx (rofecoxib)
    For management of joint stiffness and joint pain, 231-232
Vitamin and mineral options, 86, 94
    For management of acne, 287

For management of dry skin, 237
For management of fatigue, 197
For management of forgetfulness, 205-206
For management of hair loss on the scalp, 241-242
For management of hot flashes, 171
For management of insomnia, 188
For management of joint stiffness and joint pain, 228-229
For management of mood swings, irritability, depression, 213-215
For management of night sweats, 178
For management of urinary incontinence, 265
For management of vaginal dryness, 252
For prevention of Alzheimer's disease, 404-405
For prevention of heart attack, 305-308
For prevention of osteoporosis, 334-336

Vitamin A
- For management of acne, 288
- For management of dry skin, 237

Vitamin B1 (Thiamine)
- For management of acne, 287
- For management of forgetfulness, 205-206
- For management of hair loss on the scalp, 241
- For prevention of Alzheimer's disease, 404

Vitamin B2 (Riboflavin)
- For management of acne, 287
- For management of hair loss on the scalp, 241

Vitamin B3 (Niacin)
- For management of acne, 287
- For prevention of Alzheimer's disease, 405
- For prevention of heart attack, 307

Vitamin B5 (Pantothenic acid)
- For management of acne, 287
- For management of hair loss on the scalp, 241

Vitamin B6 (Pyridoxine)
- Deficiency, 308
- For management of acne, 287
- For management of mood swings, irritability, and depression, 213-214
- For prevention of Alzheimer's disease, 405

INDEX

    For prevention of heart attack, 306, 308
    For prevention of osteoporosis, 336

Vitamin B9 (Folate)
    Effect on risk of Alzheimer's disease, 403
    Deficiency, 308
    For management of acne, 287
    For management of forgetfulness, 205-206
    For management of hair loss on the scalp, 241
    For management of mood swings, irritability, and depression, 213-214
    For prevention of heart attack, 306, 308
    For prevention of osteoporosis, 336

Vitamin B12 (Cobalmin)
    Deficiency, 308
    For management of acne, 287
    For management of mood swings, irritability, and depression, 213-214
    For management of urinary incontinence, 265
    For prevention of heart attack, 306, 308

Vitamin C
    For management of acne, 287
    For management of dry skin, 237
    For management of forgetfulness, 205-206
    For management of hair loss on the scalp, 241
    For management of mood swings, irritability, and depression, 213-214
    For management of urinary incontinence, 265
    For prevention of Alzheimer's disease, 405
    For prevention of heart attack, 306
    For prevention of osteoporosis, 336

Vitamin D
    Deficiency, 318, 335
    For prevention of osteoporosis, 321, 333-334, 335, 343

Vitamin E
    For management of dry skin, 237
    For management of forgetfulness, 205-206
    For management of hot flashes, 171
    For management of night sweats, 178

    For management of vaginal dryness, 252
    For prevention of Alzheimer's disease, 405
    For prevention of heart attack, 306
Vitamin K
    For prevention of osteoporosis, 336
Vivelle, 253
Vivelle-Dot, 253
Vomiting
    As a side effect of medications, 173, 180
    As a symptom of estrogen excess, 108

W

Waist to hip ratio, 298, 302
Walking, 225, 329
Water
    For management of acne, 286
    For management of dry skin, 235-236
    For management of urinary tract infections (UTIs), 258
Waxing
    For management of hair growth in undesirable locations, 246
Weight
    Effect on acne, 286
    Effect on hair loss on the scalp, 240
    Effect on joint stiffness and joint pain, 227
    Effect on risk of breast cancer, 346
    Effect on risk of uterine cancer, 381, 382-383
    Effect on urinary incontinence, 264
Weight-bearing exercise
    For prevention of osteoporosis, 329
Weight control
    For prevention of breast cancer, 352-353
    For prevention of heart attack, 302-303
    For prevention of hair loss on the scalp, 240
    For prevention of ovarian cancer, 398

Index

    For prevention of uterine cancer, 382-383
    For prevention of urinary incontinence, 264
    Quantity of exercise for, 275
    Weight-bearing exercise, 329
Weight gain, 271-276
    As a side effect of medications, 173, 180
    As a symptom of estrogen excess, 108
    As a symptom of menopause, 76, 77, 439, 440
    As symptom of testosterone excess, 149
    Body mass index (BMI), 272-273
    During menopause, 271-272
    And HRT (Hormone Replacement Therapy), 272
    And estrone, 271
    Cause, 271-272
    Diet and lifestyle options, 273-275
Weight lifting, 225
Weight loss
    Quantity of exercise for, 275
Weight maintenance, 275
Whiskers, *see* hair growth in undesirable locations
Wild Yam (*Dioscorea villosa*), 137-138
    For management of vaginal dryness, 252
    For prevention of uterine cancer, 384
Wilson, Robert, 416
Women's Health Initiative (WHI), 420, 422, 423-434
    Analysis, 423-428
    And heart attacks, 309-310, 420, 422-434
    Estrogen alone arm, 423, 427-428
    Estrogen plus progesterone arm, 423-427
    Interpretation, 430
    Lesson from, 431-432
    Limitations, 428-430
    Purpose, 422-423
    Recommendations, 432-434
Worksheet, 5-17
Wrinkles, 233-234
    Vaginal wrinkles, see vaginal rugae

Wrist
    Fractures of, 314, 315
    Osteoporosis and, 314-315
Wu Pian
    For management of hair loss on the scalp, 241-242

Y

Yeast infections
    As a result of douching, 259
    As a side effect of antibiotics, 288
    As a symptom of estrogen excess, 109
Yoga, 171, 187, 225 226, 329, 330
    For management of fatigue, 197
    For management of headaches, 290
    For management of hot flashes, 171
    For management of insomnia, 187
    For management of joint stiffness and joint pain, 226
    For prevention of osteoporosis, 329, 330
    Pranayama breathing, 171

Z

Zaleplon (Sonata)
    For management of fatigue, 201
    For management of insomnia, 191-192
Zinc
    For management of acne, 287
    For management of forgetfulness, 205-206
    For management of hair loss on the scalp, 241-242
    For management of urinary incontinence, 265
    For prevention of Alzheimer's disease, 405
    For prevention of osteoporosis, 336

Index

Zocor (Simvastatin)
> For management of cholesterol and prevention of heart attack, 311

Zoloft (Sertraline)
> For management of depression, 218
> With aspirin, 312

Zolpidem tartrate (Ambien)
> For management of fatigue, 201
> For management of insomnia, 191-192

Z score, 326

About the Author

Barbara Taylor, M.D. is a Board Certified Obstetrician/Gynecologist. She received her undergraduate degrees in Biology and Psychology from Rice University. She completed both medical school and residency at Baylor College of Medicine. Thereafter, she practiced in the Texas Medical Center. While practicing medicine full-time, she attended graduate school part-time and received a Master's in Business Administration at The University of Houston, Clear Lake, and a Law Degree at The University of Houston, Law Center. She and her husband move frequently, living in fabulous locations around the world. Wherever she lives, Dr. Taylor gives menopause seminars, which derive from this book. Her seminars are thorough, entertaining, and quite popular. For more information on her seminars and other resources (like the slide chart), visit her website at TayloredHealth.com.

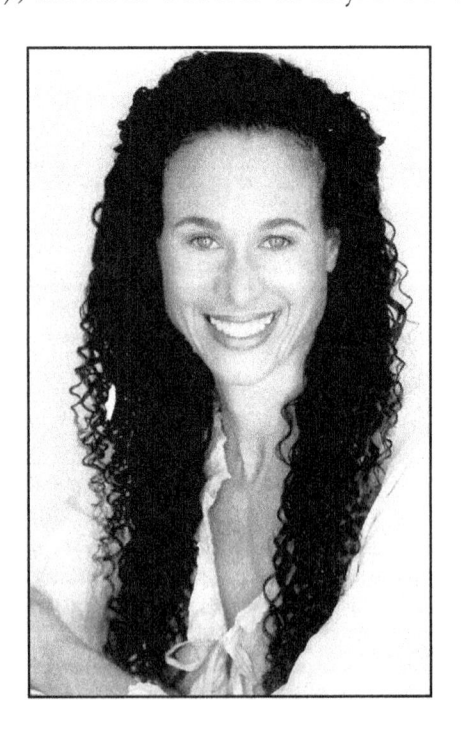

CPSIA information can be obtained
at www.ICGtesting.com
Printed in the USA
BVOW03s1434010617
485787BV00003B/4/P

9 781439 207956